THE MEDICALIZATION OF BIRTH AND DEATH

THE MEDICALIZATION
OF BIRTH AND DEATH

Lauren K. Hall

JOHNS HOPKINS UNIVERSITY PRESS

Baltimore

© 2019 Johns Hopkins University Press
All rights reserved. Published 2019
Printed in the United States of America on acid-free paper
9 8 7 6 5 4 3 2 1

Johns Hopkins University Press
2715 North Charles Street
Baltimore, Maryland 21218-4363
www.press.jhu.edu

Library of Congress Cataloging-in-Publication Data

Names: Hall, Lauren K., 1980–, author.
Title: The medicalization of birth and death / Lauren K. Hall.
Description: Baltimore : Johns Hopkins University Press, 2019. | Includes bibli-
    ographical references and index.
Identifiers: LCCN 2019010084 | ISBN 9781421433332 (hardcover : alk. paper) |
    ISBN 1421433338 (hardcover : alk. paper) | ISBN 9781421433349 (electronic) |
    ISBN 1421433346 (electronic)
Subjects: | MESH: Medicalization | Healthcare Disparities | Parturition | Death |
    Personal Autonomy | Cost Control | United States
Classification: LCC RA418 | NLM WA 31 | DDC 362.1—dc23
LC record available at https://lccn.loc.gov/2019010084

A catalog record for this book is available from the British Library.

*Special discounts are available for bulk purchases of this book. For more informa-
tion, please contact Special Sales at 410-516-6936 or specialsales@press.jhu.edu.*

Johns Hopkins University Press uses environmentally friendly book materials,
including recycled text paper that is composed of at least 30 percent post-consumer
waste, whenever possible.

To Piper, Larkin, and Juno, who give me reasons to write

CONTENTS

This book is the result of many years of thinking about my own experiences with birth and death and researching why those experiences were shaped the way they were. As a result, I have many people to thank for the book itself, however much they are in no way responsible for whatever errors are contained therein. For those I will inevitably leave out, please know your contributions were not unseen.

In the first place, I want to thank the many physicians, nurses, midwives, hospice workers, doulas, and other providers who agreed to spend their limited and valuable time being interviewed by an ignorant academic. Their experiences and wisdom helped frame many of the questions I asked at the beginning of my research and contributed in crucial ways to the solutions I propose. I also want to thank the anonymous individuals who filled out surveys about their experiences with both birth and death, which provided important background information that helped frame my research. I was assisted by the many friends, family members, and acquaintances who took time out of their busy lives to share their most vulnerable and sometimes painful experiences with me. One of the most important things I learned from writing this book is how deeply people care about these experiences and how little we actually discuss them. To everyone who shared these moments with me, thank you.

I am also grateful for the institutional support I received throughout this writing process. A good portion of the book was written during a sabbatical granted by the Rochester Institute of Technology in spring 2017, which allowed me the time off from teaching and service to interview providers and dig into the medical and public health literatures. My chair, Sean Sutton, provided research support from departmental funds and was patient with an absentee colleague over many semesters.

The Institute for Humane Studies (IHS) continued its long and unwavering support of my research by organizing and funding a manuscript workshop in Washington, DC, in spring 2018 that collected policy scholars, economists, public health scholars, and philosophers to discuss and pull apart the manuscript. One result of that workshop was the watershed metaphor that frames and provides structure to the whole work. I am extremely grateful to the workshop participants who spent many hours reading the book and an entire weekend talking about it, improving the manuscript immeasurably. Many thanks to Tim Bersak, Trevor Burrus, Yana Chernyak, Natallia Gray, Earl Grinols, Mark Hall, Rob MacDougall, Matthew Mitchell, Jake Monaghan, Nathan Nobis, James Stacey Taylor, Bradley Tipper, and the indefatigable Bill Glod, many of whom followed up in the weeks and months after the workshop with additional resources and suggestions, all of which tightened the argument and strengthened the research. The IHS also provided financial assistance for a research assistant, Jasmine Carter, who helped me wrangle hundreds of citations and footnotes as I prepared to submit the manuscript. Even more, the IHS has been a major wellspring of the vibrant intellectual community that has helped me think through complex political and social questions in a deeper and richer way, and for that they deserve a much deeper level of gratitude than I can express here.

I am also grateful to my circle of academic friends who patiently looked over various drafts in the early stages when I did not yet know what I was arguing and who pointed me in important directions for further research. Larry Arnhart, Janet Bufton, Steve Horwitz, Dan Kapust, and Sarah Skwire are among those numbers, though there are many others. Sarah Burns, as always, provided commiseration, support, and reality checks via joint writing sessions and occasional tequila deliveries.

I appreciate the support of Johns Hopkins University Press, my editor Robin Coleman, and the anonymous reviewers, whose comments all pushed the book in productive directions and clarified my thinking in a multitude of areas. Robin in particular saw potential in the project when it was not entirely clear what the project was.

Finally and most importantly, this book could not have been written without the help of my family. My husband, Brian Lilly, endured rants of frustration and provided loving care to our children during long writing days. The writing of the book coincided with the birth of our third daughter in 2017, and my parents, Robert and Deborah Hall, and my in-laws, William and Marilyn Lilly, provided invaluable herding of children and last-minute childcare. My parents also provided commentary and advice on multiple chapters of the book and on the final draft itself, and their happiness to see it published is no doubt compounded by their desire never to look at it again. My sister Marah and sister-in-law Ellen both patiently answered incessant questions about their nursing experiences at all times of the day and night, providing clinical knowledge and perspectives I would otherwise have struggled to access. Most profoundly, I am grateful to and for my three daughters. Their births changed me forever, and it was my experiences, both good and bad, bringing them into the world that motivated my belief that we can do better. For that and for their very existence, I am eternally grateful.

THE MEDICALIZATION OF BIRTH AND DEATH

The Watershed of Healthcare Decision Making

The horse is out of the barn. When you look at technology, you look at the percentage of people admitted to the ICU, the biggest predictor is having the tools. The biggest predictor of getting a CT scan is having the machine nearby. The biggest predictor of ICU admittance is ICU beds available. Changing behavior is always sticks and carrots. We have to change the incentives.
—*Palliative care physician*

AMERICANS HAVE TWO competing narratives about how healthcare decisions are made. The first narrative is that of the ideal healthcare model, the one many Americans believe exists but few will experience. In that narrative, a patient, Jane, meets with her provider, Margaret. The two women exchange information. Jane describes her goals for care, her cultural values, and the social support network in which she lives. Margaret, in turn, explains the range of current treatment alternatives and the available locations for care, their various risks and benefits, and how each might contribute to or challenge Jane's goals and values. Together, and perhaps also with input from Jane's family, Jane and Margaret create a plan for care. They meet frequently while the plan is being implemented, discussing Jane's current status, any side effects, new treatments that may be on the horizon, and how Jane's own goals may have changed during the course of treatment. If necessary, the two revise the plan to align with Jane's current medical needs and personal preferences until treatment is no longer necessary. Margaret follows up after treatment to identify any post-treatment side effects or concerns.

This interaction is the American ideal; it is characterized by respect for patient autonomy and evidence-based care, a competitive marketplace where patients and providers can choose from a range of options and where communication and trust link the interests of patients and providers together. This narrative does not, however, describe the way most Americans experience birth or death. Instead, most Americans will experience something like the second narrative. It is a narrative characterized not by informed consent and a partnership in care but instead by a tangle of regulations and reimbursement structures that constrains choice, limits the range of alternatives, and prevents communication between patients and providers. It can be best illustrated by two real-life cases, the first as a new person enters the world, the second as a person leaves it.

The first is a birth story. Miriam, a 30-year-old Manhattan woman, began researching options for the birth of her second child in 2017.[1] After her first birth ended in a cesarean section in 2015, she wanted to find a provider who would support a vaginal birth after cesarean (VBAC), both because it was the most medically appropriate birth for her situation and because it aligned with her future goals to have more children. The obstetrician who delivered her first baby, with whom she had a good relationship, said that he would not attend a VBAC but that he would be happy to schedule a repeat cesarean for her. He argued that she was not a good candidate for a vaginal birth owing to a slower-than-average dilation during her first labor, but Miriam suspected that his decision was influenced by nonmedical factors. The recommendations from the American College of Obstetricians and Gynecologists (ACOG) at the time required that her obstetrician be present in the hospital room during her entire labor; given how little he would be compensated for a vaginal birth by Miriam's insurance provider and how long he would have to be in attendance during her labor, it made little financial sense for him to attend a VBAC.

Miriam received a second opinion from another practice that deemed her a suitable candidate for VBAC and was willing to take her as a patient, but that practice was not covered by her insurance as an in-network provider, unlike her previous physician. Her private employer-provided insurance would cover hospital expenses, but not the cost of the obstetrics practice providing the care. In the end, she could choose a cesarean section with her original provider that would be fully covered by her insurance or pay an estimated $10,000 to attempt a trial of labor that might very well end in a cesarean anyway. Given her desire to have more children and her research on the compounding risks of multiple cesarean sections in subsequent pregnancies, Miriam decided to attempt the VBAC with the out-of-network practice. Her labor ended in the vaginal birth of a healthy baby girl.

To achieve a birth that was both medically appropriate and consistent with her goals, Miriam paid around $12,000 in out-of-pocket costs. Despite the positive outcome of the birth itself, she found the experience both stressful and frustrating. According to her, "the most annoying thing of all is that my previous OB couldn't admit that he just couldn't do it for [financial] reasons [or] wouldn't do it for personal reasons. Instead, he (and probably other OBs) end up exaggerating what a bad candidate you are." Apart from her own frustration, the cesarean she was encouraged to schedule would have been more expensive for the healthcare system as a whole and would also have increased her risk of serious complications in subsequent pregnancies. All available evidence supported Miriam's belief that a VBAC was the most medically appropriate option, especially for someone who wanted more children. According to Miriam, struggling with the limitations on appropriate care that she faced "came dangerously close to sucking the joy out of my pregnancy."

A similar story at the end of life was reported by the *New York Times* in 2014.[2] The article followed Maureen Stefanides as she tried to find care for her elderly father, Joseph Andrey, that would enable him to stay at home in his final days. Stefanides details how perverse incentives, poor pay for home health aides, and uncoordinated care resulted in her father's death from preventable illnesses in an institution, much against his stated wish to die at home. Stefanides could not find a way to pay for the full-time care at home that her father needed, but she discovered that insurance did pay for a variety of expensive and inappropriate care. After one hospitalization resulted in Andrey's admission to a skilled nursing facility ostensibly for rehabilitation, Stefanides was shocked to find out that the nursing home neither she nor her father wanted was charging Medicare almost $700 per day, five times more than the cost for round-the-clock home care that would have been more appropriate.

A revolving door of hospitalizations and nursing homes for "rehab" left Joseph Andrey with more and more complications, including infections and ulcers from lack of movement and inattention to skin care. The *New York Times* described the disorienting tangle of policies that Stefanides and her father found themselves in:

> Home care agencies abruptly dropped or refused high-needs cases like her
> father's as unprofitable under changes in the state's Medicaid program.
> Hospitals, eager to clear beds, increasingly sent patients to nursing homes.

The nursing homes were often too short-staffed to reliably change diapers but still drew premium Medicare rates, ordering hours of physical therapy and other treatment that studies showed was often useless or harmful. Even hospice was limited. Now mostly for-profit, hospice companies would provide supervision and visits at home a few times a week through Medicare if a doctor certified that Mr. Andrey had only six months to live. The hidden catch: He would lose all Medicaid home care, the daily help he needed to be home at all.[3]

Eventually, Stefanides was faced with the choice of taking the Medicare Hospice Benefit but losing all Medicaid home health coverage. The loss of Medicaid coverage meant that the only option for her father's care was an institution-based hospice program, which her father desperately wanted to avoid. In the end, Joseph spent three days in a hospital-based hospice program before dying of sepsis. He never made it back home, in direct opposition to his wishes. The sepsis, meanwhile, probably resulted from bedsores owing to poor care. He spent much of his last year of life cycling in and out of the institutions he was trying to avoid, despite the existence of a much more inexpensive option that was consistent with his preferences.

Overall, Medicare and Medicaid paid more than $1 million for Joseph Andrey's care in the last year of his life, most of that the result of frequent hospitalizations and complications from hospital-borne infections. In contrast, in-home care would likely have been orders of magnitude less expensive, both by avoiding the complications resulting from uncoordinated care and through lower staffing costs. While no one can be sure Joseph Andrey would have lived longer had he had quality in-home care available to him, what is known for sure is that his last year of life would have been more aligned with his wishes and would almost definitely have been less expensive than the heavily medicalized death he ended up experiencing.

Miriam's and Joseph's experiences are not rare. Most Americans will give birth and die in hospitals with high rates of interventions that produce relatively poor outcomes at great cost to individuals and insurers. In stark contrast to the ideal narrative of medical care, birth and death in America are characterized by limited choices, poor incentives, and conflicts of interest between patients and providers. Current options for birth and dying are aligned with neither evidence-based medicine nor individual preferences. The harms, both economic and moral, are alarming.

The Healthcare Watershed and the Intervention Cascade

The roots of these dysfunctional outcomes can be explored by expanding on a simple concept already in use in health research. The term "cascade of interventions" is used by medical providers and health policy scholars to describe the way in which access to medical technologies contributes to overtreatment.[4] Thinking about this cascade as part of a larger system can help craft a metaphor that clarifies the broad decision-making landscape and explains how medical decisions are limited and structured by nonmedical variables. Cascades of interventions can be thought of as part of a larger "watershed" of healthcare that includes federal, state, local, and hospital policies that structure and determine the outcome of care. Just as the geography of the landscape in a watershed directs water in particular directions—into valleys and downhill—the structure of the landscape of healthcare policies directs resources and patients downstream toward more intensive options and centralized hospitals. This intensive and centralized care contributes to more expensive and, often, inappropriate care, particularly for pregnant women, the elderly, and terminal patients, all of whom have unique needs compared to other patient populations. To see how this happens, we can explore the watershed metaphor in more detail with our ideal patient-provider dyad, Jane and Margaret.

Imagine that, in addition to patient and provider, Jane and Margaret are also kayakers attempting to navigate a river—in this case, a river of healthcare options. The river begins in various tributaries upstream and ends in hospitalization. There are dangerous rapids in places, representing cascades of interventions, inappropriate care, and overtreatment, rapids that may medicalize otherwise nonmedical events. Navigating this river and avoiding the rapids requires that both Jane and Margaret know where they want to go in order to paddle in the same direction. They also need to understand the currents and how they affect the boats. They need to have options along the shoreline, places to land safely and get out of the kayak if necessary. They also need to have an ability to communicate while in the boat and some safety gear like life jackets and emergency whistles in case things go awry.

In the simplest kind of healthcare decision in the ideal healthcare world, the main contributing "tributaries" to the river might be the disease itself and the range of available treatments. If the disease is slow and treatment and prognosis are straightforward, Jane and Margaret may have plenty of time to meander down the river and talk about options. If the prognosis is unclear or the disease "tributary" is large and fast, they may be swept along without as many options, as in the case of an acute trauma. If the "disease" is less a disease than a life event like pregnancy, with a range of possible outcomes, Jane and Margaret may be able to focus entirely on preventive care, remaining close to the shoreline, avoiding medical interventions altogether.

But in the American watershed of healthcare decisions, many other tributaries exist that affect patient and provider decision making, often in determinative ways. Instead of a simple river with the two main tributaries of disease type and available treatments, Jane and Margaret find themselves in a complex watershed with multiple tributaries dumping water in at various locations, washing away landing sites on the shore, creating an undertow, speeding up the current, forming distracting rapids, and pushing them closer and closer to the cascade of interventions at the end.

These tributaries include state regulations on providers and types of care, certificate-of-need laws that limit locations of care, corporate practice of medicine laws that restrict providers to certain care settings, Medicare and Medicaid reimbursement policies that price some locations out of existence, and professional medical association recommendations that encourage centralized care in hospitals. Together, they have the combined effect of speeding up the current and removing safe harbors on shore, spaces where Jane and Margaret could land before reaching the crisis point of the cascade, like birth centers, home care for the elderly or terminally ill, and high-quality hospice options. The strength of these tributaries creates a rush so loud that it may even prevent communication between Jane and Margaret, while the smaller rapids create a series of minor emergencies that distract them from longer conversations about long-term goals. As they navigate these rapids, different interests emerge. Margaret may worry that she will be liable if the kayak tips over, while Jane may be concerned about the financial impact on her family of whatever direction they take. Neither knows how much the options available cost because Jane relies on third-party payers. These payers do not reimburse for various landing sites along the shoreline or emergency equipment on the boat, leaving Margaret and Jane poorly prepared to navigate.

Because Jane and Margaret do not have the time or ability to communicate, and because liability fears and risk influence their goals, they paddle in different directions, unwittingly stymieing each other and preventing coordinated action. Without realizing it, they are both pulled along on a current toward what was an almost inevitable outcome: birth or death in the hospital with high levels of intensity of care. Their entrance into the rapids of hospital care strengthens the current until both Jane and Margaret fall over the edge of the cascade of interventions into a medicalized ending, victims both of medicine's success and of the watershed of healthcare policies that limit options and funnel care toward hospitals. The current is the real decision maker in the process that Jane and Margaret thought they were navigating together.

The shape of the American watershed explains the medicalization of birth and death over the past 100 years. Medicalization is the process by which human experiences or conditions come to be treated as illnesses or diseases, and it has been a particularly powerful force in birth and death.[5] In 1900 most Americans gave birth and died at home, with minimal medical intervention. By contrast, in 2019 most Americans give birth and die in hospitals. While birth and death lent themselves to medicalization because birth and death are, at least in part, medical events, the medicalization we see today is in large part the result of the historical shaping of the watershed by policies that draw patients toward the most intensive and costliest kinds of care. Evidence suggests that in addition to medicalizing birth and death, we now overtreat both. Birthing and dying people get too much medical care, inappropriate medical care, and medical care that harms them, physically, psychologically, financially, and socially.

Recent books and articles on birth and death have tried to address some of the problems of medicalization and overtreatment during birth and death by emphasizing a range of techniques physicians and patients can use to improve communication and provide better care, including birth plans, advance directives, better training in communication, and protocols within hospitals to encourage pause points in care.[6] All these interventions are the equivalent of the various kinds of safety equipment on the boat, which are, of course, very good to have. But such safety features fail to address the broader question of why the boat is moving so quickly and why the options on the shoreline, alternatives to hospital-based care, have been washed away.

Frustrating reform is that there exists no one person or institution to blame. Patients, healthcare providers, lawmakers, regulators, interest groups—each is generally operating in good faith, attempting to make decisions in their particular area, on their specific tributary, without having any idea of how those decisions contribute to a larger current that pulls patients and their providers toward costly, low-quality, high-intensity care. While there are surely some bad actors in the system, most of the actors who shape the watershed are genuinely concerned about healthcare as a crucial human good with profound outcomes. But the interests of various decision makers are often pitted against each other by misaligned incentives that fracture the provider-patient relationship and contribute to distrust and dissatisfaction on all sides.

Miriam's and Joseph's real-world experiences in the American healthcare watershed demonstrate how easily patients and providers can be caught up in currents from tributaries they do not fully understand. Both were bound up in bureaucratic rapids that prevented their desires and values from being respected. Individually, their autonomy and ability to give informed consent were seriously challenged, if not outright violated. Sociopolitically, the care they were channeled into (but that Miriam was able to pay her way out of with considerable effort) was less medically appropriate and more harmful at the same time that it was much more expensive for the relevant payers. The watershed we have is in many ways the reverse image of the ideal medical narrative we started with. The American healthcare watershed prevents individual choice, results in poor outcomes, and is catastrophically expensive.

Birth and Death in the American Healthcare Watershed

The focus of this book is on the way the healthcare watershed affects birth and death because the watershed fails birthing and dying patients in particularly harmful ways. Part of this harm comes from the fact that these life events are peculiarly vulnerable to the medicalizing effect of the tributaries involved, precisely because they are not really medical events at all. While they may (but do not always) have medical components, they have in common individual and sociocultural import that other kinds of medical events do not. While a kidney transplant may be mostly the sum of its medical parts, birth and death are much more than medical. They are composed of individual beliefs and attitudes, cultural traditions, and religious and legal practices that influence both treatments and outcomes. Birth and death are, as a consequence, much more preference sensitive than other kinds of healthcare events. They require much more input about patient preferences, many more options for care, and continuous high-quality communication between patients and providers to explore how those preferences and available options can align. Almost perversely, the American healthcare watershed creates a kind of care that ignores individual preferences, eliminates alternatives for care, and reduces or eliminates opportunities for communication all while drawing patients and their providers on a steady current toward a medicalized cascade.

As a result of our unique healthcare watershed, birth and death are now fully medicalized, and that medicalization is linked in a feedback loop with the hospitals where most births and deaths occur.[7] On many measures, medicalization has changed birth and death for the better, particularly for those births and deaths with medical complications. Maternal and infant mortality is now relatively low, with 28 maternal deaths per 100,000 births, a sharp contrast to the 1–1.5 maternal deaths out of 100 in the early days of our republic. Life expectancy is at an all-time high of 78.8 years, compared to 47 years in 1900, with much of that difference being made up by infants and children whose childhood illnesses are now treatable rather than fatal.[8] Even when medicine fails to save a life altogether, it can provide dying patients with more time and better pain relief. Birth is no longer intimately linked with death, and death is no longer a completely uncontrollable process.

Despite these obvious benefits, medicalization creates its own set of harms during birth and death, harms that originate in part from the standardization and mechanization of care in hospitals. Ninety-nine percent of American women give birth in hospitals. Almost 40 percent of those women will be induced, over one-third will have a cesarean section, and many more will have forceps deliveries, episiotomies, labor augmentation, or other interventions.[9] These intervention rates are much higher than those in comparable developed countries. Despite the high rates of interventions, and in part because of them, maternal mortality has actually risen in the past decade, and the United States continues to lose ground on crucial benchmarks like preterm birth, maternal and labor complications, and cesarean section rates. The United States has some of the worst outcomes for mothers and infants in the developed world.[10]

Similarly, while 70 percent of Americans express a preference to die at home, most Americans will die in hospitals.[11] The elderly will spend many of their final days moving from home to hospital to nursing home and back to hospital, with many avoidable readmissions.[12] A National Institutes of Health (NIH) report found that for many elderly patients who want to pass away peacefully at home, dying is characterized by "an excessive number of burdensome transitions, repeated miscommunications with the family, inadequate pain management and apparent overuse of sedation, insensitive communication with the patient, and an inordinate delay in referral to hospice."[13] Many elderly patients die in intensive care units (ICUs), subject before death to catheterization, intubation, feeding tubes, or ventilators, all meant to help them urinate, eat, or breathe.[14] Such interventions compromise quality of life and provide little to no medical benefit. Research increasingly suggests that common hospital interventions such as CPR or intubation harm elderly patients by increasing their pain and isolation without extending life in any meaningful way.[15]

Hospital-based birth and death are also expensive, both for individuals and for the healthcare system as a whole. Pregnancy and birth are two of the most expensive line items charged to Medicaid, and almost half of pregnant women use Medicaid to pay for their births.[16] Hospital-based death represents an increasingly large portion of the federal healthcare budget. Meanwhile, the 5 percent of Medicare patients who die each year account for around 30 percent of Medicare expenses, with 30 percent of those costs incurred in the last month of life.[17] Average medical expenditures amount to almost $40,000 in the last year of life.[18] Depending on how costs are measured, birth and death together account for around $300 billion of the $1.6 trillion spent on healthcare each year, close to 20 percent of all US spending on healthcare.

The History of the Watershed

The geography of the American healthcare watershed was many years in the making, but the broad strokes that created the main tributaries are relatively clear. Sociologists and anthropologists have focused on the first and most dramatic tributary, sourced by the medical advances of the twentieth century—antibiotics in the 1940s; cardiac resuscitation, open-heart surgery, and kidney transplants in the 1950s; and the creation of ICUs in the 1960s—that spurred social and cultural change.[19] As the power of medical science expanded in the twentieth century, cultural trust in doctors and medicine grew.[20] Licensing and the growing professionalism of doctors and other medical practitioners created an expert class whose authority was rarely questioned. Medical innovations involving costly machines and complicated lab work concentrated care in hospitals for teaching, research, and patient care purposes.[21] Medicine became more and more specialized, further concentrating specialists and the technology they relied on in hospitals.

Medical professional organizations, seeking to solidify their position as trusted owners of medical knowledge, facilitated centralization by lobbying to restrict the activities of other providers, in part through state legislation that required physician oversight of other practitioners like nurses and midwives.[22] Midwives were targeted by a variety of state laws that limited their scope of practice or outlawed them altogether. Nurses' scope of practice was carefully hemmed in by physician oversight, reducing the number of practitioners willing and able to visit patients in their homes. This takeover was not only a way to expand physicians' reach but also an attempt to centralize care in teaching hospitals, to further support medical research and the professionalization of medicine.[23]

Federal policies compounded the effects of professionalization in the 1950s with the combination of federal funding poured into medical research and the Hill-Burton Act of 1946, which prioritized spending on hospital construction.[24] Between 1955 and 1960, the budget for the NIH more than quadrupled, from $81 million to $400 million. The Hill-Burton Act resulted in a 40 percent increase in the number of hospital beds and an investment of $1.8 billion in hospital construction. As sociologist Paul Starr has argued, this dramatic investment in hospital construction was never justified based on medical need.[25] Part of the justification was nonmedical, as a jobs program, providing employment both in the construction of the facilities and in the staffing of the hospitals once they were operational. Crucially, the program had what Starr calls an "expansionary bias," meaning that the expectation was that hospital growth would continue over time. Some scholars trace the medicalization of birth and death directly to the growth of hospitals. The hospital architect and critic of medicalization Roslyn Lindheim argued in 1980 that "the essence of the history of the hospital in the first 80 years of this century has been its use of an ever-increasing percentage of the health budget; the growth of specialization; and the medicalization of birth and death."[26] She argued that large urban hospitals operated as "centripetal" forces, attracting medical talent, patients, and insurance and government funds, leaving rural areas badly depleted of both doctors and funding. Once the process of centralization of care began, it was difficult to stop because so many resources became bound up in hospital-based care. Both Starr and Lindheim conclude that hospital growth occurred at the expense of less costly community-based alternatives to hospitals such as primary care and outpatient clinics.[27]

These policies had dramatic effects on medical practice itself, with the strongest impacts on birthing mothers and the elderly and terminally ill. By standardizing the design of new community hospitals as a cost-saving measure, the Hill-Burton Act inadvertently calcified medical practice at its most dehumanizing. The architectural designs for new community hospitals provided by the US Public Health Service called for maternity wards where mothers and infants were separated after birth and where social support was limited.[28] These hospital designs were paired with protocols that emphasized the efficient treatment of patients and what Roslyn Lindheim called a "factory approach" to patient care, where "priorities were designed to keep the flow of patients moving."[29] According to Lindheim, the emphasis on medical technology "made space so expensive that it cannot be 'wasted' on mothers, fathers, husbands, and friends."[30] Hospitals both standardized care with strict protocols and mechanized care by replacing human providers with automated machines. Standardization and mechanization were built into the very architecture of hospitals, making it difficult for staff to institute bottom-up reforms.

Concentrating resources into medical research and hospital design and construction was only one piece of the centralization puzzle. When Medicare debuted in 1965, it compounded the Hill-Burton Act's emphasis on centralized care by focusing reimbursement around hospital-based care and providing incentives for testing and procedures under its "fee-for-service" structure.[31] Medicare's payment structure affected less interventionist providers in birth and death since "watchful waiting" and comfort care were reimbursed at much lower rates than medically intensive birth and death. Moreover, Medicare's rules for hospital payment privileged hospitals over outpatient alternatives by paying for both depreciation of hospital assets and capital reimbursement, both of which encouraged expansion of hospital facilities. This bias toward centralization continued even in the face of signals that money would be better spent elsewhere. Starr argues that in the 1960s and 1970s, "despite the widespread sense that federal policy ought to shift its emphasis to ambulatory care, the government was still putting big money behind hospital expansion."[32] Medicare essentially continued where Hill-Burton left off, privileging hospitals over decentralized medical providers and incentivizing medical technology over nontechnological approaches.

Notably, policy makers relied heavily on professional medical associations for guidance in terms of both resource allocation and specific regulatory responses. Medical organizations marketed hospital-based solutions to birth and death to both patients and policy makers not only to standardize the quality and kind of care but also "to enlarge the authority of doctors in hospitals" and eliminate competition by folk healers.[33] The guidance of professional organizations throughout the late twentieth century became the foundation for state laws and federal reimbursement policies that furthered both medicalization and centralization as more and more Americans landed in hospitals to give birth and die, even when these policies were inconsistent with medical evidence.[34] As critics like Lindheim argued, hospital-based care was "heavily oriented toward the treatment of disease, high risk care, and crisis intervention," rather than versed in handling physiological birth and death, making the centralization of these events in hospitals particularly problematic.[35] The recommendations of professional associations frequently diverged from what the medical or public health evidence suggested was the best standard of care.[36]

Centralized care in hospitals was not, therefore, driven primarily by patient desire or need, but instead by the reality that government resources were concentrated into hospital construction and outfitting, which then required that patients actually use those facilities. Alternatives to hospital-based birth and death were starved of resources and, in conjunction with protectionist policies at the state and federal level, eventually killed off almost completely. Efforts to control hospital proliferation in the 1970s, including certificate-of-need laws, were then used against hospital competitors by hospitals themselves.[37]

Birth, Death, and Medicalization

One could, very reasonably, ask whether medicalization of birth and death is really as problematic as I suggest. Before answering that question, it makes sense to provide a brief clarification on terminology. Despite the similarities suggested by the discussion above, medicalization and overtreatment are not the same thing. Medicalization differs from overtreatment in two primary ways. Most obviously, "medicalization" is a descriptive term, while "overtreatment" is a normative one. Overtreatment assumes a correct level of treatment, whether that level is determined by the medical evidence or the patient's wishes. Medicalization, on the other hand, simply describes the growth of medical intervention in and control over a particular area of life and the societal expectations that surround that medical involvement.

Another way overtreatment differs from medicalization is that in overtreatment a norm of treatment is understood to exist, wherever it may come from. Medicalization, in contrast, describes the shifting of the norm itself, as in the case of birth, where the definition of a "normal" birth has shifted dramatically in the move from home to hospital. Medicalization may make overtreatment more difficult to diagnose precisely because there is no clear norm to which to refer and because overtreatment may also shift the norm over time, driving medicalization. In what follows, I treat "medicalization" and "overtreatment" as discrete but connected terms, but I also leave the technical analysis to the sociologists and bioethicists. My goal here is not to provide a comprehensive analysis of medicalization, but instead to describe how various policy streams have shaped the American healthcare watershed in such a way that Americans give birth and die in peculiarly medicalized ways. I also make a stronger normative claim that this process comes with discrete harms, both medical and moral, that we are only beginning to grapple with.

Just as the expansion of medical science brought both triumphs and challenges, medicalization itself is neither good nor bad.[38] Medicalization can save lives, reduce stigma, and expand our knowledge of illness and disease. Scholars and policy makers can only judge its effects, both good and bad, on the individuals who experience it and the costs it creates for the healthcare system as a whole. As Peter Conrad, one of the foremost scholars of medicalization, points out, the medicalization of alcoholism—the shift from treating it as a vice to treating it as a medical condition—was considered a victory by those who struggle with the disease.[39] In contrast, the gay, lesbian, and transgender communities fought against medicalization of their identities for years, a fight that culminated in the demedicalization of homosexuality and, most recently, gender identity.[40] Defining what constitutes a disease or disorder is not itself a scientific endeavor. Instead, such definitions depend on a combination of medical advances and social and cultural attitudes about what constitutes the "norm" of a particular condition. Medicalization can be resisted and sometimes reversed.

The medicalization of birth and death is as complex and socially embedded as addiction or sexual orientation. Neither is a disease or illness on its own. It makes little sense to talk of "treating" or "curing" birth or death. Instead, parts of birth and death are subjected to medical treatment, such as when large babies are categorized as "macrosomic" or when a terminally ill person's loss of appetite is labeled "anorexia." Redefining specific aspects of these events as medical complications allows room for medical interventions and medical control: in the case of macrosomia, induction or cesarean section, and in the case of anorexia, tube-feeding. What seems clear-cut, however, is not. In both cases the definition of the medical condition requiring intervention is itself subjective, with no clear line between a "normal" big baby and a macrosomic baby or between a normal loss of appetite at the end of life and one that must be treated, in terms of either risks or outcomes. Because many of the conditions and experiences that characterize birth and death occur on a spectrum, there is no objective way to determine when medical tools are legitimately necessary and when their use is counterproductive.

The problems associated with the medicalization of birth and death result from the nature of medicine itself. Reductionism allows researchers to reduce disease to the sum of its parts, helping illuminate causes and isolate treatments. This reductionism facilitated the relatively recent explosion of innovation in the pharmaceutical and technological treatment of disease, and we see its triumphant success in plummeting mortality rates and seemingly weekly medical breakthroughs. Reductionism is why scientific progress happens. Yet because birth and death are not reducible to the sum of their medical parts, a reductionist approach creates a conflict between medical and more holistic *human* needs. Thomas Szasz, an early critic of medicalization, characterized the conflict between scientific rigor and medical compassion as an "irreconcilable antagonism between preserving and promoting dignity and preserving and promoting health."[41] For birth and death, the scientific reductionism that saved the lives of infants and mothers and extended the life span for all is the same scientific reductionism that isolates the dying from loved ones and straps pregnant women's bodies to beds during labor and delivery. Medicalization's harms are intimately bound up with its benefits because both are linked to what makes medicine successful in the first place.

Medical advances also create ethical dilemmas where none existed before. Medicalization allows us to keep extremely premature infants alive and hold death at bay for months or even years on ventilators, forcing choices between quality and quantity of life that would have been unthinkable 100 years ago. Moreover, the cultural import of birth and death and their idiosyncratic meaning for the individuals involved may increase the trauma of medical interventions by alienating individuals from themselves and their loved ones at their most vulnerable moments. At the same time, birth and death may be more susceptible to medicalization than other human events precisely because the stakes are so high and emotions are so strong.

The medicalization of birth and death—and specifically the way medicalization centralizes care in hospitals—drives its own growth by eliminating cultural knowledge about nonmedical alternatives, channeling more people into hospitals to give birth and die. Birth and death have always been intergenerational phenomena, learned by both passive watching and active caretaking. For most of human history, people reached adulthood having seen both birth and death up close, in all their complexity and confusion. Hospital-based birth and death—enclosed, isolated, and under the control of medical professionals—contribute both to fear of the events and to the belief that they cannot be handled without medical expertise.[42] Most people who give birth today will never have seen another person give birth before, apart from online videos. And most people who die or who make decisions for a loved one who is dying have never seen anyone die before. Most medical students, unlike those in past generations, have never seen a birth or death outside the hospital.[43] The loss of generational knowledge involves not only the practical side of giving birth and dying, such as how to support people in pain or what positions can make labor easier, but also a more general cultural amnesia that nonmedicalized birth and death are even possible. Both patients and providers no longer know precisely what alternatives to medicalized birth and death look like and have an even harder time supporting those alternatives in practice.

Ethical Implications of the Watershed

The medicalization of birth and death has ethical implications for both patients and providers. While this book is not about medical ethics and, as a political scientist, I would be unqualified to write such a book, I argue in what follows that the policies that shape the healthcare Americans receive create currents that result in violations of the core ethical commitments of medicine itself: autonomy, beneficence, nonmaleficence, and justice. Autonomy, seen most clearly in the commitment to informed consent, requires that patients voluntarily choose treatment and understand the relevant benefits and harms a treatment is likely to provide. Beneficence requires that a chosen medical treatment provide the most benefit possible to the patient and that treatments are not merely chosen on a whim or for financial reasons. Nonmaleficence, sometimes combined with beneficence, requires that physicians avoid harm whenever possible in their treatment of patients. And justice requires, in part, that the risks and benefits of treatments and of healthcare as a whole be fairly distributed across the population.[44] Violations of these principles do not require close philosophic analysis to unearth. They are apparent to most lay people when discussing their experiences with American healthcare.

Troublingly, powerful currents in the healthcare watershed undermine medical providers' ability to protect these principles in any robust way. And these currents originate not in unavoidable medical trade-offs or the reality of disease, but in policies at the state and federal level, influenced by interest groups and stakeholders of various kinds, that prioritize inappropriate kinds of medical care. The resulting healthcare system is one of artificial choices that not only fail to provide the best available care but also challenge informed consent, actively harm individuals, and unevenly distribute both the harms and benefits of medical innovations. The principle of informed consent itself, rooted as it is in patient autonomy, becomes almost meaningless in a complex system where no one fully understands why some interventions are available and others are not or why or how options have been artificially limited by upstream forces in the first place.

The importance of these medico-ethical principles cannot be overstated, not least because it was their violation in practice over centuries that ultimately emphasized their importance. Patient autonomy in particular emerged not from any commitments intrinsic to medical expertise (in fact, quite the opposite), but as a reaction to a wide range of abuses of medical power throughout the nineteenth and twentieth centuries.[45] These abuses—from the infamous experimentation of the Tuskegee Syphilis Study by the US Public National Health Service to the horrors of Nazi medical experimentation to the forced sterilizations of the eugenics era—emphasized, only in retrospect, the dangers of handing final authority to supposedly beneficent experts. These cases were only the most public examples of what was common practice in medicine throughout the United States and Europe. The most egregious violations of autonomy were frequently paired with violations of other principles like justice and nonmaleficence, as physicians targeted vulnerable populations with little political clout.[46]

While these bioethical principles are, to a large degree, ideals that must always be balanced, moderated, and even compromised in practice, Miriam's and Joseph's experiences demonstrate how the structure of the watershed adds artificial barriers to provider practice, barriers that make it harder to provide just, high-quality, patient-centered care. Moreover, while one might justify the violation of one principle in practice to protect the others, such as when a physician rejects a patient's claim of autonomy by refusing to provide a futile or harmful intervention, it is hard to defend a system that leads to violations of each of these principles all at the same time, as when policies incentivize low-quality, inappropriate, costly care that is inconsistent with patient preferences.

These ethical principles are most important when the stakes are the highest. Because all Americans are born, many will give birth, and all will eventually die, birth and death are most Americans' only extended contact point with the medical system. They are also profound transitions in human life, when people are at their most vulnerable, when the most is at stake for individuals and their families, and when individual preferences are the most salient. And yet most people who give birth and die in American hospitals have no clear idea how their choices about birth and death are framed, structured, and limited by policy decisions made hundreds or thousands of miles away, sometimes decades before. These policy decisions mean that Americans giving birth and dying in hospitals will experience unnecessary harms, few corresponding benefits, limited autonomy, and unequal outcomes and yet have no idea why. They are likely to never realize the full extent of the harms done to them because they are unaware that a different kind of birth and a different kind of death exist. Most Americans have no idea how or why the healthcare system is the way it is, and most will have no idea what invisible hands have structured and colored their first and final days.

Conclusion

The harms Miriam and Joseph experienced in their navigation of the American system could have been avoided altogether in a different healthcare watershed. In a different watershed, one with ample opportunities to get to shore, floating docks in midstream at which patients and providers could pause to communicate or meet up with other providers to collaborate, and plenty of small streams to be explored as alternatives to the main centralized river itself, both Miriam and Joseph might have been able to access high-quality, low-cost care that was consistent with their preferences. In a different healthcare watershed, the speed of the river itself would be slower, giving patients and providers time to make more effective decisions together, explore a range of options, and find alternatives where they exist. A slower river would also give rise to a flourishing shoreline ecosystem made up of diverse healthcare providers and locations for care that fit a wide range of individual preferences, payment abilities, and attitudes toward risk.

Restructuring the watershed to allow pregnant women and dying patients the ability to choose evidence-based care, care that aligns with their preferences, or ideally both requires rethinking many of the policy tributaries that have developed over the past 100 years and whose persistent flow channels Americans into the most medicalized options. At least in birth and death, the main cause of inappropriate medicalization is relatively straightforward, as much as reform itself may not be, because the root cause of medicalization of birth and death is the hospitalization that the combination of forces in the watershed makes almost inevitable. Moving birth and death out of hospitals, onto the shoreline of the river, improves outcomes and lowers costs. Yet for most Americans the shoreline in the watershed is not a safe haven of options, but an insurmountable cliff.

This book lays out the geography of the American healthcare watershed, with an emphasis on how the watershed challenges and constrains decisions about care at the beginning and end of life. I use a combination of interviews with providers, historical evidence, and medical and social science research to create a nautical map of sorts, one that highlights the way in which unseen political and other structural forces shape the beginning and end of life.[47] Exposing the landscape of this watershed highlights how the geography of the American healthcare system reduces available options, distorts the provider-patient relationship, and seriously compromises basic societal commitments to informed consent and justice. It also provides a clear framework for reform—and real reform will require much more than merely switching who pays the bills. By restructuring these policy tributaries, consciously creating options on the shoreline, and providing patients and providers with emergency equipment along the way, policy makers at all levels can help align the way Americans give birth and how they die with who they are and what they value as human beings. Three crucial public health outcomes of a realignment are lowered healthcare costs, more equal access, and improved outcomes. But perhaps the most important effect of restructuring the watershed is that it would grant individuals some measure of control over the most profound of human experiences: birth and death.

CHAPTER 1

Medicalized Birth and the Current of Centralized Care

I often felt like I had to go into the hospital and protect my patient, which should not be the case.—*Family practice physician*

R INAT DRAY entered Staten Island University Hospital in 2011 in labor with her third child. Dray had had two previous cesarean sections that she felt were unnecessary, and as a result of those experiences, she extensively researched area hospitals that would support a vaginal birth after cesarean. Her labor was slow, but there were no indications that anything was wrong. After she had been laboring for 30 hours, the fetal monitors she was on picked up some potentially concerning signals, though the usefulness of such evidence is strongly contested by experts. From here, accounts differ. Dray insists she was not told that the baby was in any danger, and medical experts who reviewed her file later found no signs that Dray's or the baby's life was at risk. Her obstetrician, however, insisted that a cesarean was necessary to save the life of the child. Dray begged for more time, given that her last two cesarean sections had left her barely able to walk for months, unable to care for her children.

The physician's response was placed in Dray's chart: "I have decided to override her refusal to have a C-section." Dray was strapped down and anesthetized, still resisting as she went under. Dray gave birth to a healthy baby boy, but her bladder was permanently damaged during the surgery, and she felt violated by the experience. She later sued for malpractice but lost on the grounds that the statute of limitations had expired. The case was unusual in part because Dray's physician, without consulting an ethics board or getting a court order, rejected the requirement of informed consent and subjected a patient to surgery against her will, a potentially serious ethical violation. In some ways, though, Dray's was a characteristic American birth, one where surgery is prioritized over less intensive alternatives, where communication is fraught or nonexistent, and where coercive language and actions are used to ensure compliance. Dray's story, while extreme in its outcome, is in other ways not an outlier.

The geography of the healthcare watershed in the United States molds the American birth experience.[1] A combination of tributaries including Medicaid policies, state regulations, hospital policies, and liability fears contributes to a strong current that channels women into centralized hospitals to give birth. These same tributaries churn the rapids of medicalization and overtreatment by incentivizing procedures and interventions while eliminating demedicalized and community-based options that could provide alternatives to hospital-based care for low-risk women. While the tributaries themselves will be described in later chapters, this chapter lays out the historical path toward medicalization and hospital-based birth in the United States, as well as its costs in terms of maternal and infant health, healthcare resources, and maternal autonomy. The medicalization of birth has, in turn, had profound impacts on women's and providers' attitudes toward childbirth, attitudes that undermine medicine's ethical commitments to respect autonomy, to do no harm, and to protect justice.

Medicalized Birth in the United States

American birth presents scholars, policy makers, and physicians with a puzzle. Birthing practices in the United States are some of the most medically intensive in the world, with high rates of inductions, cesarean sections, vacuum- and forceps-assisted births, and episiotomies.[2] Yet the intensity of obstetrics practice is not supported by either the clinical evidence or recommendations from national obstetrics professional organizations like the American College of Obstetrics and Gynecology. What instead seems to be happening is that the pressures and incentives created by the structure of the healthcare watershed lead obstetricians and other medical staff to intervene even when evidence suggests that such intervention is unnecessary or even harmful. Moreover, these pressures are fed by forces at all levels. While the watershed encourages centralization of care through a series of tributaries that privilege and incentivize hospitalization, the hospital environment itself creates the rapids in which a cascade of interventions occurs. The result is that location of care turns out to be more predictive of interventions than women's preferences or risk factors.[3] The hospital environment itself plays a significant, if not the determinative, role in the medicalization of American birth.

Compared to other developed countries, the American way of birth both is expensive and results in poor outcomes for mothers and their babies. A comparative study in the *Lancet* characterized American maternity care as "expensive, risky, and inconsistent" compared to less medicalized and better-integrated systems found throughout Europe.[4] Perhaps the defining characteristic of US maternity care is that almost 99 percent of births in the United States occur in hospitals, mostly under the care of obstetricians. Birth is now the leading cause of hospitalization in the United States. Perhaps unsurprisingly, location of care is strongly associated with intensity of treatment during birth. American women who give birth in hospitals are much more likely to receive a range of interventions than women who give birth either at home or in birth centers, even after researchers control for medical risk and complications.[5]

This high treatment intensity is expensive. Hospital charges for maternal and infant care during and after birth totaled almost $80 billion in 2005 and have increased since.[6] A little over 40 percent of pregnant women receive Medicaid assistance in paying for birth, which means that birth alone constitutes a large proportion of Medicaid spending.[7] In fact, pregnancy and birth are the two most expensive conditions requiring hospitalizations billed to Medicaid.[8] Per-patient expenses for birth alone are high, with private insurers paying around $20,000 for a vaginal birth and $30,000 for a cesarean section and Medicaid paying around $10,000 for a vaginal birth and $20,000 for a cesarean. These numbers are much lower than the amount hospitals charge the uninsured, with the average charges for vaginal birth hovering over $30,000 and cesarean birth close to $50,000.[9] For women without insurance even an uncomplicated vaginal birth can be financially devastating.

Despite this medically intensive and high-cost model, the United States ranks 48th in maternal mortality and 57th in infant mortality among Organisation for Economic Co-operation and Development (OECD) countries.[10] Even more troubling, the increase in medical interventions over the past decade has been paired with an increase in both maternal mortality and severe maternal morbidity. In 2014, more than 500,000 American women experienced serious complications such as hemorrhage and stroke during labor and delivery that required blood transfusions, hysterectomies, or ventilators.[11] While these poor outcomes are often linked to the worsening health, increased obesity rates, and increased age of childbearing women, severe complications are also linked to medical interventions themselves. The increase in cesarean sections is a significant risk factor for maternal death (though the absolute risk is low).[12] In 2014, 32.2 percent of women in the United States delivered via cesarean section, a rate that has increased almost every year since the 1990s.[13] In addition to increasing rates of maternal injury and mortality, cesarean sections may have long-term effects on children's lungs and immune systems.[14] Risks of cesarean sections to mothers increase with each pregnancy, making complications like hemorrhage and uterine rupture more likely.[15]

It is not only in cesarean sections that the United States leads the developed world. The United States has high rates of inductions, episiotomies, labor augmentation, electronic fetal monitoring, artificial breaking of the amniotic sac, and repairs of tears and episiotomies.[16] Yet despite this high medical intensity, the United States has been moving away from critical benchmarks of quality, including those for "low birthweight and very low birthweight, all preterm birth (live births before thirty-seven completed weeks of gestation), maternal labor and birth complications, initial ('primary') and repeat cesareans in low-risk women, cerebral palsy, and mental retardation."[17] As an indicator of overtreatment, while intervention rates have increased over the past 30 years, patient outcomes have not improved or have gotten worse.

The main professional association for obstetricians has responded to these trends with recommendations of its own to try to limit unnecessary and potentially harmful interventions. In February 2017, ACOG issued a committee report on limiting interventions in birth, including recommendations to limit artificial rupture of waters and continuous fetal monitoring (which comes with high rates of false positives and increases other interventions). The committee report also encouraged nonmedical techniques, including emotional support, nonmedical pain relief techniques, and movement during labor.[18] The drive toward increasingly medicalized birth does not seem to be supported by either medical research or the major professional organization whose guidelines obstetricians presumably follow.[19]

Apart from medical outcomes, medicalized births can be alienating and even traumatic. Many women find hospital births impersonal and invasive, characterized by unnecessary treatments and standardized care that ignores maternal comfort and preferences.[20] Medicalized birth practices such as restricting movement, use of catheters, and denial of food and fluid have no medical indications for most births and lead to both dissatisfaction with the birth experiences and worse outcomes.[21] Several studies show that women's satisfaction is higher with out-of-hospital births, though the instruments used to assess satisfaction vary dramatically across studies.[22] Increasing attention to iatrogenic "birth trauma" and what birth activists call "obstetric violence" indicates that concerns about high rates of intervention and lack of informed consent in hospitals are increasing.[23] Recent discussions of obstetric violence during birth cite examples of forced cesarean section and episiotomies, various violations of informed consent, sexual assault and sexualization of women's bodies during labor and delivery, physical restraint, and abusive and bullying conduct by providers.[24] High intervention rates and dissatisfaction with care may be associated with the development of postpartum depression and post-traumatic stress disorder.[25]

Litigation in recent years has led to high-profile civil awards against providers that go beyond malpractice concerns to accusations of fraud, violations of consent, and assault.[26] A video posted to YouTube of a doctor cutting a woman 12 times during an episiotomy that she clearly verbally refuses went viral in 2015 and resulted in a civil battery suit that was settled in 2017.[27] Another high-profile case was settled for $16 million in 2016 after nurses forcibly held an infant inside a mother's vagina for six minutes, causing permanent nerve damage to the mother.[28] Other violations such as allowing medical students to practice pelvic exams on women under anesthesia without their consent have raised concerns about women's bodily autonomy in hospitals.[29] The growth of social media and "birth activism" groups dedicated to providing advocacy for women seeking respectful, low-intervention, and consent-based birth points to an increasing divide between the person-centered care many women seek and the hospital-based birth that is the only available option for most women in the United States. Awareness campaigns like Improving Birth's #breakthesilence campaign, which collects and publicizes incidents of obstetric violence and violations of consent during birth, suggests that social media is becoming a powerful tool for cataloging the ethical concerns associated with medicalized birth.[30] These decentralized movements are in part a response to the failure of medical licensing boards to respond effectively to ethical violations.[31]

The Current of Centralized Birth

Hospital birth was not always the status quo. Until the early 1900s most American women gave birth at home. The watershed of healthcare at the time contained few tributaries, and the river of healthcare options was slow and limited. While one of the tributaries contributing to centralization of care in hospitals involved improvements in medical practices, other tributaries such as state regulations, federal funding, and professional lobbying played an even larger role in the centralization of care during the twentieth century by privileging medical providers and centralized hospitals over other types and locations of care. Once care was centered in hospitals, the proximity to medical technology and the financial incentives associated with fee-for-service care put pressure on providers that led to a cascade of interventions in labor and delivery.

One of the most important shifts in the shape of the watershed was the development of medicine as a profession and the way in which the movement to professionalize and standardize medical science affected traditional care providers. For much of medicine's history, the quality of medical education was both low and extremely variable. Professional organizations, including the American Medical Association (AMA), were created in the mid-1800s as a way for upper-class physicians to organize and strategize how to navigate and regulate an increasingly crowded medical marketplace.[32] Medical associations like the AMA realized quickly that in order to secure the status of upper-class physicians they needed to standardize medical education, eliminate folk providers, and reduce competition for patients. As medical professional organizations in America grew in power and influence in the nineteenth and early twentieth centuries through well-connected members, they exerted pressure on state legislatures to license and regulate medical providers and schools. Midwives, the primary care providers for birth, became a primary target.

Despite the claims of public campaigns at the time, the targeting of midwives was motivated by more than patient safety. Throughout the nineteenth and early twentieth centuries, outcomes of midwife-led births were on par with or even better than outcomes for births with physicians. The early wave of physician-delivered births in the eighteenth and nineteenth centuries actually increased maternal mortality owing to lack of knowledge about the spread of disease and poor hygiene. Puerperal fever, caused by poor hygiene among physicians and in hospitals, was a major cause of death for birthing women until the early 1890s and was more common in physician-led and hospital-based births.[33] Midwives had lower infection rates than physicians not because they had a superior knowledge of hygiene but because they were much less likely to intervene during labor. Rather than safety concerns, the main motivation for eliminating midwifery was the growth and professionalization of medicine itself.[34]

One strategy to eradicate midwives involved medical journals like the *Journal of the American Medical Association* (*JAMA*), which sought to emphasize the medical profession's scientific approach while highlighting midwifery's nonscientific apprentice-based training. At the same time, physicians recognized that the extent of their own medical training was limited by the fact that most women still gave birth at home, under the care of midwives. The only way to standardize maternity care education was to have exclusive access to the bodies of women giving birth. One doctor complained in *JAMA* in 1912 about the "deplorable dearth of clinical material" available to doctors, pointing to midwives as the primary competition for women's bodies and arguing that they should be rooted out.[35] Physicians successfully lobbied for state laws making midwifery illegal, even as midwives in those states had better maternal and infant mortality outcomes than competing physicians.[36]

Hanna Porn, a successful midwife in Massachusetts, was prosecuted, fined, and eventually jailed for three months in 1909 after she was reported for illegally practicing medicine without a license. According to one report, the four doctors who testified against her had infant mortality rates twice as high as Porn's. By all accounts, including testimony from clients at her trial, she was a talented and conscientious midwife with excellent outcomes. Unsurprisingly, after Porn was removed from practice, those same physicians increased the number of deliveries they attended by almost 90 percent.[37] Porn continued to practice illegally until her death, stating during her trial that she refused to stop serving women despite multiple prosecutions and many fines because "I thought the law was unjust." Porn's case highlights how state laws regulating medicine were often used, not for the purposes of ensuring patient safety or health, but to eliminate competition and provide a steady patient stream for physicians and medical schools. State laws targeting midwives removed not only safe options for birthing women but also one of the few ways in which lower- and middle-class women like Porn, who was widowed, could legitimately support themselves outside of marriage.

Medicine's alliance with wealthy donors like the Rockefellers and Carnegies solidified its legislative and regulatory power, permanently shifting American women away from midwives and toward birth in centralized hospitals. Because of the informal nature of midwifery education and the decentralized nature of most midwifery practices, midwives were ill-equipped to organize a coordinated political response. The success of the coordinated medical campaign was swift. Prior to 1900, over 95 percent of American women gave birth at home with the help of midwives who were well versed in normal low-risk births and were capable of managing common variants like breech presentation. By 1935, 75 percent of women were giving birth in hospitals under the care of physicians, though midwives persisted in poor, rural, and immigrant areas well into the twentieth century.[38] Community-based birth, owned and controlled by women, was all but eliminated by the middle of the twentieth century.

At the same time that birth was becoming centralized in hospitals, trends in medical research contributed to increasing levels of medical intervention in even low-risk births. Dr. Robert DeLee's work on forceps deliveries in the 1920s was particularly influential. DeLee argued that birth, rather than a physiological process, was instead a "pathological" condition that required almost continual intervention, and his 1920 article prescribing prophylactic use of forceps on every birthing woman became the standard of care in hospitals around the country.[39] By the 1930s most women giving birth in hospitals underwent routine episiotomy and forceps deliveries.[40] The combination of centralized care in hospitals and the belief that birth was a pathology to be treated culminated in the new American way of birth: isolated from the community in centralized hospitals, heavily medicalized with increasingly invasive interventions, all under the control of male physicians who became the new experts in women's bodies.

These forces, in turn, changed women's own attitudes toward birth. The marketing of a scientific approach to birth and better options for pain control increased women's trust in doctors even as undercurrents of dissatisfaction with the experience itself grew. Outcomes of hospital birth improved, providing new support for the originally baseless narrative of hospital birth as safer for mothers and babies. By the 1940s, physicians and hospitals had developed a better understanding of both infection and pain management. Basic hygiene like handwashing became routine, and the development of penicillin made hospital-contracted infections less likely to be fatal. Maternal and infant mortality rates dropped dramatically as a result, and women became more trusting of hospital-based care.[41] Campaigns to advertise the benefits of "twilight sleep" to mothers and babies encouraged middle-class women throughout the 1920s and 1930s to trust their births to hospitals.[42] The process of centralization of birth was finalized in the 1940s, as the new cultural emphasis on pain-free childbirth moved the cultural locus away from midwives and physiological birth and toward the medical management of labor and delivery.[43]

Government investment in healthcare infrastructure in the 1950s further standardized the medical management of labor and delivery. The floor plans for new regional hospitals under the Hill-Burton Act in 1946 calcified existing obstetrics practices such as isolation of laboring women from support networks, movement of women from room to room during labor, and separation of mothers and infants by working these practices into the very design of labor and delivery wards.[44] Changing hospital practice or individualizing care became impractical since the design of the hospital emphasized medical control. The large scale of these new modern hospitals, in turn, increased the need to efficiently coordinate the activities of many different providers and many different patients. Maternity care became increasingly impersonal and increasingly standardized, seen most clearly in the "assembly line" maternity wards of the 1960s.[45]

According to hospital architect Roslyn Lindheim, the assembly line approach to maternity care was not an accident. Hospital designers explicitly looked to factory design to increase productivity and decrease costs. A hospital design textbook from the 1960s speaks positively about a conveyor belt approach to maternity care, pointing out that the logic of factories "emphasizes the repeated transference of a mother (as in a motor-car assembly) from place to place, and also that unequal time periods at any station can render the process uneconomical."[46] As a result, maternity care from the 1920s to the 1960s emphasized standardizing women to make labor and delivery compatible with the needs of staff and the hospital itself. American hospital birth involved moving women from room to room as labor progressed, speeding up or slowing down labor with medications, and standardizing women's bodies by requiring routine pubic shaving, episiotomies, enemas, and use of catheters, even when such procedures had no scientific backing (and were later found to cause harm).[47] Practitioners also worked to standardize patient preferences, starting with prenatal examinations that emphasized obedience and that, in the words of birth historians Dorothy and Richard Wertz, "taught patients to regard themselves as objects for the impassive and well-meaning medical eye."[48] Even today, American women attend many more prenatal appointments than women in other developed countries, with some scholars arguing that after a certain point additional appointments for low-risk mothers do little more than increase opportunities for interventions.[49]

Not surprisingly, standardizing care relied on increasing mechanization of care. Birth became "the processing of a machine by machines and skilled technicians."[50] Laboring mothers were electronically monitored to track contractions and fetal heart rate, and cervical checks were used to quantify labor progress. Pitocin, forceps, and vacuum extraction were introduced if labor progress did not meet standardized expectations. In the period of "twilight sleep" in the middle of the twentieth century, women were restrained, medicated, and monitored in communal rooms. After birth, babies were whisked away to centralized nurseries, where one or two nurses could keep an eye on a multitude of babies while mothers recovered from anesthesia, surgery, or both. Such practices were later found to negatively impact maternal-infant bonding, leading to lower rates of breastfeeding success and higher rates of postpartum depression, but at the time they were seen as a way to ensure that birth was scientific, standardized, and carefully controlled.[51]

The process of centralization was solidified by the growing power of professional medical organizations like ACOG, whose recommendations for care were influenced by the needs of obstetrics as a discipline.[52]

While ACOG has, in the past five years, released a range of committee reports and practice recommendations aiming to lower intervention rates, historically it supported high-intensity care even when that care was unsupported by medical evidence. Until 2009, ACOG supported continuous fetal monitoring of women in labor, despite evidence that it provides no medical benefit for low-risk women and in fact dramatically increases intervention rates.[53] ACOG's 1999 recommendation limiting VBAC attempts to hospitals with immediately available surgical and anesthesia staff sharply reduced the number of hospitals willing to accommodate VBAC patients, despite the fact that there was little support for such a rigorous standard in the literature.[54] ACOG's recommendations also influenced state laws limiting VBAC access at birth centers and in home births, virtually ensuring that women would end up with surgical births because there were no providers legally able to oversee a VBAC.[55] Both the national and state ACOG branches actively lobbied against demedicalized options for birth, including out-of-hospital options for birth like home birth and birth centers.

While physicians and their professional associations were consolidating political and regulatory power, some began questioning the wisdom of hospital-based birth. Rogue physicians like Grantly Dick-Read expressed concern as early as the 1930s that hospital-based birth did not result in better outcomes. Increased rates of fetal injury and infection led some to conclude that interventions came with serious side effects. At the same time, medicine's ability to handle complications made maternal death less salient, encouraging women to think about the quality of the experience as a whole. By the mid-1950s, while most American women were giving birth in hospitals, increasing numbers of women expressed dissatisfaction with hospital-based birth.[56] A 1957 *Ladies Home Journal* article detailing mothers' dehumanizing experiences during hospital birth—including stories of women strapped to delivery tables, unable to move, sometimes for days—sparked a broader cultural conversation about birth. This conversation converged with a growing interest in what Betty Friedan would later call "the feminine mystique," increasing interest in natural childbirth as a way for women to regain their feminine power.[57] Grantly Dick-Read's work on natural childbirth from the 1930s was rediscovered in the 1950s as women struggled to resurrect and redefine their role as mothers in the postwar period.[58]

Despite growing interest in natural childbirth and the rediscovery of midwifery by influential providers like Ina May Gaskin in the 1970s, little changed about the actual landscape of birth over the next 40 years. Maternity wards became more attuned to cosmetic reforms such as private suite-like rooms while intervention rates continued to rise. The level of control over pregnancy drilled down even into conception itself, with the advent of genetic counseling and in vitro fertilization. Troublingly, the US approach to birth appears to be spreading to other countries, with European countries experiencing a growth in interventions.[59]

Hospital Birth and the Culture of Intervention

Once birth became centralized in hospitals, a number of factors contributed to medicalization and an increasing intensity of medical care. Interviews with hospital birth workers reveal an internal logic of control in hospitals that is largely insensitive to pressure to change practice standards, stymieing reform. This emphasis on control stems in part from the fact that hospitals were created for the sickest patients, whose needs require quick action and standardized care plans. Hospital protocol reflects the needs of these patients. Physicians and midwives who deliver in hospitals admit that the emphasis on control and activity is problematic for low-risk birthing women, who are best served by an individualized and hands-off approach. One family practice doctor explained, "We're all trained to fix a problem. Sometimes the hardest thing to do is to put your hands in your pocket and not do anything." She also reflected that the medical attitude toward birth is one where "every birth is a disaster and we're here to save you," when the reality is that most births will resolve themselves safely without any medical interventions at all, if given enough time. A hospital-based nurse midwife used the same sort of language, arguing, "We try to control a lot of what doesn't necessarily need to be controlled." A maternal-fetal specialist (an obstetrician who specializes in high-risk pregnancies) argued that in obstetrics there's a "perception that more is better and there's a lot of evidence that's just not true." Following the theories of Dr. DeLee, the hospital environment shifts all pregnancy, not only high-risk pregnancy, into a pathology that must be controlled. The alternative, known as "expectant management," involves waiting and watching, a characteristic approach of midwifery care that is difficult to achieve in a hospital environment.

The emphasis on control, whether of the environment, the process, or the patient, compounds in an environment in which practitioners interact with each other frequently and where local standards of care override evidence-based care. As large institutions, hospitals create their own unique culture of care, driven in part by administrative risk management teams, whose recommendations weigh heavily on staff members. Many practitioners interviewed felt that deviations from the norm of intervention were difficult to justify to other practitioners or in court, even when they knew that the evidence was on their side. The family practice doctor remarked, "It always felt like every time I did things that were different from the way other people were doing things, I had to defend myself. I would get anxious. So you're living with the anxiety and fear of being judged by standards that you don't necessarily agree with." The maternal-fetal specialist noted that "in general medicine has a very low threshold for deviations from the norm." This low threshold applies not only to variations in individual births, as discussed later in this chapter, but also to variations in practice within the hospital setting. Practitioners respond more to the local standard of care in their hospital than they do to evidence-based standards of care, in part because the local standard of care is both ever present and consistently enforced by the actions of nurses, physicians, and administrators.

This fear of variation from the norm of practice is exacerbated by the hierarchical environment of hospitals. A nurse midwife noted that challenges of midwives by doctors were common and sometimes hostile: "We have to know our evidence better, more thoroughly, and more intimately and make our arguments more effectively than any physician. In many cases there will be an immediate dismissal." She recalled one instance where a doctor insisted she break a patient's waters to hasten labor. When she resisted on the basis of research suggesting that artificial rupture was unnecessary and may be harmful, the doctor replied, "You're just an overpaid nurse, you do what I say." Another nurse midwife who attends home births said, "When I transfer people [to the hospital] I'm proactive if not defensive when I give report. You have to speak their language. You kind of have to learn those tricks." She recalled one nonemergency transfer where a woman in labor with a breech baby was transferred to the hospital for pain relief: "She would have been [immediately] sectioned by the crazy doctor, so I went out in the hallway and absorbed him yelling at me [to give the mother time to dilate]. It takes some creativity and sometimes manipulation to find a way to get what you need." The mother had a healthy vaginal breech delivery with another physician who arrived soon after.

Many practitioners felt that the attitude toward risk in obstetrics had changed dramatically, leading to increasing control over both patients and the birth process. Both patients and their doctors are more risk averse than in the past. One midwife described how an African patient of hers dealt with a stillbirth: "She had no expectation that just because she got pregnant she would have a new baby. We have that expectation here, and miscarriage [and infant loss] is much more difficult to deal with here." The high-risk obstetrician argued that "people want the perfect baby and no one wants to take the tiniest risk. Their doctors recommend interventions and they trust them." He also noted that this dramatic risk aversion seeps into obstetrics research as a whole: "Somehow I don't get the impression there have been major leaps forward in obstetrics in many years. What's happened instead is people have fixed on small very incremental improvements that are often associated with more interventions." Even the smallest incremental improvement is used to justify increased interventions, while the cumulative effects of these interventions or the costs to patients, doctors, and the healthcare system as a whole go largely ignored.

Perhaps counterintuitively, technology can both increase risk aversion and increase the sense of control, even if its use does not decrease actual risk.[60] Many providers identified the seemingly innocuous technology of electronic fetal monitoring as a major contributor to the cascade of interventions in birth. The maternal-fetal specialist described what he saw as a common pattern in hospital births, one that begins with fetal monitoring: "One intervention leads to another—you start with monitoring, then you do internal monitoring, then the anxiety raises, everyone is on edge, the mother starts getting concerned, and then it just becomes easiest to section." The family practice physician also singled out fetal monitoring as a primary beginning point on the interventionist path:

First it was fetoscopes, then it was hand held dopplers, then it was we could put a monitor on women all the time in all labors. Usually when you introduce a new technology you have to do randomized controlled trials, but in this case, there were so many benefits to it in terms of convenience, feeling like you were doing things, and recording things and being "scientific" and so it fed into so many different things. I would have to constantly push back against nurses hooking patients up to monitors. And there's no evidence that that's a helpful thing to do. But it's hard to step back from something once it's established.

The current consensus is that continuous fetal monitoring is unsupported in the vast majority of births precisely because its high false positive rate for fetal distress leads to increased rates of labor augmentation and increased numbers of cesarean sections.[61] Yet as of 2007, 87 percent of women reported the use of continuous fetal monitoring during their births.[62] In many hospitals, despite the fact that it provides few benefits and dramatically increases risks of other interventions, continuous fetal monitoring remains the standard of care because it allows providers to retain the illusion of control, is more convenient for staff, and provides legal cover in case of complications later. As many providers pointed out, though most physicians recognize that fetal monitoring is probably not helpful and may actually be harmful, it is difficult to stop doing it if it remains the standard of care. And, as will be discussed in chapter 6, its very existence dramatically changes practice patterns because it is also used as evidence against physicians in malpractice cases, which skews practitioners toward more, rather than less, activity. As the maternal-fetal specialist pointed out, "[Monitoring] is probably the single greatest source of malpractice suits. We monitor almost everyone and almost everyone has some not-reassuring things, so when do you intervene?"

Despite strong conformist tendencies within institutions, there exists a wide range of variation in interventions between hospitals, even within the same region, again indicating a departure from evidence-based practices. The maternal-fetal specialist pointed out that "when you look at different hospitals and you look at rates of intervention there's a wide amount of variation. I don't think case mixing [taking into account different levels of risk] makes as much difference as people think it does. It's practice habits, what your patients expect, and so on. Bottom line is there's a lot of variation in interventions and testing and not very much variation in outcomes." The fact that hospitals with higher rates of interventions do not have better outcomes for mothers and babies suggests that doctors are not responding to the risk profiles of patients, but are instead reacting primarily to their local standards of care and their own practice habits.[63] Researchers focusing on variations across hospitals found dramatic variation in cesarean section rates across hospitals, ranging from 7 to 70 percent, even across hospitals with similar patient profiles.[64] The maternal-fetal specialist expressed frustration at the level of intervention in most births: "We all want things to be the best and we are trained to think that our interventions are being done for a good reason, no matter how incremental the benefits are or how poor our reasoning. We tend to err on the side of doing things."

Technology, Standardization, and Control

The prevalence and standard use of technology in labor and delivery wards facilitate the linked tendencies to control and standardize. Perhaps not surprisingly, the mere presence of medical technology in hospitals creates a strong pull toward high-intensity care.[65] Hospitals invest in new technology to stay competitive and treat high-risk and complex patients, but the very presence of technology creates an incentive to use that technology on less appropriate patient populations, particularly when poor hospital design makes such use more efficient and convenient. Most American births occur in the equivalent of intensive care units, despite the fact that most American mothers are healthy and low risk.[66] Most of those women, regardless of their risk profile, will be hooked up to fetal monitors, their movement limited by IVs for hydration and the monitors, their labor augmented with Pitocin, and their freedom to eat and drink limited in case surgery becomes necessary, despite the fact that little evidence exists for the benefit of any of these standard practices.

As further evidence that obstetrics practices are not tightly linked to medical need, one 2017 study found that "the greatest predictor of whether a woman will have a cesarean delivery is not her personal risks or preferences, but instead the facility where she gives birth."[67] The study found that variations in hospital design contribute to medicalized births, particularly increased rates of surgical birth. Room demand, distance between patient rooms, the ratio of operating rooms to labor and delivery rooms, and distance from workstations and call rooms all correlate with increased interventions, presumably because as staff become overworked or find it difficult to easily access patients, they become more risk averse and rely more on fetal monitoring and other technologies to control the variables at play. Room demand, in particular, creates an incentive to hasten the process of labor and delivery to ensure that beds open up for new patients.[68] Providers compensate for inadequate hospital design (among other things) by using technology and automation to maintain a sense of control over the birth process.

Standardization in medicine is, of course, not always problematic. Interventions that standardize the response to a specific medical complication, such as postpartum hemorrhage, significantly improve outcomes and save lives (something, ironically, many hospitals also do not do well).[69] But advocates point out that birth itself is not a medical complication and interventions that standardize the general process of labor and delivery do not improve outcomes and may cause other kinds of iatrogenic harm.[70] As the maternal-fetal specialist pointed out in an email, many women do not respond like the average woman (by definition). The range of normal responses during labor and delivery is quite large. Additionally, he noted that "standardized protocols may be based on demonstrably positive but very small improvements in population outcomes, the tiny benefits of which may be offset by (1) the fact that most labor and deliveries will go normally without following the protocol, and (2) the subjective nature of the birth experience, and the interference that interventions impose." Standardizing birth to create incremental improvements at the population level may create dramatic harms at the individual level.

Many of these harms stem from the fact that birth resists standardization because it is heavily influenced by individual maternal and fetal variables, many of which we do not fully understand. Birth is a complex, episodic, and emergent event that requires the shifting and alignment of multiple sensitive systems in two different bodies. In the weeks leading up to labor, the cervix softens and "ripens," preparing to step back from its role as fetal guardian to allow the baby to pass through. The uterus tones itself with practice contractions in preparation for the long task of contracting the baby through the birth canal, and such practice contractions may be mistaken by women for the onset of labor. The hips widen and the joints loosen to allow the pelvis to spread further to allow the baby's large head through. The fetus is also at work, shifting and moving into position in the birth canal, flipping itself into the most efficient head-down position. During labor itself, dramatic hormonal changes occur, including skyrocketing levels of oxytocin and prolactin, hormones that facilitate contractions, help prevent hemorrhage, and assist with later lactation and bonding.[71] A woman's contractions work with the movements of the fetus to achieve ideal positioning. What to the outside may seem like "stalled" labor may be the body's way of slowing down the process until more congenial birthing conditions are achieved, a phenomenon that midwives say is common in pregnancies where the fetus is poorly positioned or where the mother feels threatened or stressed.[72] Having women labor on their backs to facilitate physician access and restricting movement to facilitate monitoring are two of the most harmful hospital policies since movement significantly facilitates the birth process and reduces pain; compounding the problem, women laboring on their backs are much more likely to need further interventions.[73] Yet these policies are standard in American hospitals owing to the prevalence of continuous fetal monitoring and the convenience of staff. Birth is standardized to fit the available technology, not the needs of women's bodies.

Apart from the complexity of the process itself, birth is notoriously difficult to predict and control and is therefore a poor fit for an environment that requires predictability and routine. Women are most likely to go into spontaneous labor in the early morning hours, an inconvenient time for staff and administrators.[74] The duration of labor and delivery frequently spans hospital shifts, leaving providers worried about handing off care to another doctor or nurse. Labor can start and stop, false or prodromal labor can bedevil women and their doctors for weeks on end, and a progressing labor can stall for hours without any apparent cause. Meanwhile, pressures like parental excitement to meet the baby, maternal exhaustion (physical and emotional), demands from other patients, scarce hospital resources, and the desire to support a laboring woman through to the end all contribute to an overwhelming tendency to standardize the process, making it predictable, controllable, and a better fit for the hospital environment.

Standardization, Control, and the Intervention Cascade

It is not surprising then that induction and labor augmentation are two of the most common interventions in birth, because each gives providers greater levels of control over the process. Around 25 percent of American women are induced, and some hospitals induce over 40 percent of labors.[75] In one nationwide survey, 40 percent of women reported that their doctors had tried to induce labor.[76] Induction of labor is a crucial component of obstetrical care, especially when it comes to serious threats to maternal or infant health like uncontrolled diabetes, poor fetal position, placental quality and attachment, preeclampsia, multiple pregnancy, and fetal growth restriction.[77] Most inductions, however, are not carried out for these reasons. Instead, the most common reasons for induction are to end a "prolonged" pregnancy past 40 weeks (around 25% of medical inductions), concerns about fetal size (around 17% of medical inductions), or elective induction at the request of the mother or doctor (as many as 35% of all inductions).[78] The most common reasons for inductions are subjective and heavily influenced by practitioner practice patterns. Inductions, even those done later in pregnancy, carry risks to both mothers and infants.[79]

A closer look at two important causes of induction in the United States—large babies (known in the medical community as macrosomia) and prolonged pregnancy, or a labor that goes past 40 weeks—demonstrates the process of medicalization, including the tendency for medical practitioners to pull aspects of pregnancy and birth toward the mean, narrowing the range of normal to create a more standard and therefore more controllable process. Both large fetal size and length of pregnancy share in common with other medicalized traits that they occur on a spectrum.[80] This spectrum includes real risk factors at the margins, including very large babies getting stuck in the birth canal or an increased risk of stillbirth in pregnancies that go beyond 42 weeks. But there is also a wide range of normal, including many mothers who happen to carry healthy babies to 42 weeks or those who happen to gestate healthy 10-pound babies. While most of these variants result in normal outcomes, hospitals do not treat them that way, instead pathologizing otherwise low-risk pregnancies. Intervention based solely on a pregnancy or labor deviating from the mean places mothers at greater risk of medical interventions without improving outcomes.

American medical attitudes toward large babies reveal how technology assists in the process of control and standardization, contributing to the medicalization of otherwise normal pregnancies. Large babies indeed come with risks, one of which is shoulder dystocia, when the infant's shoulders get stuck in the birth canal during the pushing phase. In rare cases, shoulder dystocia can result in permanent nerve damage or even infant death. Mothers of large babies may also be at greater risk of tearing and postpartum hemorrhage, though such risks are still rare. Even with those risks, there is no medical evidence supporting routine inductions for large babies, even after 39 weeks. Shoulder dystocia is actually more common in "normal"-sized babies because such babies are themselves more common than large babies, and there is no way to predict ahead of time which babies will get stuck and which will pass safely through.[81] Most large babies can be delivered vaginally without harm to infant or mother. Moreover, diagnosing fetal size (usually done through ultrasound in the third trimester) is itself an imperfect science, with high false positive rates.[82] Despite the medical evidence, the threat of a "large" baby (often defined as a baby over 8.5 pounds, though ranges vary) pushes many women toward induction or cesarean.[83]

Ironically, attempting to diagnose macrosomia may lead to worse outcomes for mothers and babies than simply assuming that the baby is of normal size. Large babies are less common than doctors think, the risks of large babies are much lower than doctors believe, and the interventions used to combat macrosomia, including induction and cesarean section, have higher risks than the vaginal delivery of a large baby.[84] Moreover, diagnosis of large fetal size is enough to change the attitude medical staff have toward a woman's labor and delivery. Mothers of suspected large babies are more likely to be diagnosed as "failure to progress" during labor, even when their progress is identical to mothers of average-sized babies with unimpeded labors.[85] One study found, ironically, that practitioner suspicion of macrosomia is actually more dangerous than having a large baby itself; births in which a practitioner suspected a large baby had more than three times the inductions, cesarean sections, and maternal complications as pregnancies where a large baby was born but not suspected ahead of time.[86] Much of the danger of large babies seems to come from the interventions large size triggers, not from large size itself.[87] Despite the conflicting evidence, large size is still one of the most common causes of induction in the United States.[88]

Standardization pressures also affect the length of labor itself. Once labor begins, physicians and hospitals place time constraints on how long laboring women can remain in each stage of labor. To keep women on this artificial clock, hospitals use a suite of interventions to hasten the process of labor from breaking the amniotic sac (or "waters"), to the use of Pitocin to augment labor, to cesarean sections when doctors determine that a labor has gone on too long. Many hospitals base their guidelines for length of each stage of labor on observational research from the 1950s, summarized in the guideline called "Friedman's curve."[89] Such policies determine how long a woman can be in active labor, how long a woman can labor after her water is broken, and how long the pushing stage can take. When women exceed these time frames, interventions like Pitocin, episiotomy, or forceps are used to bring labor length back into the "normal" range. While concern about length of labor is rooted in serious risks like infection and internal damage, many researchers acknowledge that Friedman's curve is outdated, with labors today taking longer at each stage for a variety of complex reasons.[90]

As with interventions for large infant size, attempts to standardize the length of labor cause problems of their own. One of the main reasons for primary cesarean section is what is known as "failure to progress," a term used for labors that stall or even seem to stop while a woman is in the hospital. It can also be used to describe labors in which dilation of the cervix, which occurs in stages from 0 centimeters dilated to 10 centimeters or fully dilated, continues, but too slowly for the given time frame.[91] First-time mothers, whose cervixes typically take much longer to dilate during labor than mothers who have given birth before, are at greater risk of a diagnosis of failure to progress, even though most would go on to give birth vaginally without intervention if given time.[92] Hospital protocols that artificially limit the length of labor are a primary driver of the growth in cesarean sections.

The medicalization of birth that emerged from the centralization of birth in hospitals not only has changed the experience of birth but also has shifted the very norm of pregnancy, labor, and delivery. It is no accident that the largest share of the recent increase in cesarean section rates comes from subjective indicators such as fetal size, apparent fetal distress, and "prolonged" pregnancy and labor.[93] The very logic of hospitals turns low-risk labors into medical events to be controlled, standardized, and "treated." While this movement has important medical and public health implications, it also has enormous ethical and moral implications that are rarely discussed in the literature. Medicalization makes it much more difficult for pregnant women to be treated as individuals and makes it more likely that women will receive care that is harmful, unnecessary, coercive, or all three.

Hospital Birth, Autonomy, and Control

While there has been little systematic research on how common autonomy violations are in maternity wards, examples of recently documented violations of informed consent include forced episiotomies,[94] coercive sterilization,[95] sexualized physical exams or sexual assaults during exams,[96] pelvic exams without consent,[97] denial of anesthesia,[98] and forced cesarean sections like Dray's.[99] As Miriam's case in the introduction attests, pregnant mothers are often unsure whether their physician's recommendations are the result of liability fears, hospital protocol, insurance limitations, past experiences, peculiar (and often random) clinical patterns, or some combination thereof. Widespread inappropriate use of technology like fetal monitoring further muddies the waters, triggering false positives for fetal distress and appearing to justify ever-increasing interventions. Laboring women are susceptible to being controlled by fear, exhaustion, misplaced trust, or the inability to exit a coercive environment.[100] These limitations are exacerbated by the fact that pregnancy involves two people sharing the same body and that the pregnant woman is tasked with making informed decisions for both herself and her unborn child in a situation in which her interests, while usually aligned, are occasionally at odds with those of her fetus.[101]

One of the subtlest effects of the medicalization of birth is how the emphasis on controlling the process changes the way women themselves think about their bodily autonomy. Identifying autonomy violations in labor and delivery can be particularly difficult because the language of control is so central to the culture of pregnancy and birth. Scholars have long noted that pregnancy and birth are surrounded by rules, limitations, and restrictions, many of which are arbitrary or unclear.[102] Women themselves have internalized and accepted limitations on their autonomy as part of the process of birth, regardless of whether such limitations are medically necessary or evidence based. The economist Emily Oster recounts discovering during her own pregnancy that she had "the appearance of decision-making authority, but apparently not the reality."[103] The illusion of maternal control is apparent when providers tell pregnant women what they are "allowed" or "not allowed" to do without providing reasons or asking for patient input. This language of control is sometimes paired with threats of being "fired" as a patient or of threats to involve the police or Child Protective Services, threats that are more likely for women of color.[104] During labor and delivery, providers may use language that implies that the baby is at risk, absent objective indicators of concern.[105] And for many women, their experiences and preferences are denied by the oft-repeated trope that "all that matters is a healthy baby."[106] Taking into account, in addition to this coercive language, the myriad protocols, regulations, and restrictions that come from bureaucratic forces upstream, the landscape of pregnancy and birth may be incompatible with anything like a robust view of informed consent.[107]

More subtly, medicalization and the attending environment of control impact the way women think about their bodies and the process of birth itself, making it difficult to recognize consent violations in the moment. Cristen Pascucci, an advocate for pregnant and birthing women, coined the phrase "you're not allowed to not allow me" in a blog post after hearing from women who were told they could not refuse even nonemergency procedures like inductions, IV locks during labor, and fetal monitoring, or who were told they would not be "allowed" to stand and move around during labor or eat and drink.[108] In an interview Pascucci recalled her motivation for emphasizing the language of control in birth: "It was so frustrating because it's women, too, using this internalized oppressive language and talking about their own bodies and not seeing that they're being controlled. Why does anyone think they have the right to tell people in a medical context that they're not allowed to refuse an intervention?" Pascucci found it especially disturbing that most providers and pregnant women she spoke with were unaware that pregnant women can legally refuse medical treatment. This legal right has been recognized both by courts and by ACOG's own professional guidelines.[109] Despite the legal and professional emphasis on informed consent, anecdotal evidence suggests that women rarely report violations of informed consent and physicians who violate consent during labor and delivery are rarely censured, let alone prosecuted.

Scholars have argued that the language of control in birth has gendered roots, particularly as birth shifted from being the experience of a specific and unique woman supported by almost exclusively female attendants to becoming a standardized process controlled and structured by the demands of a hierarchical and bureaucratic environment and, until recently, entirely male staff.[110] The standard language of physicians (or bystanders) "delivering" babies places the birthing woman in a passive role, if not erasing her altogether. Such language also, crucially, emphasizes a medicalized approach to labor and delivery where the birth attendant is actively involved in the birth and delivery, taking on a (or the) central role. Midwives tend to use the more passive language of "catching" a baby to emphasize their relative inaction compared to the activity and centrality of the woman giving birth. The language of medicalized birth shifts the activity and therefore decision-making power in birth away from the woman to the medical provider, who becomes the agent whose autonomous decision making takes center stage. As Rinat Dray's physician put it, "I have decided to override her refusal."

With the shift from home birth to hospital birth, birth transformed from a bottom-up, individualized event where the mother maintained as much control as the physiological process allowed to a top-down standardized one with medical staff as the locus of activity and control. While most obstetricians are now female, some scholars argue that the historical framework of the hospital as constructed around the convenience of largely male physicians and the culture of medicine that grew out of a male-dominated worldview mean that even female physicians will struggle to provide care that respects patient autonomy.[111] Sociologists such as Robert Nye argue that the entire Western medical framework is constructed around typically masculine traits like hierarchy, control, and honor, while typically feminine traits like collaboration and communication are deemphasized.[112] Some physicians have in turn argued that abuse of patients follows from the abusive and coercive nature of medical training, which is itself linked to its masculine roots as a competitive and somewhat cutthroat enterprise.[113] While over 80 percent of residents entering obstetrics are currently female, the highly hierarchical training and culture associated with gynecology and obstetrics remain unchanged. Perhaps as a result of the enduring culture of control in hospitals, intervention rates have not changed even as women become the majority of obstetrics providers.[114]

Complicating the situation, birth plans, which could elucidate women's preferences and facilitate conversations about care, have no legal or clinical status and, for a variety of reasons, are viewed with suspicion and sometimes with actual disdain by providers.[115] This attitude arises in part from the fact that birth plans are often composed without provider input. This, in turn, is due to the fact that prenatal appointments are extremely short, averaging between 10 and 15 minutes, with most of that spent with a nurse rather than the obstetrician.[116] In response to limited communication with providers, women resort to using birth plan templates available online, which may be inappropriate for a given birth setting or may directly violate hospital protocols.[117] Providers may also believe that patients with birth plans are higher maintenance or are making unreasonable requests, particularly when they decline interventions that make nursing care easier, such as automatic placement of IV ports for birthing women, even if such interventions do not improve outcomes.[118] In an expansion on a common joke in the field, a medical blog posted a satirical study that claimed to find a correlation between the length of a birth plan and the length of the resulting cesarean section scar. The implication is that women with birth plans are both high maintenance and more likely to require cesarean sections because they refuse routine care.[119]

Predictably, attitudes toward birth plans differ by provider type. Obstetricians, the most common providers in hospitals, tend to have negative attitudes toward birth plans, while midwives tend to be more positive about birth plans.[120] These attitudes align with the culture of the two disciplines: obstetricians see themselves as experts, with birth plans challenging that expertise, while midwives see themselves as partners in care. For midwives, birth plans provide them with helpful information about patient goals, rather than challenging their authority. Whatever the reasons, birth plans are viewed with skepticism by both medical providers and the hospitals in which they work.[121]

One obstetrician interviewed pointed to blogs and the internet as major barriers to realistic expectations during birth: "No one walks in with a heart attack plan—'I don't want morphine, but I want this kind of stent placement.' Because they don't have heart attack blogs." The existence of birth blogs in fact underscores two aspects of birth that, presumably, do not apply to heart attack treatments: women are dissatisfied with the care being routinely offered in hospitals, and they believe that the care being offered in hospitals is less aligned with existing medical evidence. Cristen Pascucci noted in an interview that most women construct birth plans because they are "looking for evidence-based care and the institution is saying [they] can't have evidence-based care." Poor communication, differing expectations, and intrusive third-party policies and protocols place patients and providers into relationships that are more antagonistic than collaborative. Whatever the cause of the conflict, negative attitudes toward birth plans pose a serious challenge to respecting women's autonomy both prenatally and during labor and delivery.

Women's Experiences and Preferences during Birth

Women's own experiences of labor and delivery in surveys and in interviews demonstrate complicated and nuanced attitudes toward the relationship between autonomy and birth. In the most obvious sense, interviews with women underscored that patient autonomy is not a primary value in labor and delivery wards in the United States. Jennifer, a lawyer in New York State, recounted her experience with the medical attitude toward patient autonomy during her hospital birth in 2013.[122] Jennifer was struggling with pain during a contraction, and when her midwife approached to do a routine cervical check, Jennifer verbally refused consent for the check. The midwife ignored her and forced her hand inside Jennifer's vagina while Jennifer yelled for her to stop. Jennifer later filed a complaint with the Office of Professions, reporting that she told the midwife to stop three separate times before the midwife finally pulled her hand out of Jennifer's vagina. The Office of Professions responded by apologizing that the midwife's actions had caused Jennifer physical pain. In a follow-up letter, Jennifer clarified that pain was not the issue: "The issue raised in my complaint was not simply that the vaginal exam caused me pain and discomfort. . . . Rather, the problem that led to my decision to file a complaint is the fact that a health care provider continued to touch me when I repeatedly asked (yelled) for her to stop. Consent can be withdrawn."

That neither Jennifer's midwife nor the staff at the Office of Professions noticed the clear violation of consent or found it particularly troubling indicates that expectations around informed consent in the clinical environment do not match up with the theoretical commitments to consent laid out by ACOG and the broader bioethical community.[123] Jennifer's account also demonstrates the gulf in experience between women and their providers. Her midwife denies doing anything wrong and was not censured, while Jennifer said, "I totally consider my midwife's actions to be an assault."[124] Moreover, as is common in many of the reports women provide, there was no clinical benefit to performing a cervical check on a low-risk woman in the middle of a contraction absent concerning clinical indicators. Jennifer's midwife violated her autonomy to perform a routine and (in this case) unnecessary intervention, a not uncommon narrative in hospitals.[125]

In a survey of 167 women, many expressed frustration at the limitations of the hospital environment and the way in which their basic desires, including their desire for evidence-based care, were ignored. When asked whether she felt respected during labor and delivery, one woman responded, "I was a chunk of inconvenient meat to the hospitals, (most) of the nurses, doctors, and midwives." Another responded, "Not at all. I was given a room with no tub after being told I would have a tub. Doctors performed a membrane sweep without asking. They sought medical consent while I was heavily drugged, and encouraged me to take medications while my support people were out of the room. They disappeared when I was in severe pain and left me unattended for four hours."[126]

Other respondents felt that the language used was manipulative or even coercive. When asked whether she felt she had freedom to make decisions about her care, another woman responded, "There were a lot of 'You have to . . . 's or 'we have to . . . '. No reasons given. We have to break your water now. You have to lie still. We have to take your baby to the nursery now. Things put in my [IV] that I didn't even know about until my husband mentioned it later." Another woman with a biology degree said, "Sometimes I felt as though the way that I was encouraged to make decisions was mainly through giving vague, non-specific explanations, even though I would have been capable of understanding a fairly complex breakdown of the science." Many women expressed frustration at the limits placed on even evidence-based practices such as avoiding breaking waters, allowing women water and food during labor, and allowing women to move around during labor, practices that can themselves reduce the need for other interventions.

While many women found the lack of autonomy troubling and frustrating, other women expressed trust in the hospital process and were more comfortable handing over decision-making authority to experts. When asked whether she was free to make decisions about her birthing process, one woman responded, "What decisions? Just get the baby out." Another woman, when asked if she felt as though she had freedom to make decisions about her body, replied, "No . . . and with a surgery, I don't think I should have been able to." Another woman responded,

"To the extent that I should have been. The doctors are ultimately responsible for keeping us alive, so their say mattered too." When asked how she felt about the safety of birth in general, one woman replied, "It is safe in certain conditions. I can't imagine giving birth anywhere other than a hospital."

Some women who expressed frustration with hospital limitations found that they were able to counter the controlling environment of the labor and delivery ward by simply ignoring the dictates of staff. One woman recalled, "[My wishes were respected] only because I either didn't ask for things that they would not agree to or didn't tell them. Like, I ate and drank [even though told not to], I held out as long as I could before getting the heplock, refused to stay in bed for the continuous monitoring. A lot of this was based on the first birth where I followed their rules more consistently and it was not as good an experience." Another woman recalls, "I think doctors recommend unsafe methods in order to make the prices [sic] more convenient on them, not the delivering mother. Which is awful! At the hospital with my second the doctor kept coming in telling me I NEEDED pitocin to get things started, and I kept declining because I know my body and it was doing what needed to be done." Others, like Jennifer, found that even when they declined or attempted to ignore staff, their wishes were overridden.

Many of the women who reported very positive experiences during hospital birth linked their experiences to excellent communication with staff. One woman reported that "when I first got there, the doctors asked me a bunch of questions about what I wanted and how I felt about things. They stood by what I wanted the whole time." Another woman with six children had wildly divergent birth experiences for each of her six children, linked in large part to the level of communication provided. She recalled, "#4 was the best, with no interventions; very beautiful birth. 6 was next—lots of intervention, but clearly explained in a caring environment, with epidural. 1, 2, and 3 were induced—nightmare; I still don't trust nurses as far as I can throw them. 5 was okay, but I broke down and asked for help with the pain and was given Staidol (sp.?) which did not lesson my pain one iota, but did disassociate my brain from my mouth so I stopped complaining about it. I thought that was a dirty trick."

One pattern that emerged from the surveys and interviews was that women felt the most comfortable with interventions when providers clearly explained to them why a specific intervention was being recommended. Many women were frustrated not by interventions themselves but by the fact that many interventions occurred without their knowledge or consent. One woman described her first birth: "They waited until I was on narcotics and hallucinating to ask me to sign paperwork to allow a class of medical students to watch the process, something that I expressed discomfort with beforehand. They waited until I was on my back and pushing to bring them in, so I didn't see them until I had finished birthing and could sit up again." She contrasted that experience with the cesarean birth of her third child, which she characterized as respectful, with open communication between herself and her providers. The importance of being informed about what was happening to their bodies was a consistent theme that characterized good births for many of the women in the sample.

A perhaps obvious lesson that emerges from the survey data is that the category of birthing women represents a diverse group of individuals with very different expectations, past experiences, and attitudes toward birth. Generally speaking, the women who believed that birth was a medical event felt more comfortable with hospital protocols limiting their choices than those who believed that birth can happen without interventions. At the same time, most women felt comfortable and supported when communication with their providers was clear and when staff took the time to explain what was happening. The importance of being informed is a major but unappreciated bridge for situations where patient autonomy clashes with physician autonomy or duties of care. As the bioethicist Mary Mahowhold argues, what is left in cases of conflict is the duty of "truth-telling," or the duty of physicians to "truthfulness, honesty, or veracity, that is, an attempt to communicate to others accurately and adequately."[127] Honest and open communication can be a powerful way for practitioners to protect the personhood and autonomy of patients, even when disagreements arise. In Rinat Dray's case, her physician chose coercion over truth telling, with perhaps predictable results.

Given the range of women's attitudes toward interventions, place of birth, and the birth process itself, it might seem obvious that having more options for locations and type of birth care would protect patient autonomy and the duty of informed consent by allowing women to choose providers and locations of care that are most likely to fit their needs and preferences. Yet most American women lack any options other than medicalized hospital birth. Once in hospitals, many American women lack control over even the most basic preferences and are likely to undergo unnecessary and harmful procedures.[128] As a result, the way American women give birth challenges every bioethical principle Western medicine claims to protect. The centralization of birth in hospitals puts women's lives at risk, violates their autonomy, wastes precious healthcare resources that could be better spent elsewhere, and, as will be discussed in chapter 7, contributes to racial disparities that harm the most vulnerable among us.

Conclusion

The centralization of birth and the harm it causes are due to the way policy tributaries funnel and channel resources into hospitals. Later chapters will focus on mapping the major tributaries of that larger watershed, including the combination of federal reimbursement policies, state regulations, and the liability environment. Each of these tributaries powers cascades of interventions and rapids of medicalization in which providers and patients struggle to make evidence-based decisions that reflect patient values. Demedicalizing, individualizing, and rehumanizing childbirth does not require jettisoning the medical progress that has saved the lives of perhaps hundreds of thousands of mothers and babies. It may, however, require rethinking the geography of the watershed, particularly the policies that contribute to the cascade of interventions in hospitals and the tributaries that centralize care for low-risk mothers in hospitals in the first place. Rethinking where Americans give birth can help provide the most appropriate care for different kinds of births: hospital-based care for high-risk mothers alongside community-based care for low-risk women that prevents them from being pulled into the rapids. In the rest of the book I discuss the reforms necessary for rethinking medicalized birth and reformatting and restructuring the watershed in which these decisions take place. But first, let's take a look at the other end of the life cycle.

CHAPTER 2

Medicalized Death and the Current of Centralized Care

In the hospital you have a million docs who are taking care of you, and everyone looks at their organ and orders a million tests for that organ. The default is always to do something.—*Palliative care physician*

EIGHTY-THREE-YEAR-OLD Beatrice Wiseman carefully prepared for her last days. She discussed her wishes with her husband of 57 years, crafted an advance directive, and appointed her husband her health proxy. After suffering a stroke in 2013, she was admitted to the intensive care unit and placed on a ventilator. Her husband soon determined that medical interventions were increasingly painful for her and diminishing her quality of life and that "she should be allowed to die a dignified death should her heart and/or lung function fail."[1] With the help and advice of his children, he crafted a MOLST (medical order for life-sustaining treatment) form, a legal form in Maryland that provides immunity to medical staff who forgo lifesaving interventions and protects patient wishes. Despite these precautions and preparations, when Mrs. Weisman was found blue in her bed in August 2013, staff jumped into action, and, according to a civil suit filed later, they administered "violent chest compressions, chemical stimulants to her heart, and jolted her with electrical shocks." These resuscitative effects were successful in the sense that they restarted her heart, though in the process she suffered two collapsed lungs, and she was readmitted to the ICU to stabilize her condition. Two months later she was discharged from the step-down unit she returned to because, according to the suit, the hospital "could do nothing further for her." The Weisman family tried to find a long-term care facility that would accept her, but they could not find one that would take her given her extensive physical needs and constant delirium, which required restraints.

Mrs. Weisman survived these events, but the civil suit her family filed describes her condition when she was released to her family: "Upon her discharge, Mrs. Weisman was taking Nineteen (19) different drugs, receiving nutrition through a feeding tube, had catheters in both her urethra and rectum, was disoriented and otherwise suffering from bouts of dementia and delirium, required 24/7 home healthcare and home oxygen, and otherwise could not take care of herself." Her husband William died a year after her discharge, a death his children attribute to the stress of full-time caregiving of a profoundly disabled spouse. The Weisman children sued the hospital for assault, negligence, intentional infliction of emotional distress, breach of contract, and lack of informed consent.[2] The case was settled for an undisclosed amount in 2017, and similar cases have been reported by media outlets.[3] While Mrs. Weisman recovered significant physical ability as the result of extensive physical therapy and round-the-clock care, such care was paid for out of pocket, and she continues to require extensive care at home owing to dementia.

As with Rinat Dray's case, Mrs. Weisman's experience is extreme while also symptomatic of broader patterns in how American hospitals treat dying patients, patterns that challenge the basic medical commitments to informed consent and limiting harm. Most cases of overtreatment do not stem from the kind of negligence in Mrs. Weisman's case. What is more common are disagreements among family members, poor communication, fragmented care, and patient and family member misunderstandings about the usefulness or futility of specific interventions. But what ties all these cases together is a way of dying that violates patient autonomy and causes harm to patients and their families. Despite increasing evidence that the use of high-intensity medical interventions at the end of life is harmful and costly, many Americans die in hospitals or nursing homes, often with invasive interventions that leave them restrained, sedated, or unable to eat, drink, or communicate. One physician described dying in America as "an often protracted medicalized techno-process that is hurtful to the patients and their families, and ultimately to the very fabric of our society."[4] Tributaries in the watershed, including Medicaid policies, state regulations, hospital policies, and liability fears, combine with the hope provided by new technologies and a cultural fear of death to fuel rapids of interventions that end in hospital-based death. While the specific tributaries will be discussed in more detail in later chapters, this chapter lays out the contours of American death. For the elderly or terminally ill, the promises that hospitals offer too often end in isolation, overtreatment, and poor quality of life.

Medicalized Death in the United States

Most observers agree that death in the United States is costly and traumatic for the dying.[5] The American way of death mirrors that of the American way of birth, from the location of death in centralized hospitals to the glut of procedures, the high cost of care, and the poor patient outcomes of fully medicalized death. The causes of these trends mirror those of birth: centralization of medical care in hospitals, regulations and industry capture, reimbursement barriers, and the loss of traditional caregivers and the generational knowledge of how to care for the dying. The combination of these factors makes American death the costliest and some of the most traumatic in the developed world, though the rest of the world is catching up as populations age and healthcare systems struggle to adapt.

The financial impact of the medicalization of death dwarfs the costs of medicalized births. Around 25 percent of Medicare spending occurs in the last year of life, with 30 percent of those costs incurred in the last month of life.[6] Other estimates suggest that as much as 13 percent of overall healthcare spending occurs in the last year of life.[7] While scholars disagree on whether these numbers indicate an epidemic of overtreatment or the realistic cost of treating complex patients with chronic illnesses, some of whom will recover, the overall costs to the healthcare system of treatments for seriously ill patients are high.[8] Costs to individuals are high as well, with studies finding average out-of-pocket medical expenditures of almost $40,000 in the last five years of life.[9] Many of these costs are not associated with quality of care or physical or psychological comfort. It is not even clear whether these increased costs are associated with greater length of life.

While the United States spends increasing amounts of money at the end of life, research suggests that the quality of that time has declined dramatically, with patient and family reports indicating low quality of life in the weeks before death.[10] Institutionalization at the end of life is the norm for around 75 percent of Medicare recipients, despite the fact that dying at home remains the most common desire of those approaching the end of life.[11] While the number of Medicare patients dying in hospitals has decreased over the past decade and patients have more access to hospice and palliative care, ICU use and the rate of transitions between locations of care have increased, demonstrating a fragmented system of care.[12] Surveys of dying patients and their families consistently find that dying at home is more comfortable and less traumatic for both patients and their loved ones than dying in an institution.[13] Even apart from location of care, more treatment at the end of life is not associated with better outcomes. According to one study of cancer patients, the more money spent at the end of life, the lower the quality of the experience for both patients and their families.[14] Providers have even used the term "torture" to describe what happens to patients in hospitals at the end of life, hooked up to ventilators and feeding tubes, physically restrained, and unable to communicate with family and loved ones.[15]

The now-famous SUPPORT study, published in the *Journal of the American Medical Association* in 1995, was a watershed moment in end-of-life care. The study found serious shortcomings in the way Americans die in hospitals, including high levels of aggressive treatment, poor communication between patients and providers, confusion over end-of-life wishes, and poorly controlled pain. Almost 40 percent of patients who died during the study spent over a week in an ICU. More troubling, the second phase of the study, which included interventions to improve care, had no effect on patient satisfaction or outcomes. All the interventions intended to improve the way Americans die in hospitals had failed to have any effect.[16] The SUPPORT study exposed the binary choice available to dying patients: accept either the aggressive "do-everything" care provided by hospitals or the "do-nothing" approach of hospice.[17] Many patients struggled to understand or elucidate their own preferences when faced with two extreme options that afforded little room for nuance.

One result of the SUPPORT study and the soul-searching it prompted was an increased interest in harnessing the power of medicine to serve the interests of the dying, apart from the desire to indefinitely preserve life. The relatively new specialty of palliative care, itself influenced by the much older tradition of hospice care for the dying, focused its efforts on training physicians both in the use of medical tools for the palliation of symptoms and how to individualize care for patients at the end of life. Palliative care emphasized symptom control in tandem with treating disease and worked to orient both the practitioner and the patient toward quality-of-life considerations and patient preferences rather than emphasizing life extension alone.[18] In part because palliative care emerged as a medical specialty, it gained legitimacy that calls from outside the medical community to demedicalize birth did not. Despite this medical buy-in, changing the way Americans die has proved difficult, in part because of the powerful upstream forces that centralize dying in hospitals. Physicians and authors such as Atul Gawande, Ira Byock, Jessica Zitter, and Kenneth Fischer have focused attention on the problems associated with medicalized death, highlighting the complex causes and the dearth of clear solutions.[19]

Despite the growth of palliative care training programs over the past 15 years, practitioners and advocates argue that a variety of cultural, professional, and structural currents pull patients away from palliative care and toward the rapids of medicalization, where they undergo unnecessary and harmful interventions and are more likely to die in institutions. Many of these currents have to do with the way patient expectations interact with the hospital environment. Others have to do with reimbursement structures that incentivize overtreatment, and others have to do with the culture of medicine itself. What is increasingly clear is that medicalization of death cannot be attributed to patient demand alone. Most Americans express a desire to die at home, while less than 25 percent are able to do so.[20] And the medical intensity with which Americans treat death is not the result of better care. Many of the classic medical interventions at the end of life, such as tube feeding, CPR, or ventilators, provide no medical benefit for the elderly or terminally ill.[21]

The Current of Centralized Death

Death, like birth, was not always a medically intensive event. Until the 1940s, most Americans died at home. Hospitals became the main places for dying partly because of the surge in medical knowledge in the 1950s and 1960s funded by governmental investment in the National Institutes of Health around World War II.[22] The movement of the dying to hospitals was, in many ways, the result of the success of medicine in preventing people from dying in the first place. Fewer people died early in life as a result of better primary care and the advent of antibiotics. Those who would have died later in life from chronic illnesses like heart disease or cancer were able to survive longer. The discovery of penicillin in the early 1940s changed the way Americans thought about the inevitability of death.[23] The 1950s in turn saw cardiac resuscitation, open-heart surgery, the first kidney transplants, and the advent of modern respirators. ICUs followed in 1958 as the first comprehensive approach to treating those dying from serious illnesses. The 1960s saw further waves of innovations, including heart transplants, the growth of CPR training, and refinements of these earlier innovations.

In the early days of hospitalized death, most physicians supported aggressive care at the end of life, fueled by a belief in the power of innovation that made withdrawing care seem cruel. Incredible advances could be made almost overnight, and patients could be pulled back from death at the final hour.[24] By the mid-1950s, patients were able to recover from a range of accidents, illnesses, and other conditions that would have cut short lives just decades before.[25] This burst of innovation coincided with government policies like the Hill-Burton Act, which incentivized both medical research and the creation of hospitals where that medical research would be housed and used. As Sharon Kaufman notes in her study of hospitals and dying, because of the medical breakthroughs of the twentieth century, "death today is medically and politically malleable and open to endless negotiation."[26]

Hospital-based death created momentum that further fueled medicalization. During the explosion of medical innovation in the 1950s and 1960s, labs, machinery, and other expensive technologies were centralized into government-subsidized hospitals, where specialists could have easy access to them without having to purchase them outright. Treatments like dialysis and chemotherapy originated in hospitals, and only when protocols became standardized could they be moved into outpatient clinics overseen by nurses with physician oversight.[27] The growth in the services hospitals provided and the specialists hospitals attracted created an expectation among patients and providers that much of the care related to serious illnesses would be handled in a hospital context. Hospitals moved from being passive places where people went to die without hope to centers of innovation and activity that saved lives.[28] As hospitals provided more and more care for elderly and seriously ill patients, Americans increasingly confronted the paradox of medicalized death, one that provided hope for some and an isolated and dehumanized end for others.

Demographic changes also encouraged centralization of care, further driving medicalization. An aging population encountered a greater number of chronic conditions that required new and specialized medical care. Alongside this aging population, geographic mobility increased and more women began working outside the home, leaving fewer traditional caregivers for the elderly and infirm. Between the 1930s and 1960s, increasing numbers of families sent their dying to hospitals because they could not be cared for at home.[29] Demand for institutional solutions like nursing homes and hospitals increased, and the creation of Medicare and Medicaid in the 1960s and the growth of Blue Cross and other commercial insurers meant that families could now afford intensive treatments for the seriously ill.[30] During this same period, the most common cause of death shifted from acute to chronic disease. Death from chronic disease required more intensive care over longer periods of time, creating further pressure on traditional caregivers and family doctors. Because insurers paid for medical care but not social support and caretaking, patients were funneled into hospitals not only because that was where the specialists and technology were but also because that was the only place that provided the constant care complex patients needed. Medical innovation and specialization, the changing nature of disease, a variety of state and federal policies, and a changing culture all contributed to the centralization of care for the dying and the medicalization of death.

These shifts created an explosion in the growth of hospitals from the late 1800s to the mid-1900s. In 1873, there were fewer than 200 hospitals in the United States, with a total of 35,000 beds.[31] By 1943 that number had jumped to over 6,000 hospitals, with a total of 1.6 million beds. That number stayed relatively stable until 1975, when the number of beds began dropping as a result of consolidation, cost-cutting, better access to outpatient care, and the movement of some kinds of treatments outside hospitals. As of 2017 there were a total of 6,210 hospitals, with around 930,000 beds.[32] More tellingly for end-of-life concerns, while overall hospital beds have declined somewhat since the 1970s, the number of ICU beds, the most common place of death in the hospital, has grown dramatically, with over 77,000 ICU beds in the United States alone, far more per capita than other developed nations.[33] As hospitals grew in size and number, the number of people dying in hospitals grew as well. As of 2009, 25 percent of Medicare beneficiaries died in hospitals, though this number does not include those who die in nursing homes or those who cycle in and out of hospitals and ICUs shortly prior to death.[34] While the number of Americans dying in hospitals has dropped in recent years thanks to the growth of hospice use, the short stays that characterize most hospice use indicate continued underuse.

As was the case in birth, as more people experienced dying in hospitals, an undercurrent of dissatisfaction grew with the way hospital death isolated and dehumanized patients at the end of life. This undercurrent was most obvious in the growth of the modern hospice movement, which began with Cicely Saunders's work in Britain in 1958 and spread quickly from there.[35] These two contradictory trends—a cultural belief in the importance of a peaceful and humane death and a corresponding faith in medicine that supported dramatic interventions to stave death off—led to paradoxical patterns in how Americans die. Medical expenses at the end of life escalated dramatically over the course of the twentieth century, particularly in the 1980s and 1990s, when scholars noted an important shift. Despite increasing expenditures on healthcare, life expectancy flattened in the United States.[36] The 1980s and 1990s saw an increase in intensive care for the dying, including artificial hydration and nutrition and the use of ventilators.[37] At the same time, the Medicare Hospice Benefit, signed into law in 1982, dramatically expanded Americans' access to palliative care, with hopes that hospice would be a way to limit escalating costs and rein in overtreatment.[38] Americans were actively seeking lifesaving treatments while also searching for ways to make medical care more individualized. Reversing medicalization meant not rejecting the medical innovations that saved lives but finding a way to restore the human elements to death, to balance the medical elements of death and dying against the human needs of the individuals involved.

Hospital Death and the Culture of Intervention

Part of the conflict between hospital practices and the needs of the dying relates to the obvious incompatibility between medicine and death, in terms of not only ends but also means. Most obviously, the goal of medicine is to avoid death in the first place. One palliative care physician remarked in an interview, "I would say that medicine has taken dying out of the life cycle, as something to be fought off at all costs: not just economic costs, but psychological and spiritual costs." He argued that the focus on curative treatment means that "the default is really to fight the disease to the very end." Viewing disease and death as something to be battled colors the very training medical students receive, training that emphasizes almost militaristic values of objectivity, certainty, and action. It also affects the very structure and organization of hospitals, as the training, staffing, and organization of hospital life are structured around the need to respond to acute emergencies with martial precision and discipline.

Such values are at odds with the needs of the terminally ill. Dying itself is anything but objective, certain, or active. Treatment decisions at the end of life are enormously preference sensitive, including the decision about whether to seek treatment in the first place. Ira Byock, one of the pioneers in palliative care in the United States, argued that the dying need not only symptom management but also "someone to coordinate services and appointments; consistent, ongoing, and clear communication; frank discussion of potential problems; and planning about how to prevent crises and what to do if they occur."[39] Dying requires an individualized approach that takes into account everything from the social support a person has, to her mental and physical state, to her religious and spiritual beliefs, to her short-term and long-term goals for treatment. None of these human elements are easily accessed in hospitals, which are focused on, to use Byock's phrasing, "problem-based frameworks and clinical assessment procedures."[40] This kind of intensive patient-centered approach is difficult to achieve in an environment where care is fragmented among many different providers, where time is limited, and where the routine is punctuated by a series of emergencies that require immediate action. Hospitals, created to treat acute and emergent medical crises, struggle to meet the nonmedical needs of the dying precisely because the institutional and organizational imperatives emphasize activity, intervention, and, ultimately, control.

The SUPPORT study underscored the ways in which modern hospitals struggle to meet the needs of dying patients, but these patterns existed throughout the twentieth century. At the turn of the century, patients were often separated from loved ones and subjected to invasive procedures that provided very little benefit at very high costs. By the 1950s, the growing power of medicine made hospitals even more disorienting for patients and families since providers no longer had any idea what to do with dying individuals or what the appropriate standard of care should be. One scholar described medicalized death in the hospital in the 1950s as a "strange new world of pretense, impersonal and disingenuous interacting, and carefully honed, multi-layered deception."[41] Doctors concealed terminal diagnoses from patients, isolated the dying on special "death wards," and used every possible technique and tool to prolong life, even against the express wishes of the patient.[42] The motives for such deception were a combination of concern that patients themselves could not handle a terminal diagnosis and fear that the process of dying would disrupt hospital routines. The act of dying, Roslyn Lindheim argued, "may well be perceived as a rebuke to [the hospital's] commitment to healing, as a source of guilt or shame on the part of the staff, or simply as an interference with settled routine."[43]

Death, particularly death caused by old age or chronic conditions, challenges and even contradicts the routines and protocols that make hospitals efficient medical providers. Like birth, death does not occur on a clear timetable the way a surgery does. Dying requires extensive social and emotional support that medical providers are not trained to provide. It has spiritual elements that are often starkly in contrast to the reductionist methods of medical science. It cannot be reduced to the sum of its parts because the end of a human life is, by definition, more than the sum of its parts. Medicine generally and hospitals in particular struggle with high-quality care for the dying because dying is not itself a disease and, like birth, cannot be "cured." The reductionist approach of medicine creates a barrier to holistic, individualized care for the dying. While reductionism works in patients who might recover, it harms those whose needs go well beyond what is happening on the cellular level. Almost everything about death, starting with its very existence, challenges medicine's goals and values.

This reductionism filters down into the most practical organization of the hospital environment. Hospitals were created precisely to concentrate medical knowledge and specialization in one place. Specialization, in turn, creates a barrier to the more comprehensive conversations that the end of life requires. Compared to general practitioners, surgeons and oncologists are particularly unlikely to broach end-of-life discussions.[44] Surgeons and oncologists are highly specialized, and their training emphasizes urgent, time-limited activity. Their very competence and training may contribute to a uniquely medicalized approach, one where the insoluble problem of death is particularly threatening. As physician and author Atul Gawande argues, "Your competence gives you a secure sense of identity. For a clinician, therefore, nothing is more threatening to who you think you are than a patient with a problem you cannot solve."[45] Specialization may increase that sense of threat.

Specialization creates other problems too, since dying, particularly in the elderly, may not be a single-system failure, but the failure of the entire body. One physician bemoaned in an interview that "in the hospital you have a million docs who are taking care of you, and everyone looks at their organ and orders a million tests for that organ. The default is always to do something. If you're not going to do something, not doing something requires a conversation, but because no one 'owns' these patients, no one starts the conversation, so people just keep doing things." The specialization that reductionism requires has the unintended effect of ensuring that no one provider has a comprehensive view of the patient's situation or her goals. As one palliative care doctor points out, in such a situation "no one is really running the ship."

Specialization was itself made possible by medical innovation, which changed the face of medicine from a profession of relative impotence to one of great power. While activity and intervention have always characterized medical practice, physicians before the 1950s were limited in their ability to do more than offer sympathy and some comfort at the end of life. With the explosion of medical innovations in the 1950s and 1960s, physicians not only had access to treatments for a variety of previously fatal conditions but also gained the ability to stave off death with the use of ventilators, vasopressors, various surgeries, and chemotherapy. This growth of power contributed to a corresponding change in attitude toward death and dying, changing the expectations of both patients and physicians.[46]

The hope that medical innovation fuels is particularly pernicious at the end of life, as interventions have limited impact and may cause a variety of harms.[47] One palliative care physician argued that overtreatment is fueled by a symbiotic relationship between families and their physicians: "Families have absolutely unrealistic expectations, but I think family demand is driven by docs. You can't demand anything if you don't know it's available." Physicians in turn are driven by a combination of powerful psychological biases to offer treatments that are unnecessary or even harmful. Physicians, like patients, tend to overestimate the benefits of interventions and underestimate the harms, but they also have a natural human desire to give hope to people who are vulnerable and afraid.[48] One physician reflected, "If you offer an option to a patient, you're more likely to have that patient like you. A patient will say 'I love Dr. X, because he's not willing to give up.'" Being liked not only is professionally and personally satisfying but also may affect a physician's career. One study that found that terminal cancer patients held incorrect beliefs about their prognosis also noted that "oncologists who communicate honestly with their patients, a marker of a high quality of care, may be at risk for lower patient ratings."[49] Patients prefer physicians who give them hope, and physicians prefer to be liked by their patients. The hospital contributes to this relationship with the ever-present availability of more options should one fail. Hope itself is a powerful current that fuels the cascade because it prevents patients and physicians from having honest conversations about prognosis and overall goals of care.[50]

The endless menu of options and the hope it creates contribute to one of the main drivers of overtreatment at the end of death, the failure to "diagnose dying" in the first place. While physicians no longer routinely engage in deception about a patient's status, in practice the outcome is the same. According to one ICU nurse, most of her patients never receive a terminal diagnosis, even though the signs of dying are obvious and present. A palliative care nurse practitioner described how this happens:

> Yesterday I had a talk with a family and it was a great example of how siloed treatment is. [The patient's] heart sucks, her brain is stroking, her kidneys aren't great, she has a weird GI issue and is throwing clots. But each team signed off because 'she's stable.' So the family asked me 'what's wrong with her?' And I had to do patho[physiology] 101 about how 86-year-olds start to shut down. And sometimes it's not one thing exactly that kills you, it's everything. But Neuro, Renal, Cardiac and Hematology all somehow left the family with the sense that this woman would get better. And the family was understandably confused and taken aback.

The failure to engage in honest conversations about likely prognosis prevents patients and their families from engaging in meaningful activities, conversations, and quality time that could otherwise have been salvaged if a terminal diagnosis was made earlier.

Hospital culture contributes to this problem, as scholars have noted:

"In a hospital setting, where the culture is often focused on 'cure,' continuation of invasive procedures, investigations, and treatments may be pursued at the expense of the comfort of the patient. There is sometimes a reluctance to make the diagnosis of dying if any hope of improvement exists and even more so if no definitive diagnosis has been made."[51] While diagnosing dying may seem more likely where a single care provider is addressing the needs of an individual patient, such as a primary care setting, even there physicians may be hesitant to diagnose dying because they may feel a sense of failure or a belief that they are "giving up" on a patient.[52] Primary care physicians may transfer patients to hospitals in the hopes of ensuring that patients get a diagnosis while preserving the doctor-patient bond, one possible contributor to the high rate of transfers between locations of care at the end of life.

Patients and their families contribute to this tendency to ramp up intervention in the face of death because they also are less likely to "accept defeat" given the range of available options and the pace of medical innovation. Patients share the same bias with physicians that interventions are likely to help and unlikely to harm them, which means that neither side of the physician-patient dyad is able to provide a check on the other.[53] Changes in the broader culture contribute to the narrative of hope. Media portrayals of miraculous deathbed salvations, as well as advertisements touting new treatments and cures marketed directly to patients, have changed expectations about death. Families no longer have personal experience with death, because the dying are isolated and segregated in hospitals, separate from the daily rhythms of life. Television shows like *ER* and *House* focus on heroic medical teams bringing patients back from the brink of death, but they rarely show physiological or unmedicalized deaths due to old age or terminal illness. The geography of the watershed itself also influences patient expectations, with patients accepting whatever care is covered by insurance, even if such care is inappropriate in their case.[54]

The activity bias of hospitals is aggravated by the ubiquity of medical technologies, whose use is both convenient and expected. One physician noted, "When you look at the use of technology, the biggest predictor is having the tools. The biggest predictor of getting a CT scan is having the machine nearby," even when the use of a CT scan is inappropriate or unnecessary. Access to a range of testing equipment is a major contributor to overtreatment since false positives are common and the range of normal for many tests is highly individual.[55] The elderly and those with chronic conditions are likely to have many "abnormal" tests, as a result of the gradual failure of a variety of bodily systems. While some of these failures may be treatable, many are simply the result of the aging process itself. Attempts to halt or reverse that decline can lead to unintended side effects, including treatments that trigger hospitalization and further complications.[56] Despite recommendations to limit unnecessary testing and the resulting prescription of medications, overtesting and overprescription in the elderly remain serious problems.[57] As with fetal monitoring, the use of many tests and interventions on the elderly and terminally ill became widespread largely on the basis of expected benefits that failed to materialize in a clinical environment.[58] The activity bias in hospitals combines with new innovations to standardize the use of tools that have few benefits and many potential drawbacks, particularly when used on inappropriate populations.[59] The use of ventilators, feeding tubes, CPR, and other interventions that are common in the ICU will have very different outcomes and trade-offs for young populations than for the elderly or the terminally ill.

Finally, the practical reality of hospital life makes communication difficult and fraught. Teams of multiple providers require extensive charting that eats up precious nursing shifts. Multiple providers lead to more interventions, as different specialties have their own menu of options to offer to desperate patients.[60] Patient wishes that change frequently must be communicated across multiple physicians, particularly with elderly patients who rotate frequently between locations of care, creating a fraught game of telephone. The hierarchical nature of hospitals, particularly teaching hospitals, while facilitating quick action, may be inimical to communication and collaboration, particularly when it comes to patients who are unaware of any options but those presented to them by the attending. As one physician put it, "In a hospital you're basically stuck with whatever you get. People don't even realize that there are other options. People don't realize that there are other options to being intubated." Patients accept the interventions they are offered, and physicians offer the interventions that are available, whether or not such interventions are consistent with patient goals, prognosis, or quality of life.

One way in which the culture of activity and the lack of communication in hospitals combine to create a current of overtreatment is the seemingly innocuous standard use of CPR. CPR was hailed as a major breakthrough on its invention (or rediscovery, depending on your view) in 1960.[61] Its power to save lives led to its spread, and it became the default for all patients in hospitals and nursing homes. Medicare, for example, requires CPR as a default treatment in nursing homes receiving federal funds.[62] CPR is a standard opt-out procedure in hospitals as well, in that patients who have Do Not Resuscitate (DNR) orders will not get CPR, but every other patient will.[63] As with other interventions, however, patients and their families overestimate what CPR can accomplish and underestimate the risks associated with the procedure, particularly in the elderly. While CPR will restart the hearts of around 40 percent of patients who receive it in the hospital, most of those patients will not live until discharge, and the number of successful discharges from the hospital drops dramatically as age increases.[64] Even then, those who are released may be discharged with brain damage to long-term care homes. Successful CPR requires a good deal of force, with the potential to break ribs and limit recovery and functionality, making it more likely that elderly patients will end up permanently institutionalized rather than returning home. CPR outcomes are heavily dependent on age and health status, with older patients much more likely to end up with brain damage or dependent on machines. While CPR can be avoided with a DNR order, too few people choose DNR orders in part because they misunderstand precisely what CPR can and cannot do.[65] In her book *Extreme Measures*, Jessica Zitter recounts how her excitement upon getting her first "code" as an intern turned to horror when she saw the emaciated and disease-ravaged body on which she would be performing CPR. After 30 minutes of chest compressions, the resident officially declared the patient dead, and Zitter reflected while cleaning up, "I have just assaulted a dead body."[66] The standard use of CPR on the terminally ill and elderly is much more likely to do harm than good.

Hospital Death, Activity Bias, and Palliative Care

Hospitals are not unaware of the challenges centralized care poses for the elderly and terminally ill. One attempt to address these concerns is the relatively new specialty of palliative care, which focuses on both symptom management and communication about goals of care for those with life-limiting illnesses. Palliative care teams are usually led by a specially trained physician, but they tend to be interdisciplinary, consisting of physicians, nurses, social workers, and chaplains. Research on palliative care suggests that it helps address overtreatment in part by providing patients with a kind of map of the treatment options to better understand where interventions lead while prioritizing high-quality communication to assess patient preferences.[67] Palliative care teams operate like a highly trained and coordinated sailing crew, coordinating care with specialists and assisting patients in accessing resources such as home health aides, with at least one team member in the crow's nest, keeping her eye on both where the river is taking them and where the patient wants to end up.

The interdisciplinary nature of palliative care is one way to counter the emphasis on specialists in the hospital. Nurses play a central role in palliative care teams, in part because of how much time they spend with patients and because their more generalized, holistic training in both symptom management and communication lends itself well to the palliative care approach. One nurse practitioner related that, in her experience, palliative care physicians find nurses to be more helpful in guiding patients toward end-of-life decisions than other doctors, if given the latitude to do so. She noted that "two palliative care docs have told me they would like to only hire NPs [nurse practitioners] because 'nurses get it.'" One palliative care physician supported this view, describing the resistance he gets from specialists: "I think in general the higher you go up the technology ladder, the more palliative-care averse you get." The most generalized providers who spend the most face-to-face time with patients may find it easier to see the "big picture" of patient care, which may in turn support fewer interventions at the end of life. This pattern holds particularly true in hospice, where, according to one hospice director, "most people come from nursing and social work." The more holistic training and emphasis on patient care may make it easier for these providers to identify nonmedical needs of patients and their families.

Despite general support for palliative care, the hospital environment prevents many palliative care teams from fully engaging with patients to limit overtreatment. The barriers range from subtle biases to clear protocol barriers. One palliative care provider felt that the emphasis on nursing in palliative care provokes a bias in some specialists: "Medicine is very doc heavy and very focused on curing people, while palliative care and hospice are very nurse heavy and more about what you do when nothing can be done. So there's a very strong bias [against referring patients] though I think it's unconscious." He also noted that specialists may pay lip service to palliative care but still do not refer patients until the final days or hours of life: "People will tell you they love palliative medicine, but the majority (40%–75%) of the recommendations are ignored. Forget the fact that we're not even seeing the majority of people we should be seeing."

The fact that palliative care is a specialty in the first place can create powerful barriers to better communication. Palliative care's status as a specialty makes it more difficult for physicians, particularly midcareer physicians, to get training in palliative care because the training requires going back through a separate fellowship, a significant hurdle for most established providers. But more foundationally, many of the palliative care providers interviewed expressed frustration that their specialty even existed, arguing that it makes it easier for other physicians to feel as though they do not have to learn these skills at all. As one palliative care physician noted, "It's crazy that we're being called to talk to people; why isn't their cardiologist or their oncologist doing that? If everyone were doing it you wouldn't need [the palliative care] specialty." Another physician described it as "really problematic when doctors have this attitude of 'I'll punt them out to another doc to talk to them only when there's nothing else that can be done.'" The palliative care specialization is also different from every other specialty in that its focus is knowledge all physicians should already have. As one physician put it, "Getting a palliative care consult is very value-laden. If all I do is talk and treat symptoms, that's under every doc's scope of practice. So if I'm called in and I make a recommendation, I'm saying 'I'm doing something you should have done.' That's different from every other specialty." Calling in palliative care may signal both professional and personal failure in a way other consults do not. This implicit judgment can explain why even though most specialists pay lip service to the importance of palliative care, they do not refer patients in the moment. One palliative care physician noted, "We've had two onc[ology] clinics we've closed within months because we're getting no referrals from the same people who told us they needed us."

Hospital protocols and procedures solidify these subtle and unconscious biases against palliative care. Unlike most specialist consults, which are automatic unless patients opt out of them, palliative care is usually "opt-in," meaning that patients must be made aware that the service is available and then opt for a referral. Patients are therefore at the mercy of their physician to provide them with information about the specialty, information the attending physician may have unconscious biases against providing. As a sign of this discomfort, attending physicians will sometimes limit the scope of the palliative care team's consult, perhaps as a way to avoid feeling disempowered by the process. According to one palliative care physician, "Sometimes they tell us to just come in for pain treatment, but not for disease management consultations. They'll say 'talk to the patient about pain management, but we're not ready to talk about ending treatment.' So we've been invited in by doctors who don't really want us to get into real conversations about goals of care, which makes things more difficult." The culture of activity and control explains the perverse reality that having conversations about goals of care with a trained professional is optional but CPR on elderly and terminally ill patients is standard, despite the benefits of the former and the harms of the latter.

Technology, Standardization, and Control

As with birth, death happens to discrete individuals, individuals whose subjective desires and needs play a central role in how the process plays out. For this reason, among others, death does not fit well within the hospital environment, where standardization is central to fulfilling the goal of saving lives. Standardization of care was the hallmark of even the earliest hospitals, and the most dehumanizing practices of hospital wards for the dying in the mid-twentieth century stemmed from the desire to maintain hospital routines even in the face of death and loss. Isolating the dying in special wards and purposely sending loved ones home before death to prevent emotional scenes were common throughout most of the twentieth century.[68] Hospitals attempted not just to standardize death but also to strip it of its human elements because those human elements made the precise and regulated practice of medicine more difficult.

Standardization comes in part from the need to manage risk in a complex environment. Hospital administrators defend protocols that explicitly standardize care on the grounds of limiting liability risk and risks to patients like infections and medical errors. But such standardization is damaging for populations whose needs are peculiarly preference sensitive, such as the elderly or terminally ill. When asked how his practice differed in hospitals compared to hospice care, one palliative care physician responded, "When I do palliative medicine in the hospital I often practice substandard medicine because I can't do what I think is necessary. The hospital won't allow it. For example, some meds aren't allowed on certain floors, opiates are at lower levels because people are uncomfortable with the amounts required for end-of-life care, and so on. So care is much more conservative than I would do in hospice or home hospice." Institutionalized settings such as nursing homes and hospitals, where care is limited by legally inspired protocols, have higher rates of uncontrolled pain and poor symptom management compared to outpatient hospice programs in the home.[69]

Sharon Kaufman notes in her study of dying in hospitals that the "hospital structure itself organizes and routinizes dying and life-prolongation. Individuals can only act within systems of classification that already exist."[70] Rather than having the opportunity to craft a care plan with a single provider that takes individual wishes and medical need into account, patients and their providers are swept along by currents resulting from tributaries in the watershed they do not know exist. As Kaufman discovered, "Policies, care plans, and medical algorithms are all designed to move the patient on routinized tracks of diagnoses and treatments that categorize, ameliorate, and manage disease. For many patients the tracks lead to cure and to the saving of lives. For others who are near death, the tracks move, almost inexorably, from one hospital unit to another and one treatment to another."[71] These tracks Kaufman describes create a binary approach to care that harms the elderly and terminally ill. At many hospitals, a patient is on one end of a continuum of either full code status (do everything possible) or comfort care only with a DNR order, with very little middle ground in between. Yet research increasingly shows that most patients benefit from a middle ground, one provided in part by the integration of palliative care: aggressive care when appropriate, with concurrent symptom management and frequent discussions about the goals of care.[72] Specialists and surgeons may not know what to do with patients with DNR orders in the ICU, for example, even though such a request might make sense in certain situations, such as when a patient wants to see whether a surgery might help but does not want to risk being paralyzed by CPR administration if she codes during surgery.

Despite the fact that death is in many ways a more variable process than giving birth, the broad strokes of hospital-based death end up looking very similar to hospital-based birth, particularly in the ICU, where around 30 percent of Americans will spend some time at the end of life. Access to technology and tests facilitate ordering labs and hooking patients up to monitors and machines. Patients and attending physicians usually have no prior relationship. Intensivists, as ICU physicians are called, are trained in rescue medicine and focused on acting quickly to save lives. Physicians in the ICU typically have a very short window of time for decision making and multiple patients to juggle, leaving little time for conversations about goals of care. The culture of the ICU is geared toward action above all else because that is what patients who belong in the ICU—those with a hope of recovery—need. Standardizing patients into diagnoses that can be handled with clear protocols facilitates that action. The combination of reflexive training with the reductionism of medical specialization standardizes patients themselves. Individuals with very different values, beliefs, and goals die in the ICU in similar kinds of ways. As Gawande characterized dying in America, "we have allowed our fates to be controlled by the imperatives of medicine, technology, and strangers."[73] The ICU itself represents one of the primary rapids leading toward medicalized death. The internal logic of activity and control in the hospital environment, which reaches its apex in the ICU, pushes dying patients toward the maximum level of intensity—a cascade of interventions—frequently without providing an increase in either quantity or quality of life.

The tendency to standardize contains a directional bias, originating in medicine's emphasis on action and control. Generally speaking, action is standard in the hospital, whereas inaction is not, even when medical evidence supports the less interventionist path. One palliative care physician pointed out the bias inherent in the way standard protocols operate: "There are clearly standards for who [palliative care] should be seeing. If we're going to do opt-out for every other kind of medicine, I want to know why we don't do opt-out for palliative medicine." Other physicians and nurses echoed this concern that hospital protocols make treatment the norm, while conversations about the goals of treatment are seen as secondary and usually come well after treatment begins. Studies suggest that making palliative care consults mandatory (i.e., opt-out) for all high-risk patients can reduce stays in the ICU and improve patient outcomes without increasing mortality or morbidity.[74] But few hospitals make palliative care the standard for patients with life-limiting illnesses.[75]

Comparing standard protocols for escalating and de-escalating care provides another window into the activity bias inherent in modern hospital standards. While hospitals have protocols in place to escalate treatment, they frequently lack protocols for how to de-escalate treatment at the end of life. Because the training of nurses and physicians in hospitals emphasizes quick and decisive action, not responding to a symptom or danger sign pushes against every instinct. As the physician Jessica Zitter recalls in her book, "The protocols that I crammed into my exhausted brain were always about escalating care. . . . Moreover, in the frenzy of a medical code, there are so many things to do to keep the heart beating, so many procedures to try, that it was almost inconceivable to waste time investigating whether the person even wanted to be kept alive at all costs."[76] She argues that protocols for escalation should include more standardized "pause points," or points where providers and patients can pause and have conversations about the options available before treatment is escalated.[77]

Contrast the protocols for escalating care with those for ending treatment, which are mostly nonexistent. As Zitter notes of most decisions to end treatment, "Right now, we wing it."[78] Making the de-escalation decision more fraught is that the removal of a single intervention can be done in a variety of ways, as in the case of removing mechanical ventilation. Some providers choose so-called terminal weaning, or a gradual reduction in the oxygen provided while leaving the tube in place. Other physicians opt for a complete removal of the tube (extubation), while others remove the patient from the ventilator while keeping the tube in place.[79] Each method has its proponents and detractors, and each method may be appropriate for some patients and not for others, but there is little guidance for physicians on the pros and cons of each approach. Most dying patients in hospitals are undergoing multiple interventions, and each intervention carries with it its own set of complexities and discrete decisions that must be made about each step in the process.[80] One study of decisions to end life-sustaining treatment found that, on average, almost four treatments were ended for each patient at the end of life.[81]

The lack of protocols and guidance for how to end treatment breeds moral confusion for both physicians and families, confusion that supports the bias toward continuing treatment. Zitter believes that one important function of palliative care consults is that they can provide moral and emotional support for physicians to do what they know to be the right thing (in this case withdrawing care) but may have trouble recommending owing to the moral weight and the finality of allowing someone to die. Protocols for how to end life-sustaining treatment, like maps for navigating a complex waterway, would put physicians on more comfortable moral ground while still allowing for individualization of care based on patient desires.

Providing clearer protocols for de-escalating care would also help reduce the burden on families, who are often left with decision-making power they do not fully understand. One nurse practitioner described a patient in the ICU who was intubated; was on continual dialysis; required vasopressors indicating pulmonary, kidney, and circulatory failure; and suffered from underlying cancer and strokes. A relative said in a conversation that she wished that death would happen "organically," but the ICU itself makes such a word meaningless. The nurse practitioner argued that when "treatment becomes the norm, philosophically there are very few cases of passive withdrawal. It almost all feels active. . . . This poor patient's [relative] was forced to feel like she was pulling the plug." The relative, understandably, did not want to feel responsible for ending her loved one's life. The nurse pointed out that many interventions "complicate grief for the families and the dying process for the patient" by forcing decisions of life and death onto confused and grieving family members. Moreover, the number of interventions and the associated complexity make it much more likely that patients and their families will not know how to end treatment and that physicians will shy away from having those conversations in the first place.

The combined force of these pressures in hospitals creates cascades of interventions at the end of life that do not help dying patients and sometimes (perhaps frequently) harm them. Interventions include chemotherapy for patients with end-stage cancer,[82] vasopressors to stabilize blood pressure in failing systems,[83] dialysis to filter toxins from the blood in place of functioning kidneys,[84] various pharmaceuticals to control an array of symptoms, and mechanical interventions to replace the body's most basic functions, such as artificial hydration and nutrition, breathing tubes, rectal tubes, and urinary catheters.[85] All these interventions can save lives in the young or strong, but they are often harmful in the elderly and in the terminally ill, prolonging the inevitable and adding considerable pain and suffering to the last days of life.[86] In the worst cases, such interventions paradoxically both increase suffering and shorten life.[87]

Hospital Death, Autonomy, and Control

Hospital death has ethical implications apart from the physical harm it causes, most obviously in the barriers it creates to informed consent. Complete informed consent is, of course, an impossibility. Patients can never be fully informed, and no accepted view of informed consent requires that patients be told about every possible risk, every possible benefit, or every alternative option, no matter how remote. Disease itself challenges informed consent because every prognosis is itself uncertain and because disease forces people into decisions they would never otherwise make. As one palliative care physician admitted, "disease can be pretty formidable at the very end too and it can prevent people from dying in the way they would be most comfortable." Even so, all providers interviewed pointed out ways in which the currents that hospital-based death create challenge or even violate informed consent in both avoidable and troubling ways. Particularly because decisions made at the end of life are irrevocable and terminal patients and the elderly so vulnerable, informed consent should be, if anything, more carefully guarded during this period than during any other. Yet for many people at the end of life the information they are given by providers is incomplete, fragmented, and sometimes actually deceptive.

The primary barrier to informed consent is the delay in a diagnosis of dying. This delay is the primary barrier to patient autonomy in hospitals because a terminal diagnosis is the foundation on which all other decisions are made. Most providers interviewed believed that hospitals and specialists within hospitals do not diagnose dying early enough in the process for patients to make truly informed decisions about how to proceed. This tendency helps explain why most terminal patients do not enter hospice until a few days before death. While diagnosing dying is always subject to the difficulties of disease prognosis, the combination of fragmented care and gatekeeping by specialists in hospitals makes such uncertainty worse. One nurse practitioner recalled, "I'll never forget the expression on a patient's face when she told me she was scared. And I asked her why and she said 'I think I'm dying.' She spent 45 days in the hospital before the oncologists would 'let' me discuss her poor prognosis. She stayed another couple weeks and died in a nursing home a week or two after discharge."

Patients who are not told they are dying are unable to do the most basic assessment of how to spend the limited time they have left. Dying, as one might expect, changes patient decision making, usually in the direction of fewer interventions.[88] Delaying a terminal diagnosis denies a patient the ability to come to terms with her own mortality, contact family and friends, and talk with her physician about realistic options for care. As one nurse pointed out, "dying is a process and often a downward spiral, but patients and often docs don't think or at least talk about it that way. The infections you get in the ICU are part of dying when you have underlying cancer or renal or heart failure but families are left with a sense of 'once he kicks the pneumonia then he can regain his strength.'" No one tells the family the patient is dying regardless of whether the pneumonia is cured or not, in part because each condition is treated separately and because communication between providers and between the patient and her providers is limited. Because hospitals make it difficult to diagnose dying in the first place, many patients do not have the information they need to understand the trade-offs of further interventions. Patients who are led to believe they may recover are much more likely to support further interventions than those who are honestly told that they have limited time remaining and that they should think about how they want to spend it.[89]

Apart from fragmented care, physicians have a variety of reasons—professional, psychological, cultural, legal—for failing to disclose this information to the patient or her family. Physicians feel pride in keeping patients alive and not allowing them to die.[90] Peer pressure from knowing that residents and nurses are watching every move in the hospital may also prevent physicians from diagnosing dying earlier.[91] The reflexive training of medicine, the action and activity of the hospital, the specialization of practitioners, and the hierarchical nature of hospital wards all contribute to the difficulty of diagnosing dying. One nurse argued, "What we do in the ICU is act, act, act, but what we really need to be doing [for the elderly and terminally ill] is thinking and talking and then thinking again."

Hospital-based care and the hope it provides change patient expectations about death and dying, further challenging the meaning of informed consent. It is difficult to untangle medicalization from the hope that modern medicine has provided for dying patients. Medical innovations may provide patients a reason to keep going, even if the interventions themselves provide little medical benefit or even shorten their lives. More troubling, such innovations may be attractive precisely because they offer the hope of a miracle, even if the research fails to support the likelihood of success. In one study of cancer patients, almost 80 percent of patients preferred the "hopeful gamble" treatment over the "safe bet."[92] Physicians fuel these hopes by offering treatments that they know are extremely unlikely to do any good and may in fact do harm.[93] The puzzle of demedicalization involves how to untangle patient hopes and expectations from the hospital environment that promises so much and yet, for the terminally ill, delivers so little.

More troublingly, the gatekeeping function of the hospital hierarchy makes it less likely that patients will be informed of the range of options available to them, including palliative care, where they are more likely to have robust conversations about their goals. Most seriously ill patients are never referred to palliative care at all, and when they are, it is often late in the progress of disease, too late to provide much benefit.[94] For the elderly and terminally ill in particular, conversations about wishes and values must be frequent and flexible precisely because goals change with the course of treatment. Yet unless palliative care has been called in, there is no specific person charged with having these conversations.[95] Patients who are not told the severity of their condition and not provided the opportunity to talk about their goals cannot be called "informed" in any real sense of the word.

The cascade of interventions in the hospital challenges also informed consent by placing patients on what Jessica Zitter calls in her book the "conveyor belt" of care.[96] Patients are not told the long-term risks of interventions, nor how one intervention makes another much more likely. The ventilator is a prime example of a powerful riptide that carries patients on to ever-higher-intensity care. The initial placing of a temporary breathing tube is done reflexively in the ICU to save the patient's life until she can be stabilized and assessed. If the patient does not recover quickly enough to be able to breathe on her own, as is the case with many elderly and dying patients, she will need to be switched to more permanent interventions, in this case a tracheostomy, or a hole through the neck into the windpipe (also known as a trach), and a percutaneous endoscopic gastrostomy (PEG) tube at the two-week mark. The decision to trach a patient is a critical moment in patient care.[97] Trachs and PEG tubes carry significant risks, and not only as a result of the surgery to get them in place. While they are more comfortable than a temporary breathing tube for patients, they may require restraints, increase risk of infections, and require institutionalization, precluding patients from going home to family.

Crucially, a typical informed consent document for a trach will cover the immediate risks of the procedure: reaction to anesthesia, potential to bleed, possibility of infection. But Zitter lists the risks that are rarely shared with patients before insertion: "The risk of never tasting food again. The risk of not being able to take care of your own personal hygiene. Of not being able to turn off the game show that the nurse is watching in your room. Of losing your dignity. And of a lonely death in a facility across town from your family."[98] Given these less obvious but serious risks, Zitter argues, "the two-week trach and PEG decisions should be anything but reflexive," and yet they often are.[99] In fact, long-term and nonmedical risks of most interventions are rarely discussed at all in hospitals.[100] Patients have little idea what an intervention will do or that it may cut off other options later on. The more patients know about these long-term risks of intervention at the end of life, the more they refuse them.[101] But because the long-term and nonmedical risks of interventions are not laid out, many patients and their families reflexively accept treatment in the same way the doctors reflexively offer it.

As with birth, the sheer number of interventions, their complexity, and how they affect each other in combination can make it difficult for providers and patients to have detailed and realistic conversations about what to expect, particularly when time is short. The complexity of these decisions and the number of decision makers involved contribute to a kind of treatment paralysis, where interventions continue because continuing the status quo is easier for everyone (except the dying patient) than the much more complicated and time-intensive conversations and decisions about withdrawing care. Add to this the constant barrage of tests, procedures, interventions, and new options to try that distract patients from otherwise thinking about how to spend their last days. Without a navigator to guide care and encourage pause points and conversations about care, the patient drifts along into ever more aggressive and mechanized care until the body gives out.

More indirectly, the hospital environment itself isolates patients during a profoundly important life experience, with implications for patient autonomy. Unlike an appendectomy, death is, according to one scholar, "profoundly social."[102] It marks the most fundamental change for an individual and a dramatic reworking of the social order for those who are left behind. But patients who end up in the ICU at the end of life, as well as those trapped in the revolving door from nursing home, to ICU, to skilled nursing facility, and then back to hospital, are isolated from their social and emotional support networks. Recent work in what is known as "relational autonomy" argues that social networks and the social environment contribute to and protect individual autonomy.[103] But at the most basic level, it is difficult to have a conversation if no one is there. Unfortunately, hospitals cannot be easily designed around the social needs of the dying. As one critical care nurse pointed out, "Ultimately we can't really design the ICU to be a place for people to die since really it's a place where our goal is that people don't die. Even current conversations about redesign are centered around keeping people alive."

As with birth plans, the hospital environment challenges patient autonomy even when wishes are clearly laid out and discussed ahead of time. Advance directives or DNR orders are occasionally lost in the hospital shuffle, either not making it into a patient's chart or overlooked once it is there. Even when patient preferences are explicitly discussed, the constant activity that characterizes hospital care makes them difficult to respect. One nurse described a hospital patient with liver failure who, after being intubated once, decided against future invasive interventions. She described how "two docs had it in their notes that he told them he never wanted to be intubated again and absolutely did not want a trach. He coded on the floor and in the heat of everything he was intubated and sent back to the ICU where he stayed for a couple more weeks developing new infections." Hospital protocols themselves directly challenge patient autonomy by forcing individuals to withdraw a DNR order for certain kinds of interventions, such as surgery. The current system lacks the nuance to allow patients to permit resuscitation in the event that they code during surgery, when resuscitation is often successful, but to refuse intervention if they code shortly after the surgery, when resuscitation efforts are likely to end in compromised quality of life.[104] Crucially, patients may be unsure whether an intervention is being suggested because of hospital protocol or because it is truly the best option for an individual patient, calling into question how "informed" patients actually are about the factors that are guiding their care. While the biggest liability risk is still to do nothing, recent cases of overlooked DNR orders signal that families are willing to sue for failure to respect end-of-life wishes.[105]

Patients who are isolated, unsure of their prognosis, and surrounded by activity and options will make very different decisions about care than patients who are surrounded by family and friends, provided as clear a prognosis as possible, and offered a range of options, including de-escalation of care. Hospital dying challenges informed consent by artificially limiting the options available, preventing patients from understanding the truth of their condition, and obscuring the real risks and benefits of a variety of interventions. Despite the growth in concern about patient autonomy and informed consent over the past 50 years, seriously ill patients still make decisions with little information, few or the wrong options, and almost no understanding of how their decisions are shaped and framed by forces around and above them.

Conclusion

Despite the criticism from advocates for "natural death" in the 1950s and 1960s, hospital-based death has not changed much in the intervening decades. This stasis is predictable because the hospital continues to be a perfect storm of characteristics that contribute to medicalization and overtreatment at the end of life. It is not simply that hospitals are failing to adapt to the needs of dying patients. What is more problematic is that the needs of dying patients are inimical to the goals and structures of hospitals themselves. As in birth, the complexity of the hospital environment lends itself to both medicalization and overtreatment at the end of life. The sheer complexity of hospital environments presents an information overload of constant monitoring, lab results, multiple providers, and patients moving in and out at different rates (sometimes repeatedly), alongside rigorous training based on quick action and heuristics. Dying, like birthing, does not fit well into such an environment.

The growth of palliative care teams in hospitals suggests that institutional change is possible. The growth and better integration of such teams may make dying in the hospital less isolating and less medically intensive than it once was. But there are still powerful pressures in hospitals that will always be present, no matter how skilled and integrated the palliative care side becomes. Hospitals will always be places where the primary goal is to save lives. They will (probably) always be hierarchical, and they will always be confronted by the need for quick decision making and action. They will also, crucially, always be unfamiliar to patients, with limited social support and limited freedom, and will present cultural, institutional, legal, and practical barriers to demedicalized death. It is not reasonable to ask hospitals, created to treat and to cure, to become places of peace and solace for the dying. Demedicalized death, death that recognizes and balances the individual, social, and human needs of elderly and terminal patients, is fundamentally incompatible with hospital life.

The greater puzzle is why, given the mismatch between the hospital environment and the needs of the dying, so many Americans die in hospitals to begin with. To answer that question, we must zoom out of the rapids of the ICU and the strong current of hospital-based care and focus on the broader geography of the healthcare watershed itself. In the next chapter I lay out the alternatives to hospital-based care for both birth and death, operating like docks along the shoreline providing shelter from the rapids and cascades of interventions. The rest of the book investigates how our unique healthcare watershed destroys those docks, forcing patients back into the currents of medicalized care, and how, through reimbursement policies, state and local regulations, and the medical-legal framework, patients are thrust directly into the rapids of overtreatment.

CHAPTER 3

Safe Harbors for Demedicalized Birth and Death

There's living going on. We get loud and we laugh. We don't have beeping, we're not coming in every ten minutes to check vitals; treatments are over, you don't have to worry about it. We try to get people to not look too far ahead. Get as much pleasure and joy out of it as you can. And we try to get the families to do that as well. [Our culture is] so bent on planning. [Dying] is one time you can't plan. Just like birth.
—*Executive director of a two-bed "home for the dying"*

E NVISIONING AN IDEAL healthcare watershed is relatively simple, given that patients, providers, and policy makers all agree on a basic set of principles that should theoretically guide medical care. Almost everyone agrees that the ideal healthcare system should reflect a combination of patient autonomy and choice, respect for evidence-based care and provider expertise, controlled costs, and equitable access. Mapping these ideals onto a watershed forms a geography very different from the current one. In this ideal watershed, patient choice is protected by a multitude of qualified providers and care locations, costs are kept in check by a combination of sensible reimbursement policies and competition among providers, and providers offer evidence-based medicine without fear of regulatory penalty or liability risk. The varied geography offers ample opportunities to escape from the currents of centralized and medicalized care. Such safe harbors allow individuals to pursue preference-based care, limit unnecessary interventions and prioritize primary care, provide space for social and emotional support, and prioritize evidence-based care by matching patients' needs with appropriate medical and nonmedical techniques. These harbors have access to the swift current of centralized hospital care when patient needs demand it, but otherwise they remain safely outside the currents of the main river. The ideal watershed looks something like a meandering river with docks and inlets along the way.

The geography of the US watershed, in contrast, is a canyon with sheer walls and a rushing river down the center. Because it lacks options for exit and is made up of a single rushing current leading inexorably to the same end point, it fails to protect patient autonomy, provide evidence-based care, or lower costs. At the end of this canyon is a waterfall, a cascade of medicalized care and interventions, over which birthing and dying patients are thrust by the sheer power of the current of hospital care. Pregnant women and elderly and terminally ill patients have no place on shore to land, few demedicalized providers to assist them, and no easy way to avoid the current of hospitalization that drops them over the rapids. Crucially, they often have no one in the boat with them, just a multitude of providers yelling instructions from the top of the cliffs. The lack of options and strength of the currents limit pregnant women and the dying to the most medicalized options available.

More complex watersheds can and do exist. They exist in other countries to varying degrees.[1] Inlets and safe harbors even exist in the current American watershed, accessible to a few lucky or intrepid patients. The data on these options for birth and death show that, in general, they provide patient-centered, evidence-based care at a lower cost than their hospital counterparts, though the shape of our watershed produces perverse incentives even for these providers and locations of care. These harbors accomplish low-cost, evidence-based, and patient-centered care by keeping people safely out of the river of medical options while they are supported and assessed by trained providers. When medical care becomes necessary, a variety of medical and nonmedical providers, such as midwives, palliative care workers, and doulas, can hop into the boat with their client, enter the river with them during treatment, and then assist in their safe return to shore. Shoreline options like community-based and demedicalized providers support pregnant women and the elderly or terminally ill by providing the emotional and social support these patients need while limiting the interventions that foster complications and lead to a final cascade.

Despite their benefits for patients, providers, and the healthcare system as a whole, demedicalized or community-based options, including independent birth centers, residential hospice, home birth, or home hospice, are unavailable to most people who give birth and die in the United States, owing in large part to the regulatory and reimbursement policies that shape the watershed. These strong policy tributaries generate formidable currents that push patients and practitioners toward hospital-based care, washing away community-based options on the shoreline, shaping a watershed with sheer walls and few alternatives to hospitalization. Before turning to the discussion of the policy tributaries that shape our watershed in this way, it is worth describing demedicalized providers, decentralized locations of care, and the kind of care they provide at the beginning and end of life.

Birth, Death, and the Demedicalization Movement

The almost-complete medicalization of birth and death in hospitals in the mid-twentieth century did not occur without comment or resistance. Patients and providers had concerns early on that the human aspects of birth and death, such as social, emotional, and physical needs, were being ignored in favor of reductionist medical treatments. In both birth and death, powerful descriptions of what many labeled dehumanizing practices led to a groundswell of interest in alternatives to hospital-based care. In the 1960s, mothers described themselves as "trapped animals" during hospital birth, strapped to beds, their bodies vulnerable and exposed to the whims of hospital staff.[2] The influential midwife Ina May Gaskin described the dehumanization of medicalized birth, in which "the woman becomes a passive, almost inert object—representing a barrier to the baby's eventual passage to the outside world."[3] In her groundbreaking book on death and dying in 1969, Elizabeth Kübler-Ross described the dehumanizing effects of hospitalization, arguing of the hospitalized dying patient,

> [He] slowly but surely is beginning to be treated like a thing. He is no longer a person. Decisions are made often without his opinion. . . . He may cry for rest, peace, and dignity, but he will get infusions, transfusions, a heart machine, or tracheostomy if necessary. He may want one single person to stop for one single minute so that he can ask one single question—but he will get a dozen people around the clock, all busily preoccupied with his heart rate, pulse, electrocardiogram or pulmonary functions, his secretions or excretions but not with him as a human being.[4]

Despite the pace of medical progress, Kübler-Ross believed that "dying nowadays is more gruesome in many ways, namely, more lonely, mechanical, and dehumanized."[5] Roslyn Lindheim, a hospital architect who designed some of the earliest children's hospitals, criticized the entire culture of medicalized birth and death in the 1970s, arguing that "we have allowed ourselves to rely on institutions and professional specialization to solve our most personal responsibilities toward birthing and dying. The solutions developed have been inadequate, dehumanizing, and alienating."[6]

None of these critics argued that hospitals themselves were unnecessary. All recognized the importance of hospitals for the treatment of acute or potentially serious complications during both birth and death.[7] But they believed that the medicalization of birth and death in hospitals was excessive, aimed at inappropriate patient populations, and excessively reductionist, dehumanizing patients with standardized and mechanized care. They also believed that, given the unique needs of laboring women and terminally ill patients and the absence of a discrete "disease" to be treated, the needs of many birthing and dying patients could be met in the home or an outpatient location with lower levels of interventions and greater levels of social and emotional support. The goal for most in the natural birth and death movements was and is not total demedicalization but the discovery of an appropriate mean of medicalization of birth and death, one that balanced medical need against human and individual need. In general, critics sought a way to structure demedicalized alternatives as supplements and complements to hospital-provided care, alternatives that provided options in the community for a wide array of patients with unique and individual needs.

Both movements share the conviction that birth and death, rather than illnesses to be treated or cured, are in fact physiological processes made up of discrete and predictable phases. On this view, birth and death are natural processes that most, though not all, bodies are capable of moving through with support but without medical intervention. As early as 1921, midwifery was described as being focused on "physiology rather than pathology."[8] Gaskin described the midwifery model of care as conceiving "of pregnancy and birth as inherently healthy processes and of each mother and baby as an inseparable unit," unlike the medical approach that, she argued, viewed a "woman's body as a lemon."[9] The goal of midwifery care is to support the process of physiologic birth, in which the mother's and infant's bodies go through a series of changes as the infant drops into the birth canal, the mother's pelvis shifts, and the baby spins to prepare for being pushed out into the world. Similarly, advocates for humane death like Kübler-Ross and Cicely Saunders emphasized the natural elements of death and the need to address patient comfort while working with the process of dying rather than seeking to oppose it.[10] Physiological death, they argued, is accompanied by predictable changes such as cessation of hunger or thirst, increased sleepiness, shallow breathing, and a variety of psychological and emotional changes, all of which are signs of the broader dying process.[11] Such views of birth and death are distinct from the prevailing medical view that the birthing or dying body is pathological, incapable of moving through the process on its own without medical intervention.

The problem with the medical view, according to advocates for demedicalized birth and death, is that external interventions at any stage of the process disrupt the complex changes taking place, resulting in pain or further complications, which in turn require additional interventions. Grantly Dick-Read, whose work in the 1930s and 1940s formed the basis for the natural birth movement, described what he called the "fear-tension-pain" cycle, as one example of this phenomenon.[12] Hospitals place laboring women in unfamiliar environments, force them to labor in unnatural positions, and subject them to frequent invasive checks. These standard elements of hospital-based care generate fear, which increases tension in the body. Tension inhibits labor, inhibited labor is painful, and pain causes more fear. Women's labors stall as a result, interventions are deemed necessary, and physicians arrive to save women from their "malfunctioning" bodies. In fact, the malfunctioning was caused by the environment itself. The physician John Fairbain argued as early as 1921 that the physician, with a bag of tools, is himself a barrier to physiological birth: "The frame of mind [necessary for physiological birth] is then aggravated by the wrong type of nurse and by the arrival of the medical attendant with a bottle of chloroform and a bag of clinking instruments, with their strong suggestion of a speedy ending without further effort."[13] The more mothers are poked, prodded, or given drugs, the more the physiological process of birth is interrupted and impeded and the more likely complications become.

Similarly, many interventions in physiological dying increase pain and suffering without corresponding benefits. While loss of appetite and thirst are common at the end of life, the standard medical treatment, often encouraged by family members fearful of "starving" a loved one, is intravenous fluids or feeding tubes. These interventions interrupt the physiological process of dying, in which the body responds to the inability to digest food or move fluids through the kidneys by shutting down signals for further intake. In the terminally ill, artificial hydration increases pain and swelling because the body is no longer able to process fluids efficiently. This pain and swelling must then be treated with diuretics, and the patient may be restrained to prevent pulling out the IV lines. Despite lack of medical evidence supporting its use, artificial hydration via IV at the end of life is widespread in hospitals.[14] Hospices accept lack of hunger or thirst as symptoms of a larger process and, rather than fighting the symptom, focus on keeping the patient comfortable with ice chips, moistening of the lips and tongue, or pain medications.[15]

Because both birth and death are complex and emergent processes, critics of medicalized birth and death reject the reductionism of the medical approach, instead adopting a holistic treatment plan for birthing women and dying individuals. Midwives emphasize the mind-body connection in birth and the role a woman's social, emotional, and physical environments play in reducing stress.[16] Cicely Sanders's groundbreaking contribution to treatment of the dying involved her emphasis on addressing "total pain," which included the physical, emotional, and spiritual needs of dying patients.[17] Advocates for physiological birth and death argue that because of the extreme sensitivity of individuals during birth and death to fear and stress, practitioners must minimize environmental and psychological stressors. In contrast, hospitals are unable to minimize many routine stressors, such as constant activity, unfamiliar staff, strict routines, bright lights, and constant noise, all of which generate stress that impedes these complex physiological processes.[18]

A growing body of research supports the belief that reducing stress improves outcomes for both birthing and dying patients. Evidence suggests that stress and anxiety increase pain,[19] pain and stress lower immune system response and prevent healing,[20] and treatments compound in a cascade of secondary symptoms that in turn require treatment.[21] The cascade of interventions found in hospitals is considerably less common in midwifery and hospice care in part because patient stress levels are lower and because patients have the support they need to avoid a crisis in the first place. Counterintuitively, doing less can lead to better medical outcomes. In one study of cancer patients, those who chose hospice care (and as a result gave up curative treatment) actually lived longer than those who pursued aggressive treatment, presumably as a result of lowered stress levels and fewer side effects from powerful medications.[22]

While some critics suggested reforming the hospital environment to accommodate the unique needs of laboring women and dying persons, most argued that the only real way to respect individual wishes and protect people from unnecessary stress and harm was to move care outside hospitals and back into either the home or decentralized locations like birth centers and hospices.[23] Demedicalization was almost always linked to decentralization of care because, as critics of medicalization argued, everything from the culture of hospitals, to the rigid protocol structure, to the very purpose of hospitals as locations for treatment and cure prevented demedicalized and individualized care in the hospital context. One critic summed up concerns about hospital-based death by arguing that "in a typical hospital . . . care of the terminally ill is clearly a secondary concern, and in fact its goals, methods, and values are at some deep level hostile to the very enterprise."[24] Midwives made similar arguments about hospital-based birth, arguing that the hospital environment's bright lights, multitude of staff, and continual interruptions and interventions were antithetical to the needs of physiological labor.[25] Medicine, particularly technologically focused hospital-based medicine, critics argued, was unsuitable to address the physical, emotional, and spiritual needs of those giving birth and dying. Even more fundamentally, the hospital's very purpose of curing disease made it ill-suited to handle birth and death, neither of which can be "cured" in any sense of the word.

Destandardizing Birth and Death

Critics homed in on two practical aspects of hospital-based care that increased rates of medicalization and encouraged overtreatment. Hospitals, critics argued, standardized and mechanized care as part of their mission to treat and cure.[26] These standardized protocols fostered what critics felt was an "assembly line" approach that harmed individuals during birth and death.[27] Midwives and hospice workers argued that birth and death are preference-sensitive events and will look different to each individual. Birth and death resist standardization precisely because they are not disease states and because so many of the goals of care are dependent on individual wishes and values. Yet rather than recognizing this individuality, birthing and dying patients in hospitals were tied to schedules; required to hit various milestones, such as dilation, eating, or evacuation at specified times; compelled to follow diets standardized via artificial hydration and nutrition; and isolated by strict visiting hours.[28] Such standardization emerged from the "highly authoritarian" culture of medicine in the mid- to late twentieth century, which stymied individualized approaches to care.[29]

The growth of midwifery care and hospice care as alternatives to hospital-based care for the birthing and dying coincided with the height of hospitalization in the mid-twentieth century, though the apex of both movements was probably the 1970s, when antiestablishment thinking about birth and death fit with broader cultural trends. Both midwifery and hospice linked their philosophies to much older traditions, rooted in women's traditional roles as caretakers of the birthing and dying. Both also relied on nonmedical caretakers, prioritized individual comfort rather than "cure," and located themselves in familiar environments, meeting the patient in her home and enlisting family and friends for the majority of care.

Midwifery specifically marketed itself as the rediscovery of knowledge that was lost in the battles over professionalized medicine in the early twentieth century. Much of midwifery in the 1960s and 1970s focused on relearning what the body intuitively knew how to do by looking to birthing practices in more traditional societies, where women eat, drink, and move during labor, accompanied by support people, with external stressors carefully limited.[30] Even the so-called Gaskin maneuver, which Ina May Gaskin introduced in the 1970s to relieve shoulder dystocia, was a technique learned from Central American traditional midwives.[31] Granny midwives, traditional black midwives throughout the South, emphasized "motherwit," or the combination of intuition and common sense that guided midwives for thousands of years. Onnie Lee Logan, a granny midwife for 40 years in Alabama, gave credit to the public health classes she took but said that "two-thirds of what I know about deliverin, carin for mother and baby, what to expect, what was happening and was goin on, I didn't get from the class. God give it to me. So many things I got from my own plain motherwit."[32] Midwifery relied on intuitive knowledge of women's bodies, traditional practices to support physiological birth, and a focus on the needs of the individual woman giving birth, while still accepting the need for medical intervention in some cases.[33]

Hospice advocates also saw hospice care as less an innovation than a rediscovery of older traditions about how to care for the dying. The modern hospice movement was founded in 1967 in England by Cicely Saunders, a British doctor whose work on humanizing death spanned decades. Saunders based her first hospice on a much older tradition, with roots as far back as the twelfth century. Her goal was to unite "the care of incurably ill and dying patients in traditional religious-sponsored hospices with the scientific contributions of modern medicine."[34] This combination proved powerful because it allowed patients access to the pain and symptom relief provided by modern medical techniques without the institutional environment of hospitals. Saunders rejected the medical community's attitude toward death as one of defeat, instead arguing that "the last stages of life should not be seen as defeat, but rather as life's fulfillment. It is not merely a time of negation but rather an opportunity for positive achievement."[35] Avoiding total demedicalization, Saunders argued for the appropriate use of medicine for the elderly and terminally ill, including palliative techniques that could reduce suffering at the end of life. Both midwifery and hospice treated birth and death as powerful human experiences whose medical components are merely one part of a much more complex whole and that were in some ways better supported in the past than in the present.

Perhaps unsurprisingly given the importance of birth and death in human lives and the preference-sensitive nature of the events, advocates for demedicalized birth and death have focused primarily on reforms to individualize birth and death.[36] Hospice and midwifery both contain strong individualist strains, emphasizing the primacy of the individual in the process. The creed of St. Christopher's Hospice, which animates much of the modern hospice movement, exemplifies this focus: "you matter because you are you and you matter to the last moment of your life. We will do all we can, not only to help you die peacefully, but also to live until you die."[37] Midwifery also emphasizes the individual nature of birth, trusting the laboring woman to tell the midwives how she wants to labor, what position is most comfortable, when to eat and drink, and who should be present. Because both types of care often take place in the home, the environment itself focuses care on the specific individual, taking into account all the variables in her idiosyncratic situation.

Demedicalization and Decentralization of Birth and Death

Advocates focused on reforms both within and outside of hospitals, such as increased attention to comfort measures, including pain control; attention to environmental issues like sound and light levels; access to adequate pain relief; and a general focus on patient-centered care in a robust sense of the term.[38] Other reforms focused on the social and cultural elements of birth and death, including changes to hospital protocol to allow fathers into birthing rooms and to make room for family and friends at the bedsides of the dying.[39] Practitioners also highlighted the importance of improved communication, respect for patient autonomy, and strict adherence to informed consent as ways to better assess the needs and desires of the individuals undergoing these experiences. Support for physiological birth and death required a tiered approach that involved identifying universal needs like comfort; more specific social, cultural, and religious values; and finally the individual preferences and goals of care that differ from person to person. Support for all these variables required, as a result, constant and continual communication among patients, families, and providers about goals of care.

One minor point of disagreement among critics of hospital-based birth and death regarded how far to decentralize care. The home birth movement advocated for total decentralization, in some cases rejecting the idea that birth has medical components at all.[40] More moderate advocates took a triage approach, where medical complexity would be weighed against patient wishes and where low-risk patients could give birth and die, with some medical support, outside the hospital setting. Others argued for a new institutional alternative to both hospital and home in the form of birth centers or residential hospice centers. Proponents argued that only with a real alternative to hospital-based birth could the healthcare community demedicalize birth and death to provide high-quality, low-cost, individualized, and humanized care. This institutional alternative had to recognize that for many Americans birth and death at home were not possible given the limitations of social support networks and the lack of generational knowledge of physiological birth and death.[41] For most advocates, a mix of options, like docks along the shoreline, could best provide personalized care for a wide range of individual goals and needs.

Despite the benefit of high-touch, low-tech alternatives, critics such as Gaskin, Saunders, and Kübler-Ross knew they could not rely on demand alone to fuel the growth of demedicalized options. Not only had medicalization harmed the birthing and dying, but medicalization and centralization of care in hospitals had also fostered profound cultural changes that calcified current practices and shifted the broader narrative surrounding birth and death. Medicalization had all but destroyed the generational knowledge of physiological birth and death, including traditional practices such as massage, optimal positioning for pain relief, familiar surroundings, quiet environments, and continual social and emotional support. Practitioners themselves were less familiar with physiological birth and death, meaning that physicians lacked the knowledge to care for patients who would have been able to stay at home in earlier times. Providers also centralized themselves in hospitals, doing fewer home visits and forcing patients to leave home to receive care. These changes compounded the pace of medicalization by creating two types of fear: fear of birth and death as unfamiliar and unknown and fear that birth or death could not be managed without medical intervention.[42]

Despite the visibility of the "natural" birth and death movements 40 years ago, arguments to destandardize care and allow for individualization made little traction in either birth or death. Hospitals made some changes as a result of consumer pressure, including allowing fathers in the birthing room and allowing mothers and infants to maintain close contact after birth. Changes for terminal patients were harder to achieve owing to the uncertainty of prognosis and other limitations involved in end-of-life care. Despite the dramatic growth in palliative care as a hospital-based specialty over the past 20 years, how Americans die has not changed much in that interim, even as hospice use itself has grown dramatically over that period.[43] In fact, standardization of care actually increased in the 1990s as a reaction to malpractice concerns and changes to insurance coverage.[44] For both birth and death, medicalization, centralization, standardization, and mechanization have increased rather than decreased by most measures over the past 40 years.[45] Instead of a diverse range of locations and providers of care to serve individuals with different needs and desires, most pregnant women and terminal and elderly patients are limited to hospital-based care and the cascades of intervention that follow.

Decentralized Birth and Death Today

Today, decentralized care options include home birth, home hospice, independent birth centers, and residential hospice centers. These options help limit medicalization by distancing patients and providers from medical technology and offering human-provided care and physical, emotional, and psychological support in its place. Provider background also plays a role. Decentralized care in the community involves a variety of nonmedical providers, including midwives, home health aides, hospice workers, social workers, hospice volunteers, and birth and death doulas (trained support people). Nonmedical providers take a more comprehensive and more individualized approach to birth and death because they come from nonmedical backgrounds and work within an interdisciplinary context, limiting reductive thinking. They also have different attitudes toward risk, both legal and medical, since their training is outside the standard medical model and because they operate outside the risk-averse protocols instituted by hospitals. Combining medical and nonmedical providers can provide the best of both worlds, provided that communication between providers is clear and open and that providers are trained to cooperate with one another clearly and effectively, which does not always happen (more on that in later chapters).[46]

Birth and Death at Home

Birth and death at home, once the norm of human experience, are still relatively rare in the United States. While decentralized birth and death are becoming somewhat more common as increasing numbers of individuals choose home birth or at-home hospice care, out-of-hospital births still constitute only around 1.6 percent of births.[47] Home births are the most common variant, but births in independent birth centers are growing. Out-of-hospital birth in general has almost doubled in the past 10 years, though overall numbers are still low.[48] Decentralized death is much more common, though evidence suggests that hospice in particular is still underused. While 48 percent of Medicare recipients died while in hospice care, almost 30 percent of those received less than seven days of hospice care before death.[49] Palliative care specialists argue that very short stays fail to provide the full potential benefits for patients and their families, particularly since hospice use later in an illness is often preceded by a harmful cycle of transitions in and out of institutions such as hospitals and nursing homes.[50] Home hospice is more widespread than home birth largely because it was integrated into Medicare, while home birth is rarely covered under any insurance plan at all.[51] In both cases, birth at home and death in hospice (either at home or in a nursing home) remain the most common types of out-of-hospital birth and death, partly because of policy limitations on institutional alternatives like birth centers and residential hospice.

Demedicalized providers offer a range of services aimed at keeping patients comfortable and address a wide range of needs, including social and emotional support and pain control. Home birth midwives assist pregnant women by providing prenatal care and support, assessing risk factors that might make home birth inappropriate, and then observing and providing social support during labor and delivery, intervening in cases of difficulty. Such intervention is often, though not always, nonmedical in nature. Midwives manually manipulate either the mother or the baby, encourage mothers to change positions during labor, or use props such as birth stools, squat bars, and special scarves called rebozos, all of which can help move the fetus into the optimal position for delivery.[52]

Depending on the legal restrictions on practice in a given state, home birth midwives may carry basic medical tools such as Pitocin to stop bleeding, nitrous and oxygen for pain management, and infant resuscitation equipment.[53] Even potentially serious complications like hemorrhage can, with proper training, be handled in the outpatient setting or managed until a hospital transfer can be completed. Home birth midwives also usually self-select low-risk patients, recognizing that specific complications, such as gestational diabetes, preeclampsia, and (depending on the provider) multiple births, do in fact complicate physiologic birth and require medical intervention. However, midwives believe that birth itself is not a medical event unless a separate medical diagnosis exists that endangers the mother or the infant.[54]

The philosophy and structure of home hospice are strikingly similar to those of home birth and midwifery. Home hospice workers are rarely physicians, though physicians do visit when necessary. Most care is provided by nurses or trained hospice workers and volunteers. The main principles of hospice care include a central focus on the patient and her family; a major role for nurses in coordinating care; control of psychological, spiritual, and emotional symptoms, not just physical ones; an interdisciplinary team including social workers, chaplains, and volunteers; continuity of care 24 hours a day, with follow-up bereavement care for families after; and finally a promise to provide care without regard for ability to pay.[55]

Hospice staff, like midwives, use a variety of medical tools when necessary, including pain medication, oxygen, and sometimes palliative chemotherapy or radiation (treatments that provide relief from pain but do not treat the cancer itself), though the latter treatments require temporary admittance to a hospital.[56] But they also focus on nonmedical techniques such as massage, hand-feeding, and social support. Because people die in a greater range of ways than women give birth, there exists a broader range of acceptable interventions in hospice care, provided that the goal of such interventions is palliative rather than curative. In home birth and hospice at home, individualized care is the norm. As one director of a "home for the dying" said, in the home "residents set the tone and decide what the day looks like. If someone doesn't want to take a bath or wants to eat breakfast at 2pm we let them. It can be hard for people to get used to that. People are so used to being structured, especially if they're coming from a nursing home or hospital. It's hard to give them permission to do what works for them."

The philosophy and culture of home birth and home-based death are so similar that there has been increasing interest in expanding the language of birth to that of death, with growing numbers of "death midwives" and "death doulas," whose mission is to support and guide dying patients through the process of physiological death.[57] As the founder of the "death doula" movement told the *New York Times* in an interview, "There are tremendous similarities between birthing and dying. . . . There's a great deal unknown, there's a great deal of pain and a need for support for the people around the person who is going through the experience."[58] Like midwives, hospice workers, many of whom are volunteers with no medical training, provide an array of nonmedical support for symptom relief, which can include massage, aromatherapy, music and art therapy, and social, religious, and spiritual support.[59]

The environment of home itself also mitigates stress. Research shows that being cared for at home contributes to patient comfort through the familiarity of the environment, lower levels of stress, and better access to the social support of family and friends.[60] Women giving birth at home or in birth centers report finding the familiarity of home to be reassuring and comforting. Women also highlight the freedom from hospital protocols that limit their ability to control treatment options and the high-quality communication made possible by relatively long midwifery visits as reasons they prefer out-of-hospital birth.[61] Similarly, many of the main characteristics of a "good death" found in qualitative interviews with terminal patients and their families are easier to achieve at home than in a hospital setting. These include preferences about the dying process itself (such as the acceptance or rejection of interventions like tube feeding or ventilation), adequate pain control, a connection to spiritual or religious life, emotional well-being, dignity, and the presence of family.[62] One meta-analysis identified three of the major components that make home palliative care successful, including providing care in a familiar environment, pain management, and good communication. These three components in particular are difficult to achieve in a hospital setting.[63]

Despite the benefits of deinstitutionalization, giving birth or dying at home is not always possible or desirable. Both home birth and home death require intensive support from providers and family members, support that is not always available. Home birth, for example, requires that a midwife is available to travel to the birth when labor begins, and she must stay many hours while labor progresses and through the postpartum period to ensure that both mother and infant are doing well. Because the onset of birth is uncertain, home birth midwives are limited in the number of patients they can take on, and cases of midwives missing births are not unheard of.[64] Laboring women also need partners or friends who can provide support during early labor before the midwife arrives. Finally, given the current cultural attitude toward birth, many women will be more comfortable in an environment where they feel that interventions are quickly available when needed.

Death at home requires a greater intensity of caregiving because the process can take weeks or even months. The Medicare Hospice Benefit covers four hours of care a day for average patients (more care is available for patients with complex needs, though access is limited), leaving family and friends to cover the other 20 hours of caregiving.[65] Other forms of support are limited. Unlike the comprehensive assistance provided by traditional hospice, the Medicare Home Health Benefit, for example, only covers health services and not personal care, cooking, house cleaning, or other services that are necessary to support elderly or terminally ill patients in their homes.[66] For mobile patients with family in the area, such a system may be workable, but for patients without caregivers at home or for patients who are largely immobile, death at home may not be practically possible. The uncertainty of how long a patient will live, as well as how complex care will become, can make planning for caretaking difficult, if not impossible. Caring for a loved one with a terminal illness can wreak emotional, psychological, and economic havoc on families, especially when an illness is protracted.[67] The kind of intensive social and emotional support birthing and dying patients need is inaccessible to many people for a variety of reasons.

Traditionally, midwifery and hospice provided comprehensive care in part because hospitals were not an option. Onnie Lee Logan described the way granny midwives assisted at birth: "When they go on a delivery, they didn't just go on a delivery. They do the cookin and the washin. It wasn't so much of the midwifing. They was there to he'p with anything they could do." Such comprehensive care was one reason both white and black families in the South hired midwives in addition to physicians for birth: "See the doctor's not go'n bathe that baby, not go'n dress that baby or nothin like that. That's go'n be the midwife."[68] In modern settings, birth and death doulas can provide some of this traditional support, though their services are rarely covered by insurance. While the term "doula" comes from the Greek word meaning "female helper" and is usually associated with a labor support person, the concept has been expanded in recent years to include death doulas, abortion doulas, and other cases where medical care occurs during an emotionally fraught and complex time in an individual's life.[69] Doulas make meals for families, do light cleaning, keep the birthing or dying person comfortable, run errands, and assist the family during and after birth or death has finally arrived.[70] Such support can help patients stay in the home longer and help caregivers limit time away from work, itself a serious barrier to at-home care.[71] Because the concept is relatively new, training and the kind of care doulas provide vary widely, though with increasing calls for third-party payers to provide doula coverage, more consistent standards (whether for good or ill) are likely to emerge over the next decade.[72]

Partial Decentralization of Birth and Death

Given the variety of factors at play, birth and death at home will not be appropriate for all patients. Complex patients, patients with uncontrollable pain or other symptoms, and patients who are uncomfortable with nonmedicalized birth or death may prefer a more medicalized environment. For these patients, partial decentralization is an option, though access is currently limited by an array of regulatory and insurance issues (to be discussed later).[73] Birth centers, residential hospice centers, and palliative care teams in hospitals provide a bridge between the home and hospital that reduces medicalization and improves outcomes.

Birth centers and residential hospice facilities are motivated by the same philosophies of midwifery and hospice but organized around the reality that not all patients are suitable for or comfortable with totally decentralized and demedicalized options. Birth centers are small-scale facilities, usually owned by midwives but sometimes by obstetricians, that typically host one to four birthing women at a time.[74] Most states require such centers to have transfer agreements with local hospitals, and they have a range of medical equipment on hand in case of emergency.[75] Medical equipment is kept out of sight, and rooms are intended to be comfortable and homelike. Room is provided for multiple support persons, and, unlike in hospitals, children are usually allowed, which helps mimic the environment of home and allows siblings to take part in the process of birth.

Residential hospices operate similarly. Staffed primarily by nurses and hospice aides, they are designed to be small scale, familiar, and homelike, with ample room for family and social support.[76] Equipment is more visible than in birth centers, but it is still limited to basic support such as oxygen, pain medications, and other noninvasive equipment. As with home hospice, the goal of residential hospice is to provide a homelike atmosphere where symptoms are managed in an environment that is as conducive as possible to maintaining quality of life, time with family and friends, and freedom from the sights, sounds, and smells of traditional hospital care. Despite the benefits of residential hospice care, most palliative care is provided in hospitals or at home because access to residential facilities is still quite limited.[77] Hospice can also be provided in nursing homes, which is another alternative for patients without caretakers at home, but payment limitations for nursing homes may prevent full access (discussed in chap. 5). In some regions of the country, such as Upstate New York, "homes for the dying" provide free care in a residential environment for terminally ill patients with limited time to live. These homes provide comprehensive round-the-clock care to patients and are funded entirely by donations, but their reach is extremely limited.[78]

Physician involvement in both birth centers and residential hospice programs is usually limited, with care directed by midwives in birth centers or nurse practitioners in residential hospices. While nurses provide the majority of care in both hospitals and out-of-hospital contexts, hospice nurses and nurse midwives have greater autonomy in nonhospital contexts since most physicians operate on call and there is less direct physician oversight.[79] Some states require physicians to serve as medical directors of either birth centers or residential hospices, or both, but physician involvement in day-to-day care varies widely. Moreover, the philosophy of both birth centers and residential hospice is closer to that of home birth and hospice than that of hospitals. The physicians involved are therefore usually sympathetic to the goal of demedicalized birth or death and work to limit interventions and transfers to hospitals when possible.

Such individualized and decentralized care supports a range of positive outcomes. Both home birth and birth center births have lower intervention rates than hospital-based birth, higher rates of vaginal birth, and high rates of maternal satisfaction, even when controlling for maternal risk factors.[80] As in other areas of health care, outcomes vary according to the training and quality of providers; accredited birth centers boast better safety outcomes than nonaccredited centers, and the outcomes associated with midwifery care vary based on level of training and tolerance of risk.[81] Because state laws vary dramatically on requirements for both midwife training and birth center accreditation, quality and outcomes are more uneven in the United States than in Canada and the United Kingdom, where a more uniform regulatory system and better integration into the medical system make both home birth and birth center births safer.[82] In general, though, both home birth and birth center births provide safe and demedicalized alternatives to hospital births for low-risk mothers and their babies. Decentralized birth is also less expensive overall than hospital-based birth because of its combination of lower-cost providers, lower-cost locations, and lower rates of medical interventions.

Outcomes for hospice are also positive. Patients receiving palliative care or hospice care report high rates of satisfaction with their care, and families with relatives in hospice report lower levels of stress than those whose loved ones die in hospitals.[83] Patients receiving hospice or palliative care are less likely to suffer from depression than those undergoing traditional treatment, and they report higher quality of life than those who receive high-intensity care. In some cases, patients receiving hospice and palliative care live longer than those receiving intensive curative treatment.[84] Such care may also save money; introducing palliative care into hospital care early in the process can lower length of stay in the ICU without compromising quality of care.[85] As with community-based birth, outcomes vary depending on the type of provider. For-profit hospices have come under scrutiny in recent years for, among other things, cutting corners and failing to provide expensive inpatient care.[86] Despite variation across hospice organizations, families and patients report high levels of satisfaction with both hospice and palliative care.[87]

Patient satisfaction with community-based birth and death results from the holistic approach to patient care, which includes psychological preparation during pregnancy and during the course of a terminal illness, continual social and emotional support in the form of midwives or hospice workers, medical backup by physicians for symptoms or conditions that cannot be managed without medical intervention, and ultimately a belief in the power of the body to give birth and to die without machines.[88] The combination of psychological preparation and emotional and social support helps reestablish the connection between the mind and the body that midwifery and hospice argue is a crucial counter to the reductionism of modern medicine.[89] By focusing on the entirety of an individual's experience, trained support people mitigate the fear that contributes to physical and emotional pain and suffering that triggers overtreatment. This holistic approach also allows individuals and their providers to determine the appropriate level of care for their specific situation, rather than defaulting to whatever the standard of care happens to be in a particular hospital.

Destandardization, Demechanization, and Individualized Care

As part of this comprehensive method, decentralized options both destandardize and demechanize care, making room for individual goals and preferences. Hospitals necessarily have protocols and standard treatments that work well for patients with identifiable and curable diseases but work much less well for the gray areas of birthing and dying. Hospitals also confront a very different set of regulations, liability concerns, and efficiency issues than community-based options do. Decentralized providers, because they are free from these constraints, are better able to assess the risk factors and needs of individual patients, particularly those who are at low risk to begin with.

Birth center and home birth midwives, for example, are (usually) free from hospital requirements for fetal monitoring, cervical checks, and a variety of other interventions that do little to improve the health or safety of birth in low-risk women.[90] They can also be more flexible toward length of labor, speed of dilation, and other measures of progress that vary significantly from woman to woman and do not strongly correlate with danger to the mother or the fetus.[91] Women who give birth at home or in birth centers are more likely to get individualized care precisely because they are the sole patients of their midwife or physician, and their care provider can look at the whole patient rather than becoming concerned about a single measurement. Midwives assess the progress of labor by looking not only at rate of dilation but also at the strength of contractions, how far contractions are apart, the mother's mood and pain level, and how the fetus is tolerating contractions.

Decentralization also contributes to destandardization by relying on human-provided care rather than mechanized treatments and technological monitoring.[92] Human-provided care combines treatment with social and emotional support, which, in turn, mitigates the need for further technological interventions. Midwives, for example, provide manual counterpressure to help minimize the pain of contractions, an alternative to the mechanical epidural usually found in hospitals. In hospice, hand-feeding takes the place of feeding and hydration tubes, which are painful and prevent patients from communicating with loved ones. Some hospices provide massage as a way to reduce the need for pain medication.[93] Birth centers and hospices are also more likely than hospitals to respect individual decisions about whether to eat or drink and when. One benefit of high touch care is that most of these techniques have few to no side effects, meaning that they are less likely to trigger the cascade of interventions that begins in the compounding side effects of medical interventions.[94]

Furthermore, destandardizing and demechanizing care supports the social and emotional relationships that are important for patient comfort, reversing the isolation that is endemic in hospital-based care.[95] Close proximity to family and friends not only provides social support but also engages loved ones in direct care for the individual and facilitates conversations about goals of care, improving communication.[96] Social and emotional support can dramatically improve medical outcomes, reduce stress and anxiety, and increase satisfaction with the experience of care.[97] In situations where a patient has a limited social network, birth and death doulas or other trained support persons can provide social and emotional assistance throughout the process.[98] Chaplains, social workers, and counselors may also be available in community-based birth and death, though such professionals are more common during dying than during the birthing process. Shifting reimbursement policies to support the caregivers who provide high-touch care at home can save money in the long run by reducing the likelihood of transfer to the hospital and escalation of care.[99] Because social support is so empirically powerful, some community-based options organize themselves around the social components of the process, with programs like Centering-Pregnancy, where prenatal care is provided in a support-group-like environment.[100] Such programs improve medical outcomes while also limiting medicalization, reducing, for example, rates of both prematurity and interventions during birth.[101]

Destandardization, Demechanization, and Informed Consent

Apart from medical outcomes and cost measures, decentralized care in the community protects the ethical commitments at the heart of modern medicine. While patient autonomy is important in every medical field, it may be most important in birth and death because of the unique nature of these experiences. Birth and death are highly individualized events whose outcomes are strongly influenced by a patient's goals, values, attitudes, support system, and unique medical history. Treating birthing mothers and dying patients as individuals and allowing significant freedom in choice of care, care provider, and care location lead to better diagnosis of problems, fewer unnecessary interventions, and greater satisfaction with care.[102] Perhaps unsurprisingly, respecting patient autonomy allows for better care.

Decentralized or community-based options protect that autonomy both because relationships are less hierarchical outside the hospital and because individual preferences are more salient in an outpatient environment. One palliative care physician argued that a major difference between hospital-based palliative care and home-based palliative care is that in hospital-based care the patient is generally told what limited options they have. In the home, in contrast, "you're a guest in their home. In the home, it involves a lot more conversation." A home birth midwife pointed out that relationships in a woman's home are necessarily built around trust, arguing that "the hospital treats people like they don't trust them and so patients don't trust them either. When I get to know people, I can see their labs, I know their families, I can see how they're living at home, I can get a sense of their nutritional habits, etc." The relationships built outside the hospital contribute both to better medical outcomes and to a better ability to respect patient autonomy.

Decentralized care avoids some of the major barriers to informed consent found in hospitals, where the physician is the expert, the patient is a passive recipient, and both make rushed decisions with minimal knowledge. Instead, decentralized care offers the possibility of a relationship that places patient desires and goals at the center of a horizontal relationship based on trust. Such relationships facilitate deeper conversations about goals of care, conversations that form a foundation for a more robust informed consent and less contentious patient-provider relationships. As later chapters will show, reimbursement and regulatory barriers prevent the development of the full benefits of decentralized care, and for that reason, as well as others, they pose a serious threat to medicine's ability to fulfill its most foundational ethical goals.

Conclusion

Recognizing the full humanity of birth and death does not require moving birth and death completely out of hospitals. High-quality palliative care programs within hospitals or birth centers within hospital maternity wards encourage individualizing care while still accounting for the medical limits that many births and deaths will impose. And reforms in hospitals help make birth and death humane experiences for those patients who require hospital care as a result of unavoidable complications and medical need. At the same time, demedicalizing birth and death in hospitals will always be limited. The culture, structure, protocols, and training of hospital staff are ill-suited to the embodied, physiological, and human elements of birth and death. Because birth and death are not illnesses in the traditional sense of the word, hospitals structured around the treatment of illnesses will be unable to fully address the human elements of birth and death that are essential parts of the processes.

None of this is the fault of hospitals themselves, which exist to treat acute disease and save lives. The failure is rather one of cultural expectations and the policies that grew up around and, in turn, influenced those expectations. The expectation that hospitals can treat not only disease but also the human, social, emotional, and psychological components of birth and death is both unrealistic and harmful. Such expectations burden staff to provide care they are not trained to provide and increase the strain on already-overtaxed hospital resources. Moving birth and death out of hospitals would free space and resources for hospitals to do what they do best: treat and cure disease. It would also protect the broader goals of healthcare, including patient autonomy, evidence-based care, and equal access.

Despite almost 50 years of efforts to rehumanize and decentralize birth and death, little progress has been made in fundamentally changing the way Americans give birth and die. In the second half of the book I discuss why, despite widespread recognition of the problem, demedicalization has been slow and why so few Americans have access to demedicalized options during birth and death. The explanations require knowledge of the shape of the US healthcare watershed itself, molded as it is by powerful political, policy, and legal tributaries that eliminate options for decentralized care. These policy and political tributaries promote harmful cultural expectations about the best care for the birthing and dying, while eroding generational knowledge about birth and death. They incentivize hospitals and hospital-based providers while starving out decentralized options. They stymie conversations and medical planning around these events, creating another current that pulls patients into the rapids of overtreatment. In what follows I outline the sources of the main tributaries in the watershed that centralize care in hospitals and prevent Americans who desire demedicalized options from giving birth and dying on their own terms.

CHAPTER 4

Navigating the Regulation Tributary

We have very strong opposition from the [state] Medical Association and the [state] Family Physicians. And because the physician lobby groups are so much more powerful, even though the nurse midwives have all the evidence—we have FTC [Federal Trade Commission] letters in support, a hundred different documents supporting us, [and] the physicians admitted they have no evidence—but they want to remain leaders of the team.—*Birth center owner*

DESPITE THE BENEFITS of decentralized care, a variety of forces upstream constrain individuals and healthcare providers and prevent access. One of the most powerful of these forces consists in the streams and rivers of state and federal regulations that encourage centralized and medicalized care. Monetary incentives motivate powerful interests to use state regulations to shape the flow of water, channeling federal dollars into centralized options like hospitals and corporate providers. Hospitals play an active role in shaping the watershed through relationships with policy makers and regulators and through direct lobbying against competitors like community-based providers. Physicians and other stakeholders encourage legislators to limit practitioners, locations, and treatments that could help demedicalize birth and death. The complexity of the regulatory environment and the incentives at play stymie collaboration between medical and demedicalized providers, compromising patient care and safety. As resources are stretched thin, hospitals and professional associations scramble to shape the watershed in whatever way they can, to direct the flow of resources in their direction. Meanwhile, patients and providers are isolated and confused, paddling furiously against the resulting currents, with little control over where they land.

The regulations that influence medicalization are located at multiple levels of governance, including everything from federal Medicare policies that leave gaps in hospice coverage to state laws against specific kinds of midwives to local hospital policies that create de facto bans on demedicalized options like vaginal birth after cesarean section. They take the form of specific limitations on providers such as nurse practitioners (NPs) and midwives or on locations of care such as freestanding birth centers (birth centers operating independently of hospitals) and hospices. Or they represent general regulations on the healthcare industry as a whole that inadvertently privilege centralized hospitals over community-based options, as in the case of certificate-of-need (CON) laws and limits on what is called the "corporate practice of medicine" (CPM). The immediate effect of all of these policies is that individuals who give birth or die are cut off from demedicalized options in most parts of the country, victims of a complex net of regulations. The reality of birth and death in the United States is that most patients' care is shaped ahead of time, not by their preferences, but by the region in which they live, the state laws that are in effect, the policies of their hospital, and their provider's attitude toward birth and death. These variables interact with each other to produce a vigorous current that limits patient choice, escalates costs, and lowers outcomes, pushing patients toward medicalized providers and into the rapids of medicalized care.

Regulations and Community-Based Care

Despite evidence of the effectiveness and cost savings associated with demedicalized birth and death, a combination of restrictive regulations and limited reimbursement options (discussed more in chap. 5) prevents access for most Americans. Regulatory limitations both impact and are impacted by cultural attitudes that frame how Americans think about death and dying. Cultural changes, driven in turn by the professionalization of medicine, have changed the way state legislators and regulatory bodies understand the options available for birth and death. As a result, regulators lump birth centers and hospices and the staff who work there into the regulatory framework for hospitals or ambulatory surgical centers, even though such regulations are ill-fitting and costly.[1] Regulations such as architectural requirements for gurney-width doorways (unnecessary in both birth centers and hospices), expensive resuscitative equipment (unnecessary by definition for hospice), and excessive staffing demands (such as requiring physician medical directors and social workers with terminal degrees) increase operating costs without improving patient outcomes.

Some state regulations explicitly or implicitly limit growth and competition. Birth centers in many states are limited to three or four beds total, with anything over that subject to hospital-level regulatory scrutiny, despite the fact that no medical interventions like surgery or anesthesia are provided. Many states do not know how to categorize birth centers, with some regulating them as ambulatory care centers, others as diagnostic and treatment centers, others as outpatient clinics, and some as health clinics.[2] As one birth center advocacy organization put it, "The birth center model is a maxi-home rather than a mini-hospital," but regulations rarely reflect that difference.[3] This variation in state policy environments limits the power of national advocacy organizations to make systematic changes, shifting resources away from lobbying for consistent reforms and toward a game of regulatory whack-a-mole.

Certificate-of-Need and Corporate Practice of Medicine Laws: Currents toward Centralized Care

While there are a range of regulations that make community-based care artificially costly, the most powerful currents are those that allow medical players like hospitals and physicians to prevent demedicalized providers from entering the market in the first place. Some of these regulations do not target birth centers or hospices specifically, but instead promote medicalization by eliminating competition under the guise of regulating medical care broadly. CON laws, CPM laws, and scope-of-practice limitations on advanced practice nurses all allow gatekeeping by medical providers that limits options for demedicalized birth and death. All of these laws create a powerful current at the state level that pushes providers, and eventually patients, into medicalized and centralized care.

CON laws, in states where they exist, directly prevent decentralized options from entering the market. CON laws require those who wish to open a healthcare facility or buy certain types of medical equipment to demonstrate to regulators that community need and demand for a particular service exist. Predictably, CON laws tend to limit competition. CON application fees are typically high, and the process itself often takes years, both serious impediments to small-scale providers. The process also tends to favor players that are already active in the market like hospitals by asking them to testify for or against a potential entrant's application. As one might expect, established providers and institutions are not often in favor of greater levels of competition.

CON laws are a remnant of the Hill-Burton Act of 1946, the same act that standardized hospitals and helped to centralize medical treatment. These laws originally stemmed from concerns about excessive supply of medical facilities, which lawmakers believed would artificially inflate medical prices, as hospitals raise prices to deal with falling demand.[4] Because hospitals and medical providers in general typically do not operate in a market-based system, the usual market limitations on excess supply (lowered prices) would not apply. And because prices in medical care are not transparent, patients have no way of choosing providers based on either price or quality. As a result, CON advocates argued for government intervention to regulate supply and control cost and quality. The federal government mandated CON laws in 1974, requiring that every state have some form of CON program, though this requirement was repealed in 1987, and 14 states have since eliminated their CON programs.[5]

The main arguments in favor of CON laws today are that these policies might limit spending and could assist patients in choosing quality providers. Critics argue that such laws limit competition, that they are inconsistently applied, and that they politicize economic and healthcare decisions. Because CON laws allow existing providers to protest or even veto the entrance of potential competitors, hospitals use these laws in conjunction with their economic and political clout in the community to prevent competition from small community-based options. CON laws also increase the potential for political corruption, as recent research suggests that political contributions influence the outcome of CON decisions, with higher rates of political contributions by CON applicants in states with more restrictive CON approval processes.[6] Political contributions are, unsurprisingly, associated with positive CON outcomes. Research also suggests that CON laws contribute to health disparities, in part because providers with little competition focus on wealthy white patients over lower-income minority patients. In one study, allowing more providers to enter the market dramatically reduced health disparities in access to cardiac angiographies, not because the facilities had not existed in poor areas, but because those facilities catered almost exclusively to white clientele.[7] More competition forces providers to focus on a wider range of a patient population.

Whether CON laws serve a positive regulatory purpose at all is somewhat unclear. While some studies have shown minor decreases in healthcare costs in states with CON laws, researchers have not found improvements in quality of care. At least one study found that states with CON laws were associated with lower-performing hospitals, leading the authors to conclude that CON laws actually protect poorly performing hospitals by limiting competition.[8] Both the Justice Department and the Federal Trade Commission argue that CON laws are outdated and do not provide the benefits they claim.[9] States that have CON laws on the books also tend to focus those laws on restricting the growth of outpatient facilities, centralizing care in hospitals by targeting community-based alternatives such as birth centers and hospice. At least 18 states require CON applications for new hospices, and 18 others require CON applications for obstetrics care.[10]

Another regulation on medical practice that limits community-based options for birth and death is the ban in some states on medical providers working directly for corporations. Such bans were created early in the twentieth century to prevent corporate priorities like shareholders and profits from corrupting physicians' medical opinions. CPM bans may centralize care in hospitals by making hospitals the easiest place for medical providers to work while also increasing the complexity of the regulatory environment. As of 2006, at least seven states had explicit CPM bans, while as many as nine states had case law or other kinds of guidance that also prohibited the practice. Many states provide CPM exemptions for nonprofit hospitals, teaching hospitals, and some kinds of clinics. Other states allow corporations to hire physicians so long as the corporation does not profit from the physician's activities or, in other states, does not direct the physician's provision of care. Around half of states allow hospitals to employ physicians directly, and around 60 percent of states allow physicians to form a limited liability company for the purposes of practicing medicine.[11]

Because hospitals are often exempt but community health providers like hospice agencies or birth centers may not be, CPM bans require physicians and, in some states, NPs and nurse midwives to form limited liability companies to provide care in the community. Providers get around these restrictions by working with HMOs or other exempt organizations, but many doctors and advanced practice nurses simply find that working directly with a hospital as an exempt organization is the easiest way to avoid the regulatory burdens that attach to community-based care. Both CON and CPM laws make it harder for small-scale demedicalized providers to enter the marketplace and compete for qualified providers. They also limit the spread of demedicalized options by making it difficult to spread successful models across state lines.[12] While this regulatory complexity significantly increases start-up costs, there is little evidence that such policies either improve healthcare or lower overall costs.

Scope-of-Practice Limitations: Centralizing and Medicalizing Providers

Another gatekeeping current is made up of state and federal policies that limit the scope of practice and payment options for nonphysician providers. Of particular importance are regulatory restrictions on advanced practice nurses, nurses with graduate degrees, including NPs and certified nurse midwives, the most common supervisors of birth centers and hospices. Such restrictions include limits on prescriptive authority and requirements for physician collaboration or oversight. These limitations stem from long-standing conflicts between physicians and nurses about who offers what kind of care in what context. Originally focused on routine patient caretaking, nurses now—particularly advanced practice nurses—have considerable specialized medical knowledge, including prescriptive authority and specializations in fields like midwifery and anesthesiology.[13] Physicians have responded to the growth of this pool of lower-cost healthcare providers by seeking to strengthen regulatory limits on these providers, emphasizing physicians' considerably longer training and more in-depth education.

At the same time, pressure from insurers and policy makers has begun to erode the ability of physicians to protect their primacy in the healthcare market. The dearth of primary care providers has led stakeholders to try to balance physician and advanced practice nurse interests to lower costs and improve quality of care. Such attempts, however, have been strained. A 2013 attempt by the Robert Wood Johnson Foundation to bring physicians and advanced practice nurses together to discuss primary care ended in a complete lack of consensus on issues relating to pay scale and whether advanced practice nurses can independently lead clinics. The lead author described the differences in attitude as an "interplanetary gulf" between physicians who believe that their extensive training justifies oversight of other providers and advanced practice nurses who argue that their skills and training allow them to practice independently and to assess when physician involvement is necessary.[14]

While scope-of-practice regulations ostensibly protect patients from unqualified practitioners, research suggests that there is little effect. A 2017 study on nurse midwives found that restrictive scope-of-practice limitations do not improve health outcomes.[15] In fact, states without restrictive scope-of-practice limitations on nurse midwives have lower rates of induction and cesarean section, supporting the claims of midwives that they practice less interventionist and more appropriately medicalized care during pregnancy and delivery. While scope-of-practice laws have become less restrictive over the past 20 years, high or moderate barriers to nurse midwives still exist in most states, including California, Texas, Florida, and many coastal states, affecting large numbers of women.[16]

As a result of Medicare's role in defining hospice, both state and federal limitations on NPs affect hospice providers. Medicare, for example, requires that all hospices have a physician medical director. Under federal law, NPs may be the "attending physician" in a hospice if they are allowed to do so in the state in which they practice, but they cannot replace the medical director either in name or in practice. Medicare does not allow NPs to certify or recertify a terminal diagnosis or the six-month prognosis, which delays care when the physician medical director is overwhelmed or otherwise unavailable, particularly a problem on evenings and weekends.[17] Medicare also pays NPs at a lower rate than physicians for doing the same work, without reference to experience or other relevant qualifications.[18]

Restrictions on advanced practice nurses in birth and death affect more than cost or access, touching on the provision of demedicalized care itself. Allowing hospices and birth centers to hire NPs and nurse midwives as medical directors would help ensure that the primary decision maker is one whose practice culture is actually aligned with demedicalized care. When asked about regulatory reforms, one hospice director said, "One regulatory relief that would help a lot would be if

NPs could sign the CTI [certification of terminal illness] because whether it's cultural or education, it seems like there's much more engagement with the patient and understanding of the need to move toward comfort care." A nurse midwife made a similar point, arguing that "typically midwives come at [birth] from a nursing philosophy where I am your partner and I don't know what's best for you but I'm going to try to find out how we can do what's best for you. My job is to walk beside you and your family and get you to a safe and healthy outcome." Requiring that physicians serve as gatekeepers to and overseers of demedicalized options may encourage more medicalized care.

Scope-of-practice limitations interact with other regulations to compound the complexity and increase the bureaucratic burden on community-based providers. In California, for example, efforts to expand the scope of practice for advanced practice nurses were significantly slowed when physicians insisted that nurses be subject to the same bans on corporate medicine as they were.[19] Meanwhile, conflicting state and federal laws and the variation between even Medicaid and Medicare on the status of advanced practice nurses add bureaucratic burdens for all providers. Depending on the state, a single provider treating a single patient faces dramatically different regulatory limitations and reimbursement depending on whether she sees that patient in a hospital, a nursing facility, at home, or under the supervision of a hospice agency.

Regulating Birth

The regulatory environment is particularly complex for birth in part because of the variation in midwifery practice style and education. Midwives range from fully demedicalized to fully medicalized, and this variation is rooted in deeply political debates about autonomy and control going back to the early 1900s. These debates were internally complex, with medicalized nurse midwives arguing that medical training saved lives and lent legitimacy to what had previously been a folk healing art. Traditional nonmedicalized midwives, on the other hand, resisted restrictions on previously independent practice, restrictions that might harm the most vulnerable patients such as poor, black, and rural women. Physicians added to this complexity by positioning themselves as authorities in obstetrics and therefore the rightful managers of all obstetrics teams. They resisted both traditional midwives and, ironically, nurse midwives, unless both could be placed safely under the control of expert physicians by targeted regulations.[20]

As a result of these conflicts of interest between maternity care providers, midwifery remains a heterogeneous profession. A large number of midwives lack any formal medical training. Traditional midwives carry no licensing or certification, and their education is purely apprenticeship based. Direct-entry midwives, also known as certified professional midwives, lay midwives, or licensed midwives (there are a variety of titles, depending on the state), are licensed by the state or certified by an outside organization but do not have a medical background.[21] Certified nurse midwives are advanced practice nurses with a formal graduate degree in midwifery.[22] This diversity itself has roots in physician attempts to eliminate or control midwifery at the turn of the twentieth century, using state-level regulation as a way to limit competition. Some—largely white middle-class women—joined physicians in supporting medical training for midwives. Others—often black or indigenous midwives whose practices differed radically from the medical model and whose limited resources made licensing difficult—insisted that midwives be free to practice without medical permission.

At least two ulterior motives existed for professionalizing midwifery: the first, to expand male physicians' scope of practice; the second, to centralize care in teaching hospitals, to support medical research and the professionalization of medicine. As a 1912 article in the *Journal of the American Medical Association* argued, "It is at present impossible to secure cases sufficient for the proper training in obstetrics, since 75% of the material otherwise available for clinical purposes is utilized in providing a livelihood for midwives."[23] Physicians believed that midwives were monopolizing women's bodies—the "material" on which future physicians needed to practice. Despite obstetricians being too few, less well trained, and more likely to engage in dangerous interventions, scholars note that "between 1900 and 1930, midwives were almost totally eliminated from the land—outlawed in many states, harassed by local medical authorities in others."[24] In states like Massachusetts, prosecutions for midwifery (or more technically for practicing medicine without a license) were common, with more than a dozen prosecutions of midwives recorded in a seven-month stretch between 1914 and 1915 in one town alone.[25]

Competing motives and priorities within midwifery contributed to further fragmentation. Midwives—then and now—are split on whether to join the medical community as nurse midwives and enjoy the legitimacy of state licensing (including insurance reimbursement) or whether to sacrifice that legitimacy to remain committed to providing independent and demedicalized birth to any woman who desires it. The differing priorities of nurse midwives on the one hand and direct-entry and traditional midwives on the other lead to disagreements about certification and licensure, hospital admitting privileges, and reimbursement rates. Such disagreements can become quite granular. The Big Push for Midwives, an initiative that supports licensing of direct-entry midwives in all 50 states, has been criticized both by nurse midwives for supporting what they see as untrained providers and by traditional midwives who believe that licensing laws unnecessarily limit women's options during birth.[26] Because of these internal disagreements, midwives have been less able than physicians to pursue clear legislative platforms.

Political debates about what kinds of providers are legitimate or illegitimate also affect decentralized locations for care. Birth centers rely on nurse midwives and direct-entry midwives to provide care; therefore, regulations on these kinds of providers affect birth centers directly. Most states require physician oversight of birth centers, and some even require a collaborative agreement with a physician who can serve in an on-call capacity. Until 2017, New York law mandated that birth centers must be owned by physicians, a major contributor to the dearth of birth centers in that state.[27] Midwives argue that such regulations both misunderstand the kind of nonmedicalized care that birth centers provide and place midwives under the thumb of physicians. The goal of birth centers is not to move medicalized birth into the community, but to create a triage system where medical care is limited to medical need. Nurse midwives and direct-entry midwives are trained to be able to assess laboring women and, in the event of a complication, keep them stable until transfer to a hospital can be completed. Midwives argue that regulations requiring physician oversight unnecessarily medicalize nonmedicalized options.

Such requirements may prevent birth centers from opening in the first place. In 2011 the main obstetrics organization, the American College of Gynecology and Obstetrics, issued a joint statement with the American College of Nurse Midwives that physician oversight of nurse midwives is not necessary because it does not improve safety or outcomes but does increase physician liability and malpractice costs.[28] Because oversight requirements increase liability risk for the overseeing physician, few physicians are willing to enter into such agreements. As a result, midwife birth center owners must get agreements from physicians who have powerful economic and professional incentives not to cooperate with them. Birth centers can be forced to close if their consulting physician drops the consult agreement, dies, or moves away, just as they can be forced to close if a hospital decides to rescind a transfer agreement. Birth centers, unlike most businesses, are placed peculiarly at the whim of their direct competitors in states that require such agreements.

Other regulations on midwives actually make women less safe. Traditional and direct-entry home birth midwives in many states cannot carry lifesaving medications such as Pitocin (to treat hemorrhage), IV fluids, oxygen, and antibiotics. Such tools are important for stabilizing a woman in an emergency until medical providers arrive or a hospital transfer can be accomplished.[29] In one byzantine example of regulatory confusion, as of 2017 Arizona law prohibits direct-entry midwives from prescribing such lifesaving medications, but health department regulations require them to have them on hand during home births and at birth centers. Midwives in this state must have standing orders from cooperating physicians to carry these medications, orders that are difficult to attain in rural areas or in areas where physician hostility to midwifery care is high.[30]

Requirements for physician collaboration or oversight not only make midwifery practice more difficult but also can prevent birth centers or home birth midwives from providing care at all. Physician hostility to birth centers has been a major barrier to the spread of birth centers in the United States since the first one opened in the 1970s. The Lewin Report, commissioned by the Federal Trade Commission in 1981, chronicled substantial physician opposition to the Manhattan Birth Center, including resignations from the medical advisory board (in all, 10 of the 18 Medical Advisory Board members resigned), formal opposition by physicians to insurance reimbursement for the birth center, and informal opposition in the form of unsubstantiated rumors about quality and pressure on residents at the admitting hospital to avoid cooperating with the birth center.[31]

Such opposition continues 35 years later. A survey of birth centers in 2014 found that physician opposition was a major barrier to out-of-hospital birth. One midwife in the survey contacted 16 obstetrics practices in her area, all of which refused to consult or accept referrals from the center.[32] Requiring oversight is singularly problematic in areas where a single hospital or obstetrician practice has a monopoly on physicians, preventing the collaboration mandated by state regulations. Such regulations are also costly, since some physicians demand payment for what amounts to little more than a signature. Birth centers have reported paying as much as $60,000 per year to a physician for the privilege of having a medical director in name only.[33]

While oversight agreements are burdensome, in other states non-medical providers are simply illegal and cannot operate at all. Midwifery in particular suffers from a complex licensing and accreditation environment that entails everything from an inability to bill Medicaid and insurance to threat of prosecution. While certified nurse midwives are licensed and practice legally at home or in birth centers in all 50 states, nine states prohibit direct-entry midwives from practicing at all, while five states require licensing but do not provide it, essentially outlawing such midwives.[34] The legal status of direct-entry midwives in other states is unclear. According to one midwifery organization, "in 20 states, as well as in the District of Columbia and two U.S. Territories, Puerto Rico and Guam, direct-entry midwives are at risk of criminal prosecution for practicing medicine or nursing without a license."[35] One consequence of this regulatory complexity is that women may be unaware which providers are licensed in their state and which are operating legally. Because the vast majority of midwives who attend home births and birth center births in the United States are direct-entry midwives, not nurse midwives, regulatory uncertainty primarily affects out-of-hospital birth options.

Regulations on midwives seriously limit women's options for home birth. Because many states have no nurse midwives practicing outside of hospitals and birth centers are rare, women who wish to have a trained provider at their birth must give birth at a hospital.[36] In some states, home birth with any kind of trained attendant is effectively illegal. While Alabama allowed home birth with a trained midwife or physician in 2017, restrictions on VBAC and other patients continue to limit many birthing women to hospitals.[37] Pregnant women and their midwives must resort to extreme measures to give birth outside a hospital. Some women cross the state line into neighboring states while in labor to give birth in a hotel or RV park rather than risk giving birth in an Alabama hospital, where intervention rates are markedly high.[38] Regulatory limitations on home birth make even less sense in a state like Alabama where many rural counties lack labor and delivery wards.[39] Women in these areas must drive long distances for prenatal care and during labor, distances that are themselves associated with increased rates of complications for both mothers and infants.[40] Home birth with a trained attendant may well be the safest option for low-risk women in these areas, but regulations prevent access.

Some regulations on home birth providers directly violate patient autonomy by compelling women to undergo tests or procedures in order to have any medical care at all. The Arkansas Department of Health, for example, requires all women who want midwifery care at home to undergo a health assessment at the health department, which includes a mandatory internal pelvic exam and testing for sexually transmitted diseases. Mothers who refuse to have the pelvic examination, itself of dubious clinical value, must forgo any legal providers at their birth because such providers would face prosecution. Mary Alexander, a professional midwife in Arkansas, was found in violation of state Board of Health protocols in 2018 for attending the birth of a woman who declined the exam.[41] Four women are currently suing the Arkansas Department of Health on the grounds that such requirements constitute compelled medical treatment and are therefore unlawful.[42] Arkansas, like Alabama, also bans midwives from overseeing VBACs outside of hospitals, effectively compelling women to give birth in a hospital, with a high probability of a repeat cesarean section, or forgo trained providers altogether. Tellingly, the medical director of the Arkansas Department of Health was quoted in one news source as saying that the regulations exist so that mothers "get a standard and safe health experience."[43] Since the alternatives to compelled vaginal exams with little clinical benefit are birth in a hospital with high rates of interventions or birth at home unattended, it seems at least possible that such regulations cause harm rather than improving outcomes.

Regulation of home birth is often justified by studies suggesting that home birth is more dangerous than hospital birth, though the research itself is actually quite mixed. Older studies that concluded that home birth is dangerous did not control for whether a trained provider was present or whether the birth was intentionally set at home. A major study in the *British Medical Journal* (*BMJ*) on North American home birth found it to be just as safe as hospital birth, though a meta-analysis commissioned by ACOG in response found neonatal death rates two times higher in home birth than in hospital birth. That study has come under scrutiny for incorporating outdated studies, including an older home birth study that failed to control for trained birth attendants.[44] Overall, the research regarding home birth is influenced as heavily by the politics of providers as it is by the quest for scientific truth. The *BMJ* study was paid for in part by a midwifery advocacy group, while the ACOG study was directly commissioned by an obstetrics organization. Proponents of medicalized or demedicalized birth can pick their own large peer-reviewed study to support their view of the safety of home birth. The results of both studies show that maternal and infant mortality in the United States is rare regardless of location of birth.[45]

More broadly, the question of licensing is linked to the perennial question of how to weigh maternal autonomy against infant harm. While risks to mothers are higher in hospitals, particularly when accounting for rates of unnecessary surgeries and interventions, risks to infants are higher in the home birth setting, particularly where such births are attended by direct-entry midwives without medical training. Restrictive regulations force women into choosing between the high likelihood of unnecessary interventions and lack of autonomy in the hospital on the one hand and the much rarer but serious risk of fetal or infant harm in a home birth setting on the other. Home birth advocates argue that decisions about balancing risk and autonomy are best left to mothers themselves, who have the greatest stake in both outcomes. The main professional organization for obstetrics, ACOG, has attempted to thread the needle of supporting maternal autonomy while advocating for hospital-based birth by arguing that women have the right to decline any and all medical interventions during pregnancy and delivery while at the same time rejecting home birth as a legitimate option for birth.[46]

Whether to accept riskier care that better protects patient autonomy is ultimately a matter of individual preference. Reports of direct-entry midwives who encourage risky births in inappropriate circumstances or who fail to transfer patients to hospitals when complications arise further fuel the conflict between physicians, nurse midwives, and non-medical midwives, each of whom claim that they and only they effectively balance maternal autonomy against maternal and infant safety.[47] At least some midwives who attend riskier births at home say they do so because many of the mothers they see are refusing hospital-based birth specifically to avoid coercive hospital protocols that are not evidence based.[48]

The current regulatory structure worsens conflicts between types of providers by preventing coordination between providers across care locations, leaving both women and infants more vulnerable. Home birth midwives who know that they cannot accompany their patient during a hospital transfer may wait to transfer out of a misplaced sense of loyalty. Mothers themselves may resist transferring to a hospital because of negative attitudes toward home birth transfers, including reports of bullying and aggressive behavior on the part of hospital staff. Prescriptive limits on lifesaving medications or requirements to confer with an off-site physician may prevent midwives from acting immediately when complications arise. A maternal-fetal specialist noted in an interview how the lack of integration creates poor incentives: "It's less that midwives do riskier things, but that the midwives are caught in the middle because their patients really don't want to go to the hospital. If the option is that there will be no attendant at all, the midwife may feel an obligation to do more risky births to keep the patient safe." Research shows that better integration of all types of midwives into the broader healthcare system reduces harms to both mothers and infants, including the most serious harms of maternal and neonatal death.[49]

Regulations and Medical Gatekeeping in Birth

The way regulations are used by medicalized providers to limit demedicalized options is most clear in the real-world application of CON laws. While the actual number of states that require CON laws for birth centers is unclear, in some states CON laws have all but eliminated birth centers.[50] In a letter to the commissioner of the Federal Trade Commission, the American Association of Birth Centers (AABC) noted that three-fifths of their members had had their CON opposed by their local hospital.[51] Kentucky currently has no birth centers because the most recent midwife to go through CON in that state lost her application, won on appeal, but then lost at the state supreme court. The process took four years, at least one denial, and hundreds of thousands of dollars in attorneys' and consultants' fees.[52] One obstetrician in another state described having to spend a full year's rent on an unused space while her application wound its way through the year-long CON process because the CON law required that the birth center facility be rented or purchased before undergoing CON approval. That obstetrician estimated the total amount of money she spent to open the birth center to be hundreds of thousands of dollars, much of it spent on legal fees navigating CON laws and other regulations. Given these barriers to entry, it is not difficult to understand why, despite 4 million American women giving birth every year, there are still only around 400 birth centers nationwide.[53]

One judge questioned the logic of allowing direct competitors to determine whether a potential entrant to the market can provide quality care. In the 2015 CON case for the Kentucky birth center, the judge presiding over the appeal questioned whether hospitals are "affected parties" at all and whether they should weigh in on the need for non-medicalized community-based options that directly compete with them. The judge's ruling found that alternative birth centers do not provide the same services as hospitals, because they provide a totally different birth experience and apply only to low-risk mothers, and that none of the hospitals claiming to be affected parties ran or run alternative birthing centers. Ultimately, he concluded, hospitals, like other businesses, have "no right to be free from competition."[54] The judge's final decision to grant the CON to the birth center concluded, "Expanding the options for giving birth by granting the Petitioner's CON application appears to further the purpose of the CON program by improving access to a variety of healthcare options without significantly impacting the cost of providing that care for the state."[55] The local hospital appealed that decision, however, and the case was ultimately decided against the birth center owner in the Kentucky Supreme Court. Positive decisions in CON cases are still rare. Judges in many states with CON laws continue to use testimony from medical providers, including hospitals, to judge the right of nonmedical community alternatives to exist.

Crucially, CON laws and many of the regulations discussed above rarely investigate the quality of the care being offered or the demand for a particular kind of care. Instead, regulations like CON laws rely heavily on the opinions of providers already providing care, the most powerful being hospitals and doctors. As such, they also have race and class implications in that they privilege wealthy and well-connected applicants over self-educated or low-income providers. Onnie Lee Logan, a black granny midwife in Alabama for almost 40 years, described her reaction upon receiving a letter in 1984 from the Mobile County Board of Health that her permit to provide care as a granny midwife, a traditional midwife without medical training, would not be renewed: "Nothing in my life has ever made me feel so little. . . . When my husband came home, he had to pick me up off the floor. Fact is, I'm still trying to get up."[56] The board's letter explained that granny midwives were no longer needed in Alabama, perhaps a reference to the expansion of obstetrics services throughout the state. Ironically, Alabama's maternal and infant mortality rate, today as in 1983, is one of the highest in the nation, while Onnie Lee Logan's record of safe deliveries was exemplary.[57] CON laws, licensing laws, and other regulations arbitrarily limit providers with excellent outcomes while doing little to prevent or punish established providers who do actual harm.[58] It is not accidental that licensing laws and other health regulations have operated since their inception to privilege wealthy and entrenched providers against the women, minority, and folk providers who serve primarily low-income individuals.[59]

The pregnant women who must choose from an artificially limited range of birth locations and providers typically have no idea how much political wrangling has gone on behind the scenes and how little such wrangling relates to actual evidence on safety or autonomy. In fact, evidence suggests that regulations that incentivize and prioritize hospital and physician-led birth artificially restrict maternal autonomy, are correlated with worse outcomes for mothers and infants, and perpetuate health and economic disparities in marginalized groups.[60] Such regulations therefore challenge or violate the main bioethical commitments of autonomy, beneficence, and justice for the sole sake of protecting entrenched players.

Regulating Death

The regulatory environment is somewhat less fraught in death and dying than in birth. This difference may be due to the lower risk environment of treating terminal patients, who have months or weeks to live, or to the fact that death does not involve two unique potential patients the way birth does. Whatever the reason, apart from divisive issues surrounding physician-assisted suicide, the political culture tends to be supportive of autonomy in end-of-life decisions. Still, given the numbers of Americans who die every year and the Medicaid and Medicare dollars that funnel into the system, decisions about how and where Americans die are politically contentious. Interest groups play a central role in shaping the regulatory environment, and the structure of the regulatory tributary itself reflects a variety of these conflicts of interest.

The first and most obvious way in which demedicalized options are regulated is the regulatory control over the word "hospice" itself. While hospice began as a religiously affiliated practice of providing the dying with end-of-life care, it is now a federally regulated service. The term "hospice" is regulated by Medicare policies that limit hospice providers to those recognized by Medicare under the Medicare Hospice Benefit (MHB). In order to market a location or set of providers as providing "hospice" care, one must meet certain Medicare criteria, such as requiring patients to forgo curative treatment and only accepting patients with fewer than six months to live. What was once an informal, nonmedical, and community-based type of care is now heavily regulated by centralized federal rules that constrain providers and limit access.

Physician oversight requirements affect hospices as well as birth centers. Medicare requires that a physician serve as the medical director for any palliative care organization that accepts the MHB. Medicare also limits hospices to a small per diem rate per patient, making it difficult for them to hire doctors at the market rate. As one director of a large hospice organization explained in an interview, "We're a non-profit community-based organization that can't meet the salary requirements of the hospitals, so we have trouble attracting talent. Either it has to be a real passion of yours or it's a passion that you indulge at the end of your career when you're close to retirement." Rural hospices struggle with Medicare licensing requirements since primary care doctors are rare and long travel times make physician visits to patients' homes difficult and costly. Under-the-radar options like comfort care homes, found in parts of Upstate New York and sporadically elsewhere, rely almost exclusively on medical directors who volunteer their time, though these homes do not exist in most areas of the country. When combined with scope-of-practice limitations, physician oversight requirements can directly harm patients by delaying referral into hospice, particularly on evenings and weekends or in rural areas where one physician covers multiple counties.

Hospices also struggle with unfunded mandates, including staffing requirements and care for conditions related to the terminal diagnosis. Under Medicare, hospices are required to have social workers and bereavement counselors on staff, but Medicare does not reimburse for these staff members. Similarly, hospices are required to pay for care and medications for all conditions related to the terminal condition, but what constitutes a "related" illness is unclear and can be a costly burden given the flat-fee reimbursement structure of the MHB.[61] For both community-based birth and death, Medicaid and Medicare reimbursements, where available, typically do not cover the cost of providing care, but they do impose mandates that increase the cost of providing that care. This combination of low reimbursement rates and high regulatory oversight is one reason why both hospices and birth centers struggle to compete against hospitals, which have teams of compliance experts on hand alongside higher reimbursement rates.[62]

Some providers respond to this regulatory environment by remaining out of the view of government insurers or regulators altogether. "Comfort care homes" or "homes for the dying" are found primarily in western New York and confront the conflicts between the needs of dying patients and the low reimbursement rates and complex regulatory environment that limit end-of-life care. While they provide the closest kind of care to traditional hospice care, they are not allowed to use the term "hospice" because they do not fall under Medicare's regulatory umbrella. These homes skirt state regulations by limiting themselves to two beds, thus avoiding (most) health department scrutiny. They avoid Medicare regulations by rejecting all insurance involvement and relying entirely on donations. Typically, such homes have an agreement with a local hospice agency that provides whatever care volunteers cannot provide. The hospice agency, rather than the comfort care home, bills Medicare as though the care were given in the person's home. As one executive director of a comfort care home noted, "A lot of [end-of-life care] is money driven, but that's what's nice about being here. We don't even have to talk about money. People don't realize that we're under the umbrella of the agency. We don't have to worry about any kind of reimbursement. We can just take people because they need the care." Such homes are also free from health department and Medicare requirements to purchase expensive equipment such as patient lifts and resuscitative equipment, further lowering their financial burden.

With that freedom, however, comes a degree of vulnerability. As one director noted, "All of our financing comes from donations and fundraising. We have no steady source of income. We can write foundation grants, but we don't receive any government grants [because of the strings attached]. We don't charge anything [to patients]." Donations pay for a nursing director, but the medical director operates on a volunteer basis. Staff nurses are part-time, and no one receives benefits. Directors see these limitations as the cost of providing the kind of individualized care they do. When asked whether she was concerned about regulatory oversight, the same director said, "We fly under the radar by being two beds. We're just a home. We just quietly try to do what we do. We don't try to lobby things or band together and have a march, because I think sometimes I don't think everyone knows what to think about us and do about us. And I sometimes don't want people to think too much about us." By avoiding the bureaucratic mandates of both insurance providers and government regulators, such homes are able to provide care in the community to people who need it most. This model is currently limited to a small region of the country, and it is not clear whether it will spread. It is, however, the closest to the traditional hospice model currently in place and is able to remain so largely because it avoids bureaucratic control.

CON and CPM laws also affect hospices. Given the Medicare money involved, new hospices face dramatic costs in navigating CON applications, particularly in areas with existing hospice organizations. In one CON case in Florida in 2017, a number of hospice organizations competed to determine who would have permission to open a new hospice location. Fees for each applicant started at $16,000 for the application alone. At least one existing nonprofit hospice bowed out of the process altogether, investing that money into marketing instead. The winning hospice, a for-profit corporation, spent two years and over $1 million to navigate the entire process.[63] The expense of the CON process may be one reason for the growth in for-profit hospices, now the dominant players in hospice care. Large for-profit hospices are associated with somewhat worse outcomes and higher levels of fraud compared to nonprofit providers, a concern of policy makers and hospice advocates.[64] Smaller nonprofit hospices cannot compete against corporate hospices in a regulatory environment that requires substantial financial hold-ings and legal expertise. While some research suggests that CON laws do decrease destructive competition, the effect seems small and may not outweigh the way CON laws incentivize the corporatization of hos-pice care.[65]

CPM laws in some states, meanwhile, limit how hospices contract with physicians, preventing hospice agencies from hiring physicians to provide care in the community. One hospice director in New York de-scribed how the current CPM laws in that state make it difficult for doctors to provide nonhospital care, noting that "the only reason our doctor can see patients is because we negotiated a contract directly with the insurance company." Insurance companies in many states are ex-empt from the CPM laws, but hospice agencies in many states, even nonprofit ones, cannot hire physicians directly. While the Department of Health in New York issued guidance saying they would not prosecute a hospice for such a consult, the director noted that uncertainty over the law "has stopped everyone from moving forward." Such confusion increases the bureaucratic burden on already-strained organizations.

Perhaps the most powerful regulatory stranglehold on hospices is not state regulations but the complexity and restrictions of the MHB itself. Hospices, originally small community-based organizations, must now familiarize themselves with constantly changing and ever more complex regulations, many of which open them up to audits years later. Predict-ably, this complexity has led to growth in secondary organizations de-voted to helping hospices comply with regulations. More troublingly, the MHB limits the kinds of patients who are eligible for hospice care, requiring that patients have both a terminal diagnosis and six months or less to live. One palliative care physician pointed to these limitations as perhaps the greatest limit on the benefits hospice can provide: "Most people, myself included, think that when someone is ready for a hos-pice philosophy, and they and their families are ready, say for example if the person has dementia, they won't qualify for hospice anyway. What we can provide then is acute care, which isn't what they need. [Many] dementia patients in particular won't qualify for hospice because they'll live too long." The MHB limitations on patients who qualify for hospice were a significant cause for concern among hospice advocates when the MHB was first created in 1983.[66] Cicely Saunders herself strongly rejected the inclusion of these limitations on hospice care in the original MHB, arguing that they would serve as barriers to care for all but the most obviously terminal patients, which has indeed proven to be the case.[67]

Moreover, Medicare has responded to the growing expense of caring for an increasingly elderly population by shifting more of the costs of caring for terminal patients to hospice organizations. One particularly burdensome regulatory change came in 2015 when Medicare expanded the way hospices must think about conditions that are related to the terminal diagnosis. The change imposed an additional requirement that made hospice organizations responsible not only for care related to the terminal diagnosis but also for the costs of care of all "related" diagnoses themselves. This change meant both dramatically increased costs of care and administrative headaches for hospices. Since hospices must cover all terminal care for patients on the same per diem daily rate, a more expansive understanding of what constitutes a "related diagnosis" can dramatically increase what hospices must pay for. Meanwhile, the vagueness of the regulation opens hospices up to audits because the requirement to cover "related" diagnoses is completely subjective. One commenter on a website devoted to hospice compliance pointed out that a hip fracture from falling could be related or unrelated to a dementia diagnosis, but the determination would be completely dependent on one's point of view. Another pointed out, with gallows humor, that given the mortality of all humans, everything is "related" to our terminal diagnosis in the end.[68] Determining the meaning of the single word "related" has caused significant consternation in the hospice community in part because the change fails to recognize the dramatic way the end-of-life landscape has changed since the MHB was created in 1983. As more expensive drugs for a variety of complex conditions have become available, hospices must, under the MHB, cover those drugs for any condition "relating" to the terminal diagnosis. The cost of drugs hospice must cover has increased over time, while Medicare continues to expand the breadth of conditions for which hospice must provide drugs. Reimbursement rates have, however, remained relatively flat.

The low per diem rate hospices receive, alongside the complexity of the requirements, creates incentives for various kinds of manipulation of documentation, sometimes constituting outright fraud. A Department of Health and Human Services (HHS) investigation in 2016 found that hospices engaged in a variety of troubling practices, including billing some drugs they are supposed to cover to Medicare D (drug coverage), admitting patients to hospitals or skilled nursing facilities for uncontrolled symptoms when the condition does not warrant such an admittance, and failing to provide care that was billed for.[69] The HHS report found both that for-profit hospices were more likely to bill in "creative" ways and that they represent the largest growth area for hospices nationwide. Such hospices have the resources to absorb fines and fees from noncompliance and the incentives to maximize reimbursement under MHB, unlike small-scale providers. One palliative care physician described the incentives hospices face under the MHB and how these incentives skew care: "[Hospices] make money on longer stay patients, they lose money on short stay patients and they lose money at the very end when the needs get more complicated." It should come as no surprise that some hospices respond to these incentives through the choices they make over what kinds of patients they take and how they coordinate care for those patients.[70]

Whatever the broader economic costs, regulations on hospice ultimately have unintended consequences for patients themselves. In the current system, the well-being of individuals at the end of life is weighed against the needs of third-party payers and a strained system that requires top-down bureaucratic oversight over both individual providers and the fast-growing hospice industry itself. As with birth, trade-offs among expense, risk, and autonomy or choice create an opening for political jockeying and lobbying by different parties who each claim they can best limit risks while providing dying and elderly patients with high-quality, low-cost, and individualized care.

Hospitals and Professional Organizations as Lobbyists

While it is tempting to assume maleficent intent on the part of lobbyists and interest groups, centralization of care and limited patient options are often rather the unintended consequence of a tangle of state and federal regulations that interact with each other in unpredictable ways, feeding off the competing interests of healthcare providers amid competition for scarce healthcare dollars. Some of these laws, like CON and CPM laws, are holdovers from earlier eras when the rapid expansion of medical research and medical care seemed to require government regulation and planning to protect both the public as patients and the public as taxpayers. But others, like restrictive legislation on practitioners and places of care, arise from lobbying efforts by hospitals, professional organizations, and medical practitioners, who presumably view their interests as aligned with those of patients. Hospitals may view lobbying against decentralized options as a way to preserve scarce resources for their lifesaving functions. Physicians may see their medical authority grounded in years of rigorous training as the best way to protect patients from harm. In both cases, perverse incentives in the regulatory framework combine with more beneficent motives to limit patient options.

Both hospital and professional medical associations are major players in shaping the regulatory tributary.[71] Hospital associations spend significant amounts of money lobbying at both the state and federal levels, for understandable reasons. Most hospitals struggle with narrow margins, and they rely on maternity care as a loss leader and end-of-life care as an important source of income. Hospitals are extensively regulated but also rely heavily on government payers like Medicare for funding. They therefore have a complicated and codependent relationship with regulators and policy makers. They are also under increasing pressure from outpatient providers: the percentage of care that occurs in outpatient settings has increased every year and the number of hospitals has been declining since 1974.[72] As hospitals respond by consolidating into large conglomerates or expanding into outpatient care themselves, they increase lobbying efforts to ensure adequate reimbursement and regulatory relief. At the state level, lobbying affects birth centers particularly, since they compete directly with hospital maternity wards.[73]

Alabama again provides a case study for the role physicians and hospitals play in regulating community-based providers. Prior to the passage of the bill in 2017 that allowed direct-entry midwives to practice in Alabama, women in the state were limited to hospital-based obstetrics care if they wanted to give birth with a trained provider. Alabama hospitals, meanwhile, had some of the highest intervention rates in the nation, and many women had limited access to any maternity care at all, given closures of rural maternity wards.[74] Despite evidence on the safety of home birth with trained attendants and the benefits of expanding access to prenatal care for both maternal and infant outcomes, the bill to legalize and license trained midwives was opposed by the

Alabama Hospital Association, the Medical Association of the State of Alabama, the Alabama branch of ACOG, and the Alabama State Society of Anesthesiologists.[75]

One of the hospitals that opposed the bill, Brookwood Medical Center, had a cesarean section rate of 43 percent at the time, the highest cesarean rate in Alabama and one of the highest in the country.[76] The same hospital was later sued and ordered to pay a record $16 million judgment after nurses reportedly held a baby in a woman's vagina for six minutes until a doctor could arrive, causing permanent nerve damage to the mother.[77] In one exchange during debate over the bill, the executive director of the Alabama Medical Association argued that it was "unfair" for hospitals to have to treat women who were transferred from home births without advance notice. A state legislator sensibly responded that people who get shot do not know ahead of time that they will be shot, concluding that hospitals have a duty to treat everyone, even if their illness or injury is self-caused or the result of poor decision making.[78] Despite significant evidence that maternity care in Alabama is highly interventionist, is difficult to access, and has relatively poor outcomes, hospitals, physicians, and medical associations opposed the home birth bill multiple times over many years before the bill finally garnered the support of key state legislators and the governor in 2017.

In states where midwifery is legal, hospitals, physicians, and state medical boards work to limit midwives in other ways, lobbying state legislators to pass laws that restrict VBAC, for example, to hospitals.[79] Most hospitals, however, do not support VBAC at all, as the number of hospitals with de facto VBAC bans grew dramatically in the first decade of the 2000s.[80] Bans on VBACs in out-of-hospital birth therefore constitute de facto bans on VBAC across the board in many states.[81] In one study in California, fully 44 percent of hospitals did not allow a trial of labor after cesarean at all, and the rest placed restrictions on VBAC labors such that surgery was almost inevitable. While research suggests that VBAC success rates should be around 70 percent, the VBAC success rate across California hospitals is 10 percent.[82] The unusually low VBAC success rate in California hospitals suggests that restrictive hospital policies incentivize repeat surgeries.[83] Hospital VBAC bans are, in turn, driven in large part by a 1999 ACOG Practice Bulletin (to be discussed in more length in chap. 6) that recommended such restrictive guidelines for VBAC that almost no physician or hospital could practically meet them.[84] Women in many states with bans on VBAC in home birth and birth centers are caught in a regulatory paradox where their only legal option for a VBAC is in a hospital that does not allow one.

In South Carolina, where a recent controversy over midwifery licensing threatened all birth centers in the state, hospital lobbyists and physician groups, including the South Carolina Medical Association, the South Carolina branch of ACOG, and the South Carolina Hospital Association, were major players in opposing birth center expansion. One nurse midwife described attending a meeting on a bill: "I walked up to the meeting and there were the hospital and medical association lobbyist talking to the sponsor of the bill in the hallway. They can stop any bill at any time. They just say 'We don't like it, pull it.' And that's what happened with one of our compromise bills." She also pointed out that many legislators who pass health regulations do not have any medical expertise and rely on the hospital associations and medical associations as the "experts" in demedicalized birth. She noted wryly, "When the chair of the medical committee for the state legislature is a tow truck driver, you have a lot of educating to do." During hearings, one South Carolina legislator expressed bewilderment that any woman would want to give birth outside a hospital in the first place.

Hospital lobbying is influential with state legislators in part because hospitals have successfully marketed themselves as lifesaving entities and centers of medical expertise. While hospitals position themselves as a major cause of lowered maternal and infant mortality rates, epidemiologists argue that the fall in perinatal mortality is due less to hospitalization than it is to overall improvements in quality of life such as "better housing, better nutrition, and family planning."[85] In fact, evidence suggests that the flattening of perinatal mortality rates since the 1990s is due in large part to the medicalization of childbirth, which actually increases risk of prematurity and other risk factors, much of which is linked to hospital practices.[86] Despite this reality, the primacy of hospitals as policy players and their resistance to community-based birth are primary reasons for the failure of community-based birth options. One birth center owner argued that "birth centers are traditionally midwife owned entrepreneurial small businesses and that's our problem. It's hard for that to be sustainable when you're up against the Hospital Corporation of America."

Lobbying by hospitals and professional associations rarely affects hospices as significantly as it affects birth centers, in part because hospitals do not see hospices as directly competing with hospitals for business. The palliative care hospitals provide at the end of life is, under current reimbursement structures, poorly reimbursed, and many hospitals lose money on that care, which provides an incentive to support hospices that can take over less profitable patients.[87] While the interests of palliative care and hospice are not perfectly aligned and conflicts exist between the medical and nonmedical providers in the field, the conflicts that do exist are more minor than those in birth.[88] Hospice care has also been more successfully integrated into the healthcare system, owing in large part to the MHB, and the federal nature of that regulation means that hospice and palliative care providers face less regulatory fragmentation than maternity care providers. Hospice is also much more culturally accepted, both by the general public and by the medical community, than community-based birth. Hospice is now involved in the care of around 40 percent of people who die in America (albeit in often very limited ways), while birth centers and home births, on the other hand, still account for fewer than 2 percent of American babies born each year. The MHB, while restricting and problematic in many ways, protects hospice by providing credibility to decentralized death that decentralized birth so far does not have.

Perhaps not surprisingly, now that hospice agencies have become more entrenched as stakeholders in policies surrounding death and dying, they now wield the same regulatory tools that hospitals use to avoid competition. An attempt in Florida in 2017 to repeal CON laws in that state ended up exempting nursing homes and hospice organizations, with the Florida Hospice & Palliative Care Association arguing that CON laws were necessary to manage the growth of hospice and prevent damaging competition.[89] One hospice vice president argued that CON laws are necessary precisely because so much of hospice funding comes from the federal government. His comment, perhaps unintentionally, demonstrates how existing players use state laws to channel federal dollars.[90] The hospice exemption is likely to further consolidate hospice programs in the state, particularly among large-scale for-profit providers, who are better able to navigate the expensive and time-consuming CON process. For-profit corporate hospices are outcompeting small providers in many states because they are the only agencies capable of paying for the lawyers needed to navigate the CON process.[91] Hospices in the original sense of the term—small community-based organizations staffed by volunteers—may very well disappear.

While birth centers have considerably less lobbying clout than hospices do, one can expect lobbying in the coming years over CON laws and Medicaid and insurance reimbursement, particularly as conflicts between accredited and unaccredited birth centers grow. The South Carolina example discussed below gives a taste of what the future may hold. Given the incentives provided by federal dollars and the regulatory tools provided by states, one can predict that early arrivals will use the regulatory toolbox at their disposal to limit new entrants to the field. It is yet unclear whether lobbying by palliative care and hospice organizations and birth center associations will result in greater access to demedicalized alternatives or will result in these options being subsumed by the broader medical model (as in the case of hospital birth centers), or consolidated into large-scale corporate alternatives (as in the case of for-profit hospices).

Physicians as Gatekeepers and Lawmakers

Medicalized approaches to birth and death are also more likely to be represented in state legislatures precisely because physicians are more likely to engage in legislative work than community-based providers. Physicians' higher salaries and formal educations presumably make them more likely to have connections to political parties and donors. Historically, physicians as a group have been both entrenched in the political community and highly respected by that community.[92] While physicians remain a small minority of legislators at the state and federal level, their participation is disproportionate to their numbers nationwide.[93] While little research exists on physician's positions on healthcare as legislators, there are characteristics of physician-legislators that may be relevant. Most physician-legislators are Republicans and male. Physicians in general tend to be more conservative than the general population and may therefore be less likely to support reforms, particularly reforms that focus on demedicalization. On the other hand, both birth centers and hospice agencies have the potential to provide substantial cost savings, so fiscally conservative physicians might find such programs an attractive alternative to expensive hospitalization. At this point, the data do not exist to analyze physician preferences overall.

Anecdotal evidence from legislative fights over demedicalized options shows that physicians in positions of political power do advocate for higher levels of restrictions on demedicalized options for birth and death, though how often this happens is not clear. In Alabama, for example, the sponsor of a bill (HB344) that would have licensed midwives while severely restricting their scope of practice is the director of business development for a local medical center, while also serving as the chair of Alabama's House Health Committee.[94] Her husband is a medical director at Blue Cross Blue Shield (BCBS) of Alabama. In South Carolina, a proposed bill to require birth centers to have a written agreement with a hospital within 45 miles was sponsored by Representative Robert Ridgeway, who was chief of obstetrics at an area hospital before serving as a state legislator.[95] A similar bill introduced in Utah that would have heavily regulated direct-entry midwives was sponsored by a state senator who is a former labor and delivery nurse. Her husband is a retired obstetrician. The bill, among other things, would have banned women with prior cesareans from giving birth with professional midwives, either at home or in birth centers. The bill failed to pass.[96] Legislation introduced in Arizona in 2014 that would substantially limit midwives' ability to attend births, including VBAC and multiple pregnancies, was sponsored by Senator Kelli Ward, a physician. As evidence of the need for more oversight of midwives, she cited discredited research on home birth safety while introducing the bill.[97] Decentralized and demedicalized providers like midwives or hospice nurses are almost never represented in state legislatures.

Physicians and hospitals also play a major gatekeeping role as members of insurance company advisory boards and state licensing boards. The Lewin study of the Manhattan Birth Center found that physician interference with community-based birthing options may involve indirect pressure on insurers and licensing boards rather than direct legislation. The report noted that letters of opposition to the birth center were sent to BCBS, the insurer debating whether to allow reimbursement for birth center birth, by "District II, American College of Obstetricians and Gynecologists; the National Committee on Fetus and Newborn, American Academy of Pediatrics; the local Committee on Fetus and Newborn, American Academy of Pediatrics; the Commissioner of the New York City Public Health Department; and the chiefs of obstetrics and gynecology from six of New York City's seven teaching hospitals," all arguing that the birth center was "an unsafe alternative." However, the report concludes, "after considerable reflection, the Board of Directors [of the insurance company] nevertheless voted to reimburse the Child-bearing Center on an experimental basis because, according to one BC/BS executive familiar with the situation, these allegations [about safety] were unsubstantiated."[98]

The decision by BCBS in the Manhattan Birth Center case is all the more surprising, since the professional advisory committee was made up entirely of practicing physicians. While the professional advisory committee ultimately supported the proposal, "debates were heated," in the words of one participant. The success of the proposal depended in large part on its being championed by a "highly placed BC/BS executive" and billed as an "experimental" policy subject to continual and careful review.[99] Without influential support from an insurance executive, it is likely that the birth center would not have been approved.[100] Precisely because of barriers like these, birth centers tend to be heavily reliant on personal connections with people in positions of power. The anticompetitive tendencies of physician advisory boards have been described by the Federal Trade Commission, which has argued against the physician monopoly on licensing boards and advisory boards for years, to no avail.[101]

The experience of the Manhattan Birth Center 40 years ago closely parallels current battles over birth centers today. An obstetrician-gynecologist who opened a birth center in 2013 found that when it came to opening her birth center, her success in fulfilling all of the major regulatory requirements depended entirely on personal relationships she had as a physician. Her connections enabled her to finally get a transfer agreement with one of the two hospitals in town after six months of initial denials, and her reputation as an obstetrician allowed her to get a facility fee from a small insurance provider after all other insurance companies refused payment. She said of the experience, "It all traded on personal interactions." As an obstetrician in practice since the late 1980s with connections with physicians and insurers, she expressed doubt that a less connected person could have successfully navigated either the red tape of regulation or the agreements that were required with hospitals and insurers. Even with substantial connections, the approval process took five years and many tens of thousands of dollars. The experiences of community-based providers cast doubt on whether regulatory bodies can function as impartial protectors of community and patient safety, particularly in oversight of competitors.

South Carolina Birth Centers and the Current of Regulations

Perhaps more troubling than the role regulations play in preventing entry into the market, shifting regulations or their interpretation by regulatory agencies can have devastating effects on existing businesses, particularly small entrepreneurial community-based options with limited cash reserves. Recent legislative gridlock over the fate of all five of South Carolina's birth centers demonstrates how the politics of birth providers collides with regulatory capture to imperil demedicalized options. The South Carolina case hinged in part on the distinction between accredited and nonaccredited birth centers, as well as the distinct and contradictory ways different types of midwives are regulated. Of South Carolina's five birth centers, three are accredited by the main national birth center accrediting body, the Commission for the Accreditation of Birth Centers (CABC), and two are not. Of the nonaccredited centers, both are run by direct-entry midwives, while nurse midwives run two of the three accredited centers. A series of infant deaths at one of the nonaccredited centers run by a direct-entry midwife in 2014 and 2015 led state regulators to look more closely at birth centers in general.

The trouble began prior to 2013, with disagreements about the South Carolina requirement for physician oversight of birth centers. It was compounded by the differing interests of nurse midwives and direct-entry midwives in the state. Under South Carolina law, nurse midwives are more heavily regulated than direct-entry midwives, despite their greater level of training. Nurse midwives are regulated largely through the licensing board, which at the time required close physician oversight of nurse midwives, including those who own and operate birth centers. Direct-entry midwives, however, did not have the same oversight requirements in South Carolina since they have no relevant licensing board, even though they have substantially less education overall and have no formal medical or healthcare training. The result is two different sets of birth centers: accredited centers run largely by nurse midwives with strong safety records and heavy regulatory burdens through the licensing boards, and nonaccredited centers run by direct-entry midwives who answer primarily to the health department.

Infant deaths at a nonaccredited center run by direct-entry midwives triggered the state health department to notify all birth centers that it was reinterpreting the physician oversight regulation, requiring that in addition to a consulting agreement with a physician, that physician would also have to be available to visit the birth center in case of an emergency. Apart from being redundant, since birth centers transfer women to hospitals for emergencies, such a regulation can be interpreted as requiring birth centers to wait for physician input before transferring, a requirement that would delay emergency care. More problematic for the centers themselves, however, such an agreement violates most physicians' malpractice insurance contracts, which do not cover care provided in a birth center. No physician would sign such an agreement even if he or she were sympathetic to the birth center's mission. State regulators were requiring birth center owners to comply with a regulation that is, practically speaking, impossible to comply with. The result was imminent closure of all five birth centers in South Carolina unless legislation was passed to clarify the regulatory environment. Because direct-entry midwives did not want tighter regulation, they opposed the compromise bills nurse midwife groups reached with physicians' groups.

In the end, the legislature changed the restrictions for all advanced practice registered nurses in the state, including nurse midwives, removing the physician oversight requirement and requiring a more flexible collaborative agreement instead. Despite nurse midwives winning greater freedom to practice, this regulatory quagmire had enormous impacts on birth center owners. Some birth centers, particularly those owned by direct-entry midwives, are still in limbo. Others lost tens of thousands of dollars in legal fees fighting the initial regulatory change. Leslie Rathbun, a nurse midwife and the owner of a birth center threatened with closure, said that before the regulation was reinterpreted by the health department her birth center was so successful that she was planning on expanding and was ready to put down an offer on land: "I had $180,000 put aside as building funds, but every penny has now been spent on this legislative fight."[102]

When interviewed while the conflict was still active, she lamented that "it's just so wrong that in this country built on capitalism you can have a health provider with high patient demand, high quality, excellent outcomes, and low costs, and yet due to regulatory burdens we can't grow—or even survive." Before the legislative decision that saved her center in early 2018, she feared that her only option was to sell her practice to a hospital, which would mean that all her midwives would be forced to move out of state because there would be no midwifery jobs available outside of hospitals anywhere in South Carolina. In the end, her birth center was saved, at the cost of her entire savings and years of legal wrangling. The fallout from a seemingly minor reinterpretation of a seemingly minor regulation can be dramatic. Such experiences may be enough to deter potential small business owners who fear such regulatory volatility.

Cases like South Carolina's are not rare. Between CON laws, scope-of-practice and licensing laws, and regulations that make providers dependent on their direct competitors, the tangle of regulations poses enormous barriers to entrepreneurial community-based birth. The alternative is a corporatized approach to demedicalized care, already found in some states.[103] A for-profit corporatized approach is already the status quo in hospice care.[104] While some states have resisted corporatization by limiting for-profit, corporate hospices in various ways, such limits fail to address the incentives that create corporate hospices in the first place: a regulatory environment that makes it all but impossible for small-scale community-based providers to start up and succeed.

Conclusion

Regulatory restrictions that centralize and consolidate care harm patients by both compromising care and limiting options. The regulatory current pushes options for birth and death in two different directions that nevertheless both end in medicalization. The first is birth or death in a centralized hospital. The second is the gradual corporatization of demedicalized providers. Corporatized and centralized care entails not only a loss of the innovation and competition among entrepreneurs that could help solve America's most entrenched healthcare crises. It also leads to a loss of the individualized care that independent providers can offer, making it more difficult for patients to find care that aligns with their unique needs. As demedicalized options become corporatized in response to the demands of regulatory bodies, financial, compliance, and liability pressures will push providers toward standardized care. The main characteristics of demedicalized care, its high-quality communication and individualized approach, will be weakened, if not lost altogether. The regulatory tributary becomes even more forceful when it is combined with the tributary of reimbursement, which more directly constrains patient options, like a riptide pulling patients toward centralized providers and locations of care. That tributary is the subject of the next chapter.

CHAPTER 5

Swept Away on the Reimbursement Headwater

There are financial barriers to hospices being able to sustain themselves. The per diem daily rate is not enough to sustain most hospices and in order to keep a hospice afloat you have to have a large number of patients who live a long amount of time, but ever since the Medicare [Hospice Benefit] was put into effect that length of stay has not budged. But the cost and the amount of services that government requires of hospices continues to grow and yet government continues to decrease the reimbursement.—*Hospice director*

A huge issue is there's no [insurance] code for home birth and as our society dictates, we worship technology and we worship codes.—*Home birth midwife*

D ESPITE THE POWER of state- and federal-level regulations, insurance and reimbursement policies create the largest and most powerful tributary in the healthcare watershed because they guide the flow of resources and support or restrain different models of care. In effect, they control the absolute volume of water in the watershed. Reimbursement policies determine the kinds of providers and locations of care patients can access. And because they determine which kinds of treatments and interventions are reimbursed and at what rate, they mold the standard of care over time. Much of the power behind reimbursement policies is due to the unique way Americans pay for healthcare, where third parties—either private insurance or government programs—pay for most care.

Because a few major payers control so much of the payment landscape, providers of all types have incentives to manipulate and shape the regulatory and reimbursement policy environment in order to maximize payments. Outdated government reimbursement policies created long before the leap in innovation of the past few decades create perverse incentives to maximize procedures and interventions. Meanwhile, insurers starve community-based or demedicalized providers of resources with artificially low reimbursement rates, limiting patient options and inflating the cost of healthcare generally. Patients rarely know how much their treatments cost, what forces shape their access to care, and how little control they have over what their insurance covers. The result of all these forces is a resource flow toward high-intensity care that washes away alternative providers. These currents are particularly problematic for pregnant women and dying patients, both of whom benefit from individualized care that the current system does not support. These reimbursement decisions are themselves linked to the broader political conversation about what kinds of providers and locations are legitimate and which should receive public dollars, a debate that has been ongoing since the advent of medical professionalization.[1]

The US reimbursement framework creates high costs that are not tightly correlated with positive outcomes. The United States spends a much higher percentage of gross domestic product (GDP) on healthcare and yet has lower life expectancy and ranks lower on other primary health measures than other Organisation for Economic Co-operation and Development countries. As of 2011, the United States spent close to 18 percent of GDP on healthcare, while the Netherlands, the next-highest spender, spent just 12 percent.[2] This number has remained consistent through 2017 but is expected to increase to almost 20 percent over the next 10 years.[3] While the United States leads the developed world in medical innovation, it lags behind in the appropriate use of that innovation, with analyses suggesting that medical innovations are increasingly used in inappropriate populations, which is in turn linked to the way large payers like Medicare structure payment policies.[4] The growth in US healthcare expenditures is due in part to the unique structure of the American healthcare payment system, which combines the emphasis on third-party payers with a lack of the usual rationing and cost-effectiveness policies that keep costs down in other countries.[5] The United States represents in some ways the worst combination of private and government control. The healthcare system lacks true market prices that would provide information about supply, demand, and quality to patients and providers, but it also lacks a central authority to control supply or demand through rationing.

In addition to rising costs, reimbursement policies have serious implications for individual choice and control over healthcare decisions. Patients are limited by both the treatment options covered by their insurer and the incentives insurers provide to physicians to offer certain kinds of care. Available options do not always align with either individual preferences or the best standard of care. Lobbying efforts far upstream by state and national medical associations, insurance groups, and various other interested parties combine to create medicalized rapids that trap patients and physicians into costly, substandard care. Patients often have no idea what alternatives exist and cannot freely choose between alternatives even if they do know. The constraints insurers place on patients and their providers call into question the usefulness of principles like informed consent that require both knowledge and voluntary decision making on the part of patients.

Payment policies also create disparities and unequal access to care, as the benefits of medical innovation are spread unevenly across the population. Low-income and minority populations are peculiarly vulnerable to restrictive insurance policies that fail to cover the kind of individualized care that supports good outcomes during birth and death. Higher-income individuals can work around Medicare's limitation on community-based providers by paying out of pocket for home health aides and other supports, while low-income Americans are more likely to end up in the current of centralized care during birth and death. Some community-based options respond to perverse incentives in the system by refusing certain types of patients who are too expensive or for whom reimbursement is too low, further limiting access. As a result, the majority of Americans do not have access to high-quality patient-centered demedicalized options for birth or death, and low-income and minority populations are the least likely to have access.

Reimbursement policies also restrict providers. Physicians feel forced into providing care that does not benefit and even harms their patients. The demands of third-party payers privilege and prioritize procedures over conversations about care, locking patients and their physicians into cycles of costly testing, drugs, and procedures. The bureaucracy of third-party insurance requirements leads to complex coding systems with skyrocketing administrative costs alongside low reimbursement rates.[6] The demands of charting and coding mandate that physicians spend more time on administrative tasks and less on patient care.[7] Reduced face-to-face time with patients drives distrust between patients and providers, heightening dissatisfaction on both sides. Rather than copilots in the boat on the river, physicians and patients feel pulled in different directions, unable to coordinate treatment goals and successfully navigate treatment options together. Frustration with the current reimbursement system has led to increasing rates of physician burnout, much of which can be linked to the structure of healthcare financing.[8]

Perhaps the most obvious consequence of reimbursement policies on how Americans give birth and die is the centralization of care in hospitals. Pregnant women and the dying are channeled into centralized hospitals because such hospitals are the only reimbursable provider in a given area. Hospitals are then reimbursed based on a fee-for-service model that incentivizes procedures over other kinds of care. Meanwhile, reimbursement for primary care, nonmedical caregivers, and communication across the care team is either inadequate or not provided at all. Care is fragmented across multiple care locations and multiple providers with few or no incentives to integrate care. Americans do not receive the individualized, community-based care at the beginning and end of life that research indicates they both want and need.

The Costs of Medicalized Birth and Death

Medicaid (for low-income Americans) and Medicare (for the elderly and disabled) are the primary payers for birth and death, though private insurance plays a large role in birth as well. Almost 50 percent of women receive Medicaid or Tricare (military healthcare) during pregnancy and birth.[9] Meanwhile, Medicare covers more than 75 percent of individuals at the end of life.[10] For both experiences, government policies dictate type and location of care, and private insurers often follow the government's lead in deciding what to fund and how. The combination of payers, different reimbursement policies across payers, and the fee-for-service payment structures supported by most insurers create inefficiencies in care and confusion for patients and their families. It is often not clear ahead of time what treatments will be covered, which providers will be covered, and which combination of provider and setting of care is in-network and covered. Often, the cost of procedures is unknown to either providers or patients, or both. More troubling, the cost insurers pay may not reflect the actual cost of the care provided. When asked how rates were set by hospitals, one veteran of the industry was quoted in the *Wall Street Journal* as saying, "There is no method to this madness. As we went through the years, we had these cocka-mamie formulas. We multiplied our costs to set our charges."[11] Not only do doctors and patients not know how much procedures cost to patients, but hospitals themselves frequently do not know how much a single procedure actually costs the hospital in terms of time, equipment, and staffing. Changes to federal law in 2018 that required hospitals to publicly disclose their charge lists have led to confusion rather than transparency, as most patients will not pay the listed rate for any given intervention.[12]

Birth and death create substantial costs for both public and private insurers, precisely because they affect every American at some point in their lives. Birth and death are, for many people, the most intensive and most expensive interactions they will ever have with the medical system. They also make up substantial portions of healthcare expenditures each year. In the case of birth, costs for pregnancy and delivery totaled around $111 billion in 2010, with costs increasing since then.[13] Around 50 percent of these costs were hospital fees, with the other 50 percent made up of provider fees, radiology and imaging, drug costs, and lab work. In the case of death, around 13 percent of total healthcare costs are spent on those in their last year of life, with totals for the last year of life around $205 billion in 2011.[14] Birth and death together make up around $300 billion of the $1.6 trillion spent on healthcare each year, or around 19 percent of total US spending on healthcare. Overall, hospital services make up around 32 percent of total healthcare costs.[15]

The costs of giving birth and dying, like other medical events, have increased dramatically since the 1970s. While some of these increases stem from new technologies and procedures that save lives, in general higher costs have not been associated with better outcomes for either the birthing or dying, with maternal and infant outcomes worsening in recent years, even as costs rise.[16] American maternity care struggles with some of the highest infant and maternal mortality in the developed world, and American end-of-life care is beset by low patient satisfaction rates, poor pain control, and inadequate social and emotional support.[17]

It is no surprise that hospital costs play a major role in payments for birth and death, since the vast majority of Americans now give birth and die in hospitals. Over 98 percent of women in the United States give birth in hospitals, and one in five Americans spend time in the intensive care unit at the end of life.[18] Inpatient hospital stays accounted for 50 percent of Medicare spending for the elderly in 2006, with hospice and home healthcare totaling just under 14 percent.[19] Around 73 percent of deaths of the elderly occur in hospitals.[20] Both birth and death are costly and overwhelmingly hospital based.

A significant contributor to these costs in hospitals is the widespread use of medical technology on inappropriate populations. In the case of birth, routine ultrasounds, continuous fetal monitoring, and other common procedures not only are unsupported by the evidence but also may lead to other unnecessary interventions.[21] In the case of death, providers point to the overuse of interventions such as CPR, feeding tubes, and admission to an ICU. One recent analysis found that as many as 42 percent of Medicare recipients will receive an unnecessary test or procedure in any given year. These tests added up to around $8.5 billion in healthcare costs, though the actual costs of unnecessary care are probably significantly higher since the study only looked at a subset of unnecessary procedures.[22] Moreover, while Medicare has some rules in place to limit unnecessary testing, it frequently fails to enforce those rules, even when unnecessary care harms patients.[23]

In addition to costs to insurers and the healthcare system as a whole, birth and death have significant financial impacts on families, as almost every birth and death involves unreimbursed expenses, whether in the form of out-of-pocket costs or lost wages. Reimbursement policies in the United States are characterized by confusing policies, gaps in coverage, and fee-for-service plans that encourage high-intensity care. Many women will owe thousands of dollars after childbirth, even with "excellent" private insurance coverage.[24] The average out-of-pocket cost for women after childbirth in a hospital is $3,400, which makes home birth and birth center birth, even when not covered by insurance, seem comparably inexpensive for a more personalized experience.[25] In death, the numbers are significantly higher. One study found that average out-of-pocket costs for Medicare beneficiaries in the last year of life were around $12,000, while another study found that those costs ballooned to close to $40,000 for the last five years of life, though there is substantial variation in these numbers, with some individuals spending much more than others.[26] More troublingly, the high price families pay does not correspond with patient desires or good outcomes.[27]

Paying for Birth

The way American women give birth is heavily influenced by insurer policies. The births of around half of American women are paid for by government providers, including Medicaid and Tricare. The other 50 percent or so are covered by private insurers, with around 6 percent of women paying out of pocket for birth. Even when policies cover home birth and birth centers, coverage can be confusing and require multiple levels of appeal.[28] Like with death, the costs of birth vary dramatically across regions and even from hospital to hospital. A cesarean section averaged $13,943 in Louisiana in 2010 but $21,307 in California in the same year.[29] Birth center births and home birth are the least expensive options, with average prices ranging from $2,000 to $6,000, including prenatal care. Different third-party payers also pay substantially different rates. Medicaid pays around $9,000 for a hospital-based vaginal birth and $13,600 for a cesarean section, while private insurance pays around twice that, with average costs of $18,000 and $28,000 for vaginal and cesarean births, respectively. Cost sharing can range from almost nothing in the case of Medicaid and some private insurers to tens of thousands of dollars for high-deductible plans or for care provided by out-of-network providers. Costs continue to rise, with hospitals charging more for everything from cesareans to pain relief.[30] But for both Medicaid and private insurers, the costs of medicalized hospital birth are significantly higher than demedicalized options.[31]

The way American women give birth is structured and channeled by reimbursement policies that many women do not fully understand. In most areas, the only reimbursable provider under most insurance plans is a hospital. Once in a hospital, women are channeled into unnecessary interventions by a fee-for-service maternity model that prioritizes high-intensity care. While less intensive approaches that limit interventions like midwifery may not be provided or even allowed owing to restrictive hospital policies, some of the most common standard interventions for low-risk births are unsupported by medical evidence, including continuous fetal monitoring.[32] As is the case with vaginal birth after cesarean policies, the financial incentives created by insurers may combine with liability concerns to push providers and hospitals to prioritize cesarean sections over vaginal birth.[33] Overall, the United States has some of the most expensive maternity care in the world, alongside some of the worst outcomes for mothers and infants.[34]

Lack of price transparency makes planning for the cost of birth difficult, if not impossible. Pregnancy can be handled on either a global billing system, intended to slow the growth of maternity-related costs, or the traditional fee-for-service system. In a global fee system, hospitals are generally reimbursed at a standard rate for uncomplicated vaginal births and another standard rate for cesarean sections, which usually includes epidural anesthesia.[35] Even with global fees, however, hospitals may add on individual charges for specific items or for providers who are out-of-network, including providers like anesthesiologists, whose fees can be thousands of dollars. Women and their families may not know ahead of time which interventions or aspects of birth are covered, resulting in unexpectedly large bills after birth. Moreover, many women find themselves trapped in confusing or poorly structured insurance policies, paying high deductibles before any coverage kicks in, being responsible for high co-pays for each service, and then wrestling with multiple bills for services from months before while they recover from birth, when they are least able to handle sorting through duplicate charges and ensuring proper payment.[36]

Poor incentives also abound. While the standard rate for cesarean is higher than that for vaginal birth, surgery is usually much quicker than a vaginal labor and delivery (and may actually be cheaper for hospitals to perform). Many worry that this disparity between payment and time providing care creates incentives to hasten vaginal delivery with induction and labor augmentation or provide scheduled cesarean sections for relatively low risk women.[37] One benefit of birth center births is that because they cannot provide cesarean sections or any kind of medical induction, there are few direct financial incentives or medical means for staff to hasten labor.[38] At the same time, providers who support demedicalized births are financially penalized under the current system.[39] A variety of state regulations and professional organization recommendations contribute to these problems by increasing the risk perception of specific kinds of births, like VBAC and breech birth. While such births can be safely attempted vaginally, hospitals have financial incentives to move women quickly through the maternity ward, and obstetricians have incentives to do surgery. Vaginal breech birth and VBAC are rare in many parts of the country because hospitals use older recommendations to justify protocols requiring cesarean sections.

Another factor contributing to medicalized childbirth is the way in which reimbursement structures interact with other regulations. Licensing, for example, is usually linked to reimbursement eligibility, tangling payment options in broader political debates. Patients who want insurance to cover midwifery care outside a hospital may find that their insurance will only reimburse for home births or birth center births with a nurse midwife, while the number of nurse midwives who provide community-based birth is relatively small. In 2014, for example, over 94 percent of births attended by nurse midwives occurred in hospitals.[40] Families seeking demedicalized birth may have to pay for home birth providers out of pocket or use insurance to pay for hospital-based midwives, whose scope of practice and independence may be dramatically limited by hospital protocols and oversight requirements.[41]

Even home births with nurse midwives are subject to wrangling over payment given that most insurance companies lack the codes to adequately reflect the care that home birth midwives provide. One nurse midwife described in an interview how she bills for a home birth: "The only bill I can submit is the same coding as the hospital for a midwife, but the code is one number different for home. They say 'here's what we give a midwife in a hospital for catching a baby: $1700.' What I charge, around $5500, is ten months of care, blood tests, etc. But there's no code for that, no way for me to get reimbursed for that care. That's how they speak. 'There's no code for that.'" In her case, all her clients pay out of pocket until 37 weeks, "and then I bill insurance and code it for the delivery itself, which has been hell, to be honest, and then [the family] submits it and then we argue with the insurance company for a long time. I just got payment from an insurance company for a birth in December 2016 yesterday [December 2017]." Because so much of insurance reimbursement is standardized via codes developed originally for hospital-based care, decentralized options must get creative about billing to provide even minimally individualized care. The gaps that such unorthodox billing creates are shouldered directly by families.

The Affordable Care Act (ACA) shifted the landscape somewhat by requiring Medicaid and insurance coverage for all licensed medical providers in their states, including direct-entry midwives where states allow them. However, state implementation of this requirement has been slow.

As of May 2019, just 14 states allowed Medicaid reimbursement for direct-entry midwives, with some states adding restrictions such as requiring them to provide care within a birth center overseen by a physician or nurse midwife.[42] Even with the ACA requirement, reimbursement remains limited in most cases to midwives who practice in hospitals. While 33 states require private insurance to cover nurse midwives, such policies leave a substantial coverage gap for births outside hospitals. In the majority of states, women still cannot use insurance to pay for birth with direct-entry midwives, the most common type of out-of-hospital midwife. Midwives in states that do not license or certify direct-entry midwives are excluded from formal reimbursement structures altogether. In response, many women who want to give birth at home pay out of pocket for a home birth with a direct-entry midwife (in states where direct-entry midwives are legally allowed to attend births), since the cost of $2000–$6000 either is considered a reasonable price to pay to avoid interventions or would be close to the deductible for a hospital-based birth on many insurance policies.[43] Either way, women who want to use a direct-entry midwife for birth do so without insurance reimbursement in most states. Even in states where reimbursement is possible, like California, the process is so burdensome that many midwives simply refuse to participate. As one direct-entry home birth midwife explained, "I charge a flat rate [and do not accept insurance] and most out-of-hospital midwives don't take insurance because it's a full time job to get it."

Medicare and Medicaid further prioritize medicalized options by offering artificially low payment rates that do not reflect the care being provided. While physicians and hospitals also bemoan the low rates provided by government insurers, these practitioners are reimbursed at higher levels than community-based care providers for the same care. Birth centers and midwives struggle with Medicaid rates that are often too low to support operations. Variations across states not only affect how much individual women pay but also indirectly affect their access to qualified professionals. Some states reimburse nurse midwives at 10 times the rates of other states, leading to a dearth of midwives in those lower-paying states.[44] Midwives in New Jersey, a particularly low-paying state, are paid just $371 for attending a vaginal birth that can take many hours.[45] Many midwives and birth centers in New Jersey and other low-reimbursement states respond by not accepting Medicaid at all, limiting access and overwhelmingly affecting low-income women. As mentioned above, some midwives eschew insurance altogether because the combination of low reimbursement rates and high levels of paperwork makes it more profitable to operate as a boutique provider.

Birth centers also struggle with payment structures that privilege hospital-based birth over community-based birth. Medicaid's reimbursement model, depending on the state, reimburses only for physicians or nurse midwives, but not for direct-entry midwives or other birthing support. Some states offer a flat global fee that fails to take into account how long a mother labors or how much staff attendance she requires. Some states reimburse birth centers at half the rate for hospital-based vaginal delivery, which makes birth centers more cost-effective on paper but prevents them from making enough money to stay in business. A Nebraska birth center owner said of the reimbursement rate of $325 per birth in that state, "We can't even turn on the lights for that." Birth centers in many states also suffer when a woman needs to transfer to a hospital, since under some states' Medicaid models only labor and delivery are reimbursable events. Birth centers in those states are not reimbursed for any of the prenatal or labor care provided to the mother before the transfer.[46] Such policies, while limiting costs on one side of the ledger, increase costs in the long run by channeling women into higher-intervention hospital-based birth.

While the number of accredited and nonaccredited birth centers has been growing steadily since the ACA mandated coverage in 2012, there are still just over 400 birth centers in the United States as of 2019.[47] Given that there were almost 4 million births in the United States in 2018, the number of available birth centers cannot meet the needs of even a small fraction of low-risk mothers.[48] Moreover, government insurers like Medicaid and Tricare usually will only reimburse birth centers accredited by the Commission for the Accreditation of Birth Centers, a restriction that affects the majority of birth centers in the United States. Insurers therefore do not reimburse for the most common type of community-based midwife or for the most common type of birth center. As of January 2019, there were 122 birth centers that were accredited by the CABC or were in the process of receiving accreditation, with most of these centers located on the coasts.[49] The majority of American women do not have access to an accredited birth center that their insurance will cover.

Specific kinds of patients also find that insurance limits their options for birth, as state regulations on community-based providers and settings limit whom providers can see. Accredited birth centers, the only kind reimbursed by Medicaid, generally do not allow high-risk pregnancies, including twin or multiple pregnancies, vaginal breech babies, VBAC, chronic high blood pressure, diabetes, and placenta previa. While midwives agree that many of these risk factors require hospital monitoring, they differ with the American College of Obstetricians and Gynecologists on whether twin pregnancies, breech births, and VBACs can safely take place in outpatient birth centers. Some argue that these variants can be handled safely by trained personnel even outside a hospital, with evidence supporting those claims.[50] Women with these concerns who give birth in hospitals are likely to have a cesarean delivery owing to restrictive hospital policies and a lack of training in vaginal birth for higher-risk mothers, including twin births and breech babies.[51] Insurers may rely on regulations to set their reimbursement policies, despite the way these regulations were themselves molded by interest groups.

Finally and perhaps most foundationally, payment policies, like other kinds of policies in healthcare, demonstrate a bias toward activity and treatment. Insurers are more likely to pay for medical procedures than for nonmedical care, even when such procedures have no positive effect on patient outcomes. Continuous electronic fetal monitoring in hospital-based births again provides a helpful example. Insurance companies, as well as Medicaid, cover continuous fetal monitoring as a standard maternity care practice in hospital birth, despite substantial evidence that such monitoring actually does harm as a result of its high false positive rate for fetal distress and its association with higher rates of interventions.[52] ACOG has recently released recommendations to limit the use of continuous fetal monitoring, favoring instead intermittent monitoring that allows women freedom of movement and has lower false positive rates.[53]

Yet reimbursement policies have not followed suit. The medical evidence does not support many of the most common interventions during birth, including artificial induction, augmentation of labor with Pitocin, IV fluids, and breaking of the waters, for routine use in low-risk mothers.[54] One obstetrician admitted that he was puzzled by insurers' willingness to pay for procedures: "Essentially there's no real penalty for over ordering. I'm sometimes surprised that insurers pay for the things they do." He thought that insurers could play a more active role in refusing to reimburse for unnecessary interventions, though he acknowledges that "the line between directive and adversarial is really thin." Insurers may shy away from seeming as though they are questioning physician judgment, a major critique of restrictive managed care policies in the 1990s.

The bias toward activity is evident when one contrasts reimbursement for fetal monitoring with that for doulas. Doulas, trained labor support people, provide both physical and emotional support and can provide assistance in communicating with medical providers. Research accepted by ACOG and other major medical associations found that doula support during labor lowers intervention rates, especially cesarean sections.[55] One analysis found that out of a range of different birth interventions (including a variety of medical interventions), doulas were one of only three to receive an "A" rating in that they provide dramatic benefits with no negative side effects and very little cost.[56] Yet despite that supporting evidence, insurance and Medicaid rarely, if ever, reimburse for doulas or other nonmedical support people. Oregon and Minnesota are the only states in which Medicaid reimburses for doulas.[57] Commercial insurance rarely does, though women in some plans can use health savings or flex accounts to pay for doula coverage.[58] Women who would like doula support before, during, and after birth typically pay out of pocket for such care, which can range anywhere from $300 to $5000, depending on the doula's experience and geographic region.[59] Low-income and minority women are at increased risk of interventions and benefit the most from doula support and yet have the least access to these providers because Medicaid does not cover them.[60] Troublingly, while more women are demanding access to evidence-based care, many women do not even realize the way in which the biases of their insurance providers funnel and channel their care toward the most medicalized options. They therefore do not even know to ask for alternative modes of care because they are unaware such care exists. The reimbursement tributary affects the dying in similar ways, as we will see.

Paying for Death

Payment for care for the elderly, who make up the large majority of those who die, is generally split between Medicare and Medicaid, with some private insurance coverage as well. All Americans over age 65 are eligible for Medicare, while only low-income Americans qualify for Medicaid. Medicare covers medical and acute-care expenses, as well as short rehabilitative nursing home stays. Medicaid covers nursing home care and some other kinds of assisted living care for the low-income elderly, though policies vary dramatically by state. More than 60 percent of nursing home residents in the United States are covered by Medicaid.[61] A small percentage of Americans have private insurance or long-term care insurance, but the majority of the elderly who die in America are covered by some combination of Medicare and Medicaid. Around 9 million Americans are what is known as "dual eligible," meaning that they qualify for both Medicare and Medicaid, though this number includes younger disabled Americans as well as the elderly.[62] Some Americans "spend down" assets at the end of life to qualify for Medicaid coverage of nursing home care, which increases the numbers of dual-eligible individuals.[63] Despite the government roots of both Medicare and Medicaid, these systems are not coordinated. Medicare is administered by the federal government, whereas Medicaid is administered by the states, which share costs with the federal government. This lack of coordination contributes to the high rates of hospitalizations in the elderly in a few ways.

The way insurance policies medicalize death is somewhat clearer than the way they medicalize birth, since Medicare covers 75 percent of individuals in the United States at the end of life, and Medicare policies are uniform across all 50 states, unlike Medicaid policies. Despite this uniformity, there exists wide regional and geographic variation in how Americans die, and expenditures vary widely as well. Individuals in North Dakota spend less than one day in an ICU before death on average, while those in Miami spend more than 10 days in intensive care.[64] Rates of hospice use and palliative care use also vary widely. Some of this variation is cultural, but some is also the result of different state-level regulatory frameworks for hospice and palliative care (discussed in chap. 4). Medicare spending on end-of-life care thus varies widely by state and region. Most of this variation derives from differences in the use of post-acute care after a hospitalization, which can include skilled nursing facilities, home healthcare, hospice and various kinds of palliative care, or long-term hospitalization.[65]

Even with uniform Medicare reimbursement, the mix of payers for the dying can still include Medicare, private insurance, and Medicaid.

Medicare payment policies are complex, are often inefficient, and tend to emphasize centralized and mechanized care over community-based human care as a result of the "fee-for-service" model that provides codes for each part of a physician's activities and pays accordingly. These codes display the same activity bias as policies in birth do. According to one study, physicians are paid between 3 and 5 times more for procedural care or care involving testing, surgeries, and so on, than they are for what is called "cognitive" care, which involves diagnosing problems, counseling patients, and coordinating care.[66] Unsurprisingly, this model increases costs, hospitalizations, and high-intensity, low-quality care at the end of life and also drives physicians toward more procedural specialties. By encouraging interventions but effectively penalizing conversations and coordination of care, the procedural bias discourages the very kind of care that is most beneficial to elderly and dying patients.

The fee-for-service model and mix of payers also create more troubling incentives. As many have noted, reimbursement policies are largely responsible for the "revolving door" of hospitalizations at the end of life, where patients move from hospital to nursing home and back again.[67] Medicaid's payments for nursing homes are relatively low, but Medicare's reimbursement for skilled nursing care is relatively high.[68] Because Medicaid pays a lower rate for nursing home care than it does for the skilled nursing care that is only available after a hospitalization, Medicare creates an incentive for nursing homes to hospitalize patients in order to reap the higher skilled nursing facility payment rate. One study found that almost one-quarter of Medicare patients were readmitted to a hospital within 30 days after spending time in a skilled nursing facility.[69] Researchers have also found that nursing homes that also contain skilled nursing facilities have a pattern of hospitalizing dual-eligible patients, presumably to take advantage of the higher skilled nursing reimbursement rate.[70] A recent study documented disturbing rates of orders for intensive rehabilitation in nursing homes for very elderly or dying patients, rehab that research suggests provides no benefit but that allows nursing homes to bill at a much higher rate.[71]

Transfers between locations of care are expensive, as a result of transportation costs and the costs associated with admissions and discharges.[72] But more importantly, uncoordinated multisetting care adversely impacts patient health. Medical mistakes are higher when patients move from facility to facility, and frequent moves also cause stress, slow down recovery, increase the likelihood of miscommunication, and distract patients, families, and providers from important conversations about care.[73] Changing this landscape requires better coordination between Medicare and Medicaid, since they each create potentially perverse incentives for the other. According to one analysis, nursing home investment in reducing hospitalizations saves money for Medicare, which pays for hospitalizations, but not for Medicaid, which pays for the longer resulting nursing home stays.[74] States that have higher Medicaid nursing home payment rates have lower rates of rehospitalization, presumably because nursing homes do not feel as much financial pressure to hospitalize patients for the skilled nursing benefit rate in those states.[75]

Medicare and Medicaid policies share in common that they provide little support for elderly and terminally ill patients prior to a crisis, support that could prevent hospitalization in the first place. Eight hours of home health aide coverage costs around $168, while the cost of an ICU stay ranges from $1500 to $3500 per day, but only the latter is covered by Medicare.[76] Medicaid covers more through its home healthcare benefit, but recipients must be classified as low-income and meet other requirements that vary dramatically by state.[77] Much like insurance refusal to cover doulas, the bias toward procedures over human care incentivizes hospitalization. Compounding this bias, poor coordination between Medicare and Medicaid leads to gaps in coverage that again channel patients into hospitals.

While hospice workers are better integrated into the payment system than midwives, there are still significant coverage gaps that prevent individuals at the end of life from accessing community-based care. Perhaps the major barrier to hospice use is that Medicare hospice coverage is limited to individuals in nursing homes or those who have dedicated caregivers at home. Since neither Medicare nor most private insurers reimburse for residential hospice except for very short "respite" stays to give caregivers time away, dying patients without caregivers at home are unable to take advantage of hospice care in their final weeks and months of life. While at-home hospice providers who are reimbursed through the Medicare Hospice Benefit provide care for four hours a day, a family member is still required at home most of the time to do routine care. Hospice providers also typically do not help with tasks like bathing and toileting, which families can find the most difficult to manage, though Medicaid may cover personal aides if the individual meets the income requirements.[78] Many people who would benefit from hospice end up in hospitals not because of medical need but because they lack social support at home.[79] While some regions have "homes for the dying" or "comfort care homes" that do not charge for care and that run on donations from churches and private givers, such options are not available in most areas.

Broader coverage for routine residential hospice or coverage for non-medical care providers like home health aides would decrease the emotional and financial burdens on families, which provide most of this care. According to one estimate, 92 percent of those who require long-term care in the community rely on unpaid help to remain at home, usually family members. Only 13 percent of the total receive paid help from any source, though the elderly are more likely to receive paid care than younger populations.[80] At the same time, expanding coverage for residential hospice, in conjunction with regulations like certificate-of-need laws (discussed in chap. 4), may create other unintended consequences, driving corporatization and a different kind of institutionalization.[81] As one palliative care nurse practitioner noted with frustration in an interview, "Insurance companies will cover third line chemo [which is very unlikely to help] for $40,000 but won't cover SNF [skilled nursing facility] room and board or home aides for a patient on hospice." The chemotherapy, she argued, would destroy the patient's quality of life, while the home health aides would dramatically increase it. Paying for home health aides is the most direct way to keep patients who wish to remain in their homes out of institutions of all kinds.

Despite less variation in payment rates than is the case with birth centers, hospices also struggle with payment rates that do not adequately cover expenses. Medicare reimburses hospices with a flat-fee per diem rate that starts at $187.54 for the first 60 days and then moves to $145.14 thereafter.[82] Such flat fees do not take into account the extra care that complex patients require, which leads as many as 78 percent of hospices to limit eligibility for complex patients in some way.[83] On top of the relatively low per diem rate, Medicare requires hospices to comply with a complex array of regulations to qualify for coverage. These regulations were discussed in more depth in chapter 4, but they include requirements to own a variety of resuscitative equipment (unnecessary in most hospice contexts) and provide a variety of support, including bereavement support, nurses, social workers, volunteer coordinators, and other care providers that they are not reimbursed for. The combination of low, flat reimbursement and nonreimbursable mandates means that many hospices, particularly small nonprofit ones, rely heavily on volunteers. It is not surprising again that the greatest growth of hospice care is in larger for-profit hospices, which, through economies of scale, are better able to absorb the unfunded mandates and low reimbursement rates provided by Medicare.[84]

Physicians themselves express frustration with the way the payment system limits their care of elderly or dying patients and creates perverse incentives for treatment. One physician pointed out that "most of the money in medicine comes from doing procedures. There's a tremendous incentive economically to do things to people." Palliative care as a field is at odds with the economic incentives that drive much of medicine. As one practitioner noted, "That conversation [about end-of-life goals] is not very well reimbursed and if we do decide to stop treatment all the money to all those providers dries up." Another physician concurred, arguing, "Part of the problem is money, which is that once you talk to patients about their goals and values, very often they won't want things done, and the second that happens you've taken money out of someone's pocket."

The payment bias toward testing and treatments is exacerbated by policies that limit conversations about end-of-life care. Until 2015, Medicare did not compensate doctors for conversations about end-of-life care, largely as a result of the mischaracterization of such conversations as "death panels" by Sarah Palin and other opponents of the ACA. While reimbursement for such conversations was provided in 2015, Medicare compensates doctors much less for communication, outreach with other providers, and coordinating care than it does for medical procedures.[85] Many doctors also do not feel they have the time to have extended conversations with patients about treatment goals, in part because they are not adequately compensated for such conversations. They may then resort to tests and interventions as a way to stay psychologically connected with patients.[86] The burden of unreimbursed communication is high in elderly and terminally ill populations, since reaching providers across multiple care settings and communicating with sometimes far-flung family members can be time intensive and difficult. Accurate and detailed charting and record keeping for complex patients are rarely fully reimbursed. Doctors report spending significant amounts of time at home charting, while nurses frequently stay well past the end of their shift to complete charts.[87]

Nowhere are the effects of the combination of these various perverse incentives clearer than in cancer treatment. Cancer is the second-leading cause of death in the United States, and around 60 percent of cancer patients are over the age of 65.[88] Treating cancer constitutes a significant portion of healthcare and Medicare spending, with total costs of $147.3 billion in 2017, not including cancer screening.[89] Cancer care represents 1 out of every 12 dollars spent by Medicare by some estimates.[90] Costs continue to rise in part because of new breakthroughs and the growth of personalized medicine. Yet even taking recent innovations into account, many observers acknowledge a pattern of overtesting, overtreatment, and lack of coordination of care, largely as a result of the way Medicare policies shape physician behavior.[91] In an open letter on a health blog in 2009, a well-known oncologist argued that perverse incentives in cancer treatment contribute to overtreatment in terminally ill patients.[92] He pointed out that conversations about care are not billable events; the office employees who coordinate care, schedule appointments, and provide various kinds of patient support are not billable staff; and the main way in which all oncology practices make money is by selling chemotherapy drugs. In order to have an office staffed in a way that adequately supports patient care, oncologists must sell more of the most expensive kinds of chemotherapy drugs. He concluded, "I think that the incentives are so mis-aligned and the temptations are so great that docs have a tough time making the right decisions."[93]

Research into financial incentives for chemotherapy supports his belief, with evidence suggesting that oncologists lead patients away from treatments for which they get paid less.[94] Simply changing the policies does not always work, as physicians respond in a variety of unforeseeable ways to reforms. One study found that changing Medicare's policies to promote less expensive outpatient cancer care simply increased the number of procedures done on bladder cancer patients in the outpatient facility, without lowering costs.[95] Crucially, the United States does not use cost-effectiveness analysis to determine when to reimburse for care, so oncologists can and do suggest a variety of treatments that do not take into account the life expectancy of the patient, the cost comparison of other available drugs or treatments, or other relevant factors for care.[96] These incentives cause harm to terminal cancer patients, for whom chemotherapy often provides no benefit but seriously compromises quality of life. These are also the patients who would benefit most from comfort care surrounded by loved ones.[97] Given the way financial incentives interact with the psychological and emotional factors involved in cancer care, reimbursement policies channel the terminally ill into centralized and medicalized care, doing real harm to individuals in the process.

Medicare rules compound these problems by limiting patients' access to hospice until later in the course of an illness. Most palliative care under Medicare is covered under the MHB, which requires that patients have less than six months to live and that they forgo all "curative" treatment. The six-month limit was created in the early days of hospice, largely as a response to the needs of cancer patients, for whom prognostication about the end of life is more accurate than for other kinds of illnesses.[98] Other kinds of patients with unclear prognoses, such as AIDS patients or dementia patients, may be excluded. Moreover, requiring patients to forgo curative treatment draws a line between curative and palliative treatments that many physicians argue does not exist in practice.[99] And many terminally ill patients, particularly younger patients, do not want to forgo curative treatment until all options are exhausted.[100] The policy also excludes most nonterminal patients or those who have more than six months of life left from the comprehensive support hospice offers, including social, psychological, and spiritual support; pain relief; and protection from unnecessary treatments.[101] Moreover, the Medicare skilled nursing benefit cannot be claimed at the same time as the hospice benefit. Residents must choose between rehabilitative care and hospice care, a false choice since both may be necessary. Medicare's restrictions limit hospice care to those who are well into the course of a terminal illness, with most hospice users enrolled for only a few days before death, usually after an ICU stay.

Medicare's policies on end-of-life care also show a bias toward payment for hospital-based care. While palliative care, as opposed to hospice, can be offered alongside curative treatment, palliative care teams are most commonly found in hospitals, and reimbursement under Medicare is limited to hospital patients. Medicare inadvertently incentivizes hospitalization for patients who do not qualify for community-based care but whose palliative care in the hospital would be covered. This policy persists despite evidence that community-based palliative care can lower costs and improve outcomes for patients by avoiding hospitalization in the first place.[102] Medicare therefore prevents patients from accessing community-based palliative care options until much later in their illness, when research shows it has less impact. Medicare has recently acknowledged some of these limitations, rolling out small-scale concurrent care programs, which allow both curative and palliative treatment at the same time, in 2011. Many private insurance companies already allow for concurrent care with demonstrable success.[103]

Finally, the very structure of Medicare tends to push patients toward hospitals, sometimes explicitly. Some Medicare policies require hospitalization, such as Medicare's rule that ambulances must transport a patient to a hospital in most cases in order to be reimbursed for responding to a call.[104] Since many calls are not emergencies, allowing first responders to assess the patient and communicate with a primary care doctor or facilitate follow-up care by a visiting nurse would prevent hospitalization, particularly of the elderly.[105] Medicare also typically does not reimburse for the support professionals who can keep patients comfortable and at home. A dying elderly person does not need medical interventions so much as high-quality primary care, social workers, home health aides, physical and occupational therapists, bereavement counselors, clergy, and other caregivers. Research demonstrates that support professionals can help avoid unnecessary hospital admittances, prevent wasted resources related to uncoordinated care, and ease the anxiety of patients and their families.[106] Overall, there is a wide consensus among doctors and policy analysts that greater access to *human* care in general, including but not limited to both palliative care and hospice care, would eliminate many of the trade-offs the dying confront in their final days.

Demedicalized Providers and the Politics of Reimbursement

In addition to the ways hospitals monopolize scarce resources, a growing concern among demedicalized community-based providers is the way hospitals are now marketing themselves as providers of demedicalized care. Hospital maternity wards describe themselves as "birth centers," while growing numbers of palliative care clinics provide hospice-like care within the hospital itself. Hospitals argue that they are providing more options for patients and that these options can help prevent escalation of care even when hospitalization is necessary. Critics, however, contend that these options are frequently lower quality, less integrated, and much more restrictive on patient choices than community-based care. Further, they believe that the hospital environment itself promotes medicalization even against patient wishes. Perhaps more fundamentally, community-based options view hospital-provided community-based care as an existential threat to care that they believe can and should remain in the community. Hospital competition may destroy or take over independent community options, replacing truly demedicalized providers with medical providers, with the result that truly demedicalized care is lost altogether.

Community-based providers point to reimbursement policies as a primary way this takeover begins. In the case of hospice, the six-month diagnosis and the requirement to forgo curative treatment prevent hospices from competing with more flexible hospital-based palliative care programs. As one hospice executive noted, "Hospitals are trying to expand their palliative care programs [into the community] and own the outpatient setting and with the new Medicaid redesign there's a potential for them to redesign what the community already has." She pointed out that competition between community-based options and hospitals "is getting ever more present as the dollars are shrinking." Yet community-based options struggle to lay claim to a fair share of resources. She mused, "I think it's also about resources and about the ability to fly your flag, claim your space, put money and time into academic publishing. The access to the research [dollars] lies in the hospitals, it doesn't lie in the community. And then you're competing with the same groups for grants and funding." Hospital-based programs, by virtue of their research and lobbying power, stamp out demedicalized outpatient options simply by competing more effectively for the government dollars that drive the system. Hospital-based programs also have more flexibility, since palliative care in hospitals will generally be reimbursed by Medicare regardless of whether a patient has a terminal condition. In short, the artificial restraints the MHB creates prevent community providers from competing with hospital practices.

Demedicalized options that attempt to compete directly with hospitals are also hamstrung by the artificially low reimbursement rates set by government payers. In the case of birth centers, facilities fees from Medicaid and private insurers are much lower than those of hospitals, they lack the ability to negotiate lower medical malpractice rates for their practitioners, and they cannot average the costs of such rates across multiple medical specialties as hospitals can. Obstetrics malpractice insurance rates continue to rise, and many birth centers rely heavily on outside donations to offset these costs. Malpractice costs are one of the main reasons otherwise successful birth centers are forced to close. In the Manhattan case, malpractice insurance rates increased by 400 percent in one year, a cost the birth center could not absorb.[107] Malpractice insurance costs currently threaten successful birth centers for low-income women in places like Washington, DC, leaving vulnerable women without access to low-intervention birth in an area where in-hospital cesarean section rates top 40 percent.[108] Home birth midwives and some birth centers do not carry malpractice insurance at all because they cannot afford it when paired with low reimbursement rates for care. Overall, the costs of insurance, combined with low reimbursement rates, pose probably the most serious barrier to community-based options for birth, while hospitals have more flexible facility-fee charges and greater bargaining power with insurers.[109]

If hospitals provided higher-quality or lower-cost demedicalized options than outpatient options in the community, there would be less cause for concern. But the incentives within the hospital and the goals of hospitals themselves—providing acute, legitimately medicalized care—will always pose a barrier to their provision of demedicalized care. In many cases, the success or failures of demedicalized options affiliated with hospitals are limited not by patient demand or the success of the program but by the protocols and budget needs of the larger hospital organization, as was the case when the sole birth center in Rochester, New York, closed after its affiliated hospital determined that its services were "redundant" with the medicalized maternity ward the hospital provided. At the same time, demedicalized options offered in the hospital are limited by protocols designed for sicker and more complex patients or by restrictions on providers of demedicalized care such as midwives and palliative care physicians. More troubling is that, given the fee-for-service structure of most insurance policies in the United States, hospitals simply do not have incentives to do demedicalized care well. The least medicalized options are the first to be cut precisely because they do not provide the same profit possibilities as medicalized care. Because of the way reimbursement policies promote procedures over human-centered care, demedicalized options like palliative care and hospital-based birth centers do not generate revenue for hospitals and actively prevent the lucrative procedures and interventions hospitals make the most on.[110] The incentives reimbursement structures create simply do not support true demedicalization in the hospital context.

The Human Costs of Paying for Birth and Death

Unsurprisingly, patients and their families report significant frustration with the payment options available for both American birth and death. In a short survey, participants answered questions about their experiences with insurance coverage of various sorts during birth or death. Generally, those who had given birth showed much more familiarity with their insurer and with the out-of-pocket expenses associated with birth than those at the end of life. Those surveyed who had helped a loved one through the dying process were much less likely to know how the care was paid for or were more likely to assume that costs were generally covered by Medicare. The major exceptions to this pattern were those whose loved one was not elderly. These respondents had private insurance and expressed anger at significant out-of-pocket expenses.

For families that welcomed a new baby, many noted that their birthing choices were sharply limited by what their insurance would cover. Women who seek nonhospital birth find themselves particularly limited by insurance policies. One respondent had an unassisted home birth (a birth with no midwife or medical assistance) because paying for coverage in between returning from abroad and the start of her new job was financially prohibitive: "Looking back, I'm very frustrated that I didn't have better choices given our financial constraints, and feel incredibly blessed that all went very smoothly." Another woman who paid out of pocket for a home birth reported, "I felt incredibly grateful that we were able to pay for the home birth and was keenly aware that was an incredible privilege. Yet, at the same time, I was frustrated that the system didn't give us a home birth option covered by insurance. So, it was bittersweet, but totally worth it for us."

Women with private insurance giving birth in hospitals found the process stressful, confusing, and surprisingly expensive. Another woman with a high-quality employer-based private plan reported that the payment process "wasn't straightforward and we are still dealing with it and paying for it months later. At first they were charging too high of co-pays, then not charging a co-pay at all. Nothing made sense." Another woman with private insurance who had a hospital birth said, "It seemed ridiculous that we were still getting bills two years later." The women who were most satisfied with the ease of payment were generally federal employees, Medicaid recipients, or privately insured women with well-structured global fee policies. Women who chose birth center birth also expressed satisfaction with the transparency of costs given the simple global fee system most birth centers use. One woman who had both hospital and birth center births said of her experience, "Our hospital birth ended up costing substantially less [out of pocket] than our birth center birth, but billing has been a nightmare. For the birth center, we received a payment plan up front, with all costs clearly outlined, and had it all paid for by the time our daughter was born. For our hospital birth, we're still receiving bills over a year later, we've had multiple instances of being billed incorrectly, been owed hundreds in overpayments, that were automatically deducted from our HSA, and just generally had a difficult time in getting a clear and outlined invoice. It's been extremely frustrating." Because so many women pay out of pocket for birth center births and home births, and because costly interventions are lower, the overall cost for decentralized birth is usually much more transparent. Birth centers and home birth midwives are often able to charge a simple flat fee on a payment plan as a result, another reason some women prefer such care.

While Medicaid recipients reported being happy with the ease of Medicaid coverage, they also expressed frustration at how Medicaid limited their birthing options to hospitals. One woman who gave birth in Oregon before Medicaid coverage for home births began in 2013 reported, "I had Medicaid, but opted to pay out of pocket in order to have a home birth (not covered by Medicaid), which is a frustrating choice to have to make. My midwife's costs were reasonable, but it seems silly that Medicaid is willing to cover hospital births that are on average $7,000 a pop and not consider home births that are much much cheaper." Most states still do not reimburse for home birth or birth center birth with Medicaid. When asked generally about how they felt about the American maternity care payment system in general, many respondents wished for more flexible alternatives.

In contrast, a similar survey on insurance coverage at the end of life found that many of the patients' families surveyed do not fully know or understand how reimbursement works at the end of life. For those directly involved in payment, some mentioned the difficulty of paying for services at home. One noted out-of-pocket expenses totaling around $5000 for "home health aides, equipment and supplies to accommodate mobility issues." Another noted that limitations on hospice enrollment meant that the family was forced to pay out of pocket for supportive care at home in the final days of life: "The home care aides seemed obnoxiously expensive, especially once we realized how little help they really provided, but at the time we brought her home (and at the time of her death), she wasn't enrolled in hospice—they couldn't process her claim quickly enough. My biggest bureaucratic issue was that hospice couldn't get her enrolled Thursday-Sunday (when she died)."[111] Making it easier for patients to be admitted over weekends would significantly help families where decline is rapid and death is imminent. Others pointed out that policies create artificial barriers to more appropriate care at the end of life, such as the respondent who said, "I believe that the fact that Medicare covered hospice but not long-term care influenced the decision to transfer my father to hospice rather than a rehabilitative facility."

The two respondents whose relatives died while covered under private insurance expressed the most frustration with the process. One respondent whose infant died shortly after birth from a congenital heart defect noted that the combination of payers (private insurance for most of the care, Medicare for hospice) compounded the confusion and extreme distress of the tragedy. The respondent described the experience as "terrible, very confusing, during a very hard time in our lives." This respondent also estimated out-of-pocket expenses of around $67,000 at the time she took the survey, with more likely coming, remarking, "It was awful. Insurance did everything in their power to refuse payment for many many things." For both birth and death, government insurers seem to provide some of the clearest reimbursement policies, while satisfaction with private insurance ranges widely and was seen by most respondents to be the most confusing and least transparent. In both cases, people expressed frustration at the way all kinds of reimbursement policies limited the options for care at the beginning and end of life.

Conclusion

The American system of healthcare payment represents in many ways the worst of all possible worlds. Viewing it from the perspective of the overall watershed, the system lacks the locks and dams to control water flow that would normally be provided either by market prices or by rationing and cost-effectiveness measures. Medicare pays for interventions even it says it should not, patients do not have access to basic care that everyone agrees they should, and the overall costs of healthcare erode individual and government budgets. Payment structures funnel patients into the rapids of medicalized care without an integrated medical team to help them navigate the current or determine what the desired landing site should be.

A crucial part of the problem—and one that is unlikely to change—is that most Americans pay for birth and death through third-party payers whose incentives do not align with individual patient needs and desires. Insurers, because they must cover a broad swath of individuals, cannot individualize care. And individuals, because they are not paying directly for their care, cannot demand individualized care or access alternative options. The cycle is a vicious one: insurers listen to physicians to determine the standard of care, but physicians are in turn responding to poor incentives in the insurance policies themselves about what to cover, all of which, according to the Federal Trade Commission, "restrict[s] the range of choices and trade-offs that consumers may desire."[112]

Hospital-based birth and death are primary drivers of medicalization, but the causes of centralization of care in hospitals can be traced back up the watershed to the tributary of insurance policies that determine who gets paid for what kind of care. In effect, American reimbursement policies create a powerful current that drives individuals and their providers, through a variety of perverse incentives, toward higher levels and intensities of care. Fundamentally, the way in which Americans pay for birth and death seriously challenges the claimed commitment to principles such as autonomy, justice, and the promise to do no harm. Given the restrictions from third-party payers, as well as the way in which reimbursement policies have shaped the healthcare watershed, Americans have very little choice about their healthcare, have unequal access to that healthcare, and are frequently harmed by inappropriate care. While alternative payment systems exist that could respect patient autonomy, improve outcomes, and lower costs, there is little evidence that American policymakers have the political will to change an entrenched and complex system.[113] The most dramatic changes may, as discussed in the conclusion, come from those who opt out of the centralized reimbursement framework altogether.

CHAPTER 6

Caught in the Riptide of Risk

I think a big part of what drives the C-section rate is that you're afraid you're going to get blamed or criticized. You don't practice in a vacuum. You don't get blamed for doing an unnecessary C-section and it's really hard to just sit there and do nothing.—*Family practice physician*

JUST AS the rivers of reimbursement and regulations meet to create powerful currents that push patients toward medicalized care, a third tributary in the watershed enters the river of healthcare to create its own riptide, changing practitioner behavior and creating powerful eddies when combined with currents from the regulatory and reimbursement streams. This tributary consists of the complex constellation of risks that physicians and other healthcare practitioners face while providing care. The most powerful of these risks include legal risks such as malpractice concerns, criminal penalties, and administrative and professional sanctions that are intended to protect patients against negligent or intentional harm by physicians, nurses, and other practitioners. The incentives these risks create unite with other forces in the watershed to shift physician behavior and steer patients toward more medicalized care in centralized hospitals.

Despite efforts to protect patients from medical harm, insurers and policy makers inadvertently increase harm to patients by encouraging overtreatment and penalizing demedicalized providers. Meanwhile, legal remedies for actual harm done fail to provide accountability or compensation for most medical negligence and malpractice that occurs and feed the rapids by stoking practitioner fear of lawsuits. The hospital environment heightens these fears, distorting patient care in a way that undermines patient preferences and evidence-based care in favor of reducing legal liability. These fears all compound to drive overtreatment by incentivizing testing and procedures to hedge against legal liability. Meanwhile, patients and most providers face very different perceptions of and kinds of risks, creating conflicts of interest. Rather than navigating together to traverse the river of treatment options, patients and providers paddle in different directions with different goals in mind, inhibiting providers' ability to offer individualized and evidence-based care.

Medicine and Risk

A major risk facing medical providers of all kinds is liability for negligence or malpractice. Physicians and some policy makers contend that the malpractice environment prevents physicians from practicing medicine in a way that is consistent with best practices and patient preferences, driving both medicalization and overtreatment. Physicians argue that the cost and frequency of malpractice claims constitute a malpractice crisis. The American Medical Association and other professional organizations have argued for various kinds of legislative reforms, including caps on awards and limits on noneconomic damages.[1] While the malpractice crisis story line is compelling, research suggests that the situation is much more complex than a surplus of litigation.[2] The actual cost of malpractice claims on the healthcare system as a whole is relatively low.[3] While practitioner perception of liability risk is very high, the risk of litigation for any one practitioner is comparatively low, and malpractice costs remain a minor contributor to healthcare costs overall. Medical staff also tend to ignore reforms to their practice style that would actually reduce their liability risk, such as improving communication and trust with patients and lowering the number of medical errors. They instead focus efforts on legal reforms that have little impact on reducing medical harm or improving patient outcomes. What does seem clear is that physician *perception* of liability risk encourages behaviors that are not in the patient's best interest, including those that actively violate patient preferences. Physician responses to perceived liability risk may, perversely, increase risks to patients such as poor medical outcomes and emotional trauma, while doing little to actually limit the risk of litigation. Physician and hospital strategies to limit legal vulnerability also pose serious barriers to patient autonomy and informed consent, by creating protocols or framing options in a way that limit legal risk, whether or not the offered options are good for patients or in line with their preferences.

Liability risk is, of course, not the only kind of risk practitioners face, and in the complexity of clinical medicine physicians juggle different kinds of risks simultaneously, often under tight time frames, all while trying to incorporate patient wishes, hospital protocol, and the current medical evidence. Avoiding one type of risk increases other kinds of risk, and different kinds of risks compound on one another. Risk of liability, for example, is often related to a patient's level of medical complexity, which is in turn related to the patient's risk of serious illness, injury, or death. Maternal-fetal medicine specialists, those who deal with higher-risk and more complicated pregnancies, are sued at higher rates than general practice obstetricians, largely because they deal with a population that is more likely to encounter serious problems during pregnancy, labor, or delivery. Midwives, on the other end of the spectrum, typically serve low-risk women and are at the lowest risk of being sued.[4] In general, the more medically complex a physician's practice, the greater the legal risk.[5] The relationship between medical risk and liability risk is one reason why hospital practitioners frequently perceive both liability and medical risk in different terms than their community-based counterparts.

Adding to the complexity, medical and legal risks are not the only risks physicians face during diagnosis and treatment. Decisions to treat or not treat are not themselves simple risk calculations. Physicians face a range of concerns about risk when suggesting courses of treatment, from the risk of undertreatment, including failure to diagnose an illness, to the risk of overtreatment, including risks associated with treatments themselves, such as pharmaceutical side effects or risks of damage or death during surgery. Much of medical research deals with population-level risk, making it difficult for providers to translate the risks of a treatment or lack of treatment into concrete risks for a specific patient. Medical risks to patients are intimately bound up in other kinds of risks providers face.

Physicians also operate in a complex legal and administrative environment that includes civil, criminal, and administrative liability, each with their own treatment standards, due process protections, and burdens of proof.[6] In the case of administrative involvement, physicians can face a range of accusations and a range of punishments, including reprimand, censure, fines, sanctions, suspension of practice, restrictions on prescribing or surgical privileges, or mandated supervision.[7] Though such actions are probably much rarer than the incidences of malpractice or negligence, physicians believe their risk to be relatively high.[8] These administrative bodies themselves operate as legislators, setting the standard of care, but they also operate as judge, prosecutor, and jury. Physicians report confusing evidentiary standards and no clear due process, which stokes both fear and uncertainty over what the accepted standard of care is in an individual case. The civil and criminal system is similarly complex, and while the courts support physicians in the majority of civil cases, the stress of an investigation and reputational concerns cause considerable fear and heighten perceptions of the risk of suits. Moreover, malpractice insurance typically does not assist in administrative or criminal defenses, leaving practitioners to shoulder the burden of such investigations on their own.[9]

As a result of the combination of liability risks, reputational risks, risks of administrative or other actions, and risks to the relationship between the physician and the patient, physicians rarely make decisions on the basis of medical risk alone. More frequently, they are cobbling together, often unconsciously, a sort of risk portfolio that includes social, legal, reputational, ethical and moral, and medical components. The salience of any one of these components at any given point in time, including how to balance risks to the patient and risks to the physician, will depend on the personality of the doctor, her personal history with a patient, her history as a physician (including experiences with lawsuits or administrative action), her age, and the environment in which she practices, among other things.

Legal Risk in Birth and Death

While all these other kinds of risks are important for understanding practitioner behavior, legal risks represent a central link between medicalization, centralization of care, and the political and policy framework of healthcare. In both birth and death, legal fears over both civil and criminal penalties influence practitioner behavior, pushing medical care away from best practices and even warping the standard of care over time.[10] Additionally, the coincidence of different kinds of risks compounds physician fears in ways that escalate under- or overtreatment, as in the case of vaginal birth after cesarean, to be discussed further in the next section. Understanding the legal environment physicians face, as well as the broader political context for that legal environment, is therefore crucial in understanding why treatment intensity and practitioner behavior vary so dramatically across care settings. It turns out that perception of legal risk plays an important and underanalyzed role in determining how patients give birth or die.

Interviews with doctors, nurses, and other practitioners demonstrate substantial concerns about liability and malpractice, and physicians argue that a primary way they limit liability is through practicing defensive medicine. Proponents of this view argue that defensive medicine drives medicalization, as physicians are forced to use high-intensity medical care to prevent or defend themselves from malpractice litigation.[11] Overtreatment is much harder to sue for than undertreatment, the narrative goes, so doctors have little incentive to practice conservatively, even if conservative treatment is the best option for an individual patient or condition, as is often the case in birth and death. Advocates for tort reform argue that medical malpractice litigation is a major factor in rising healthcare costs in general and a major cause of poor outcomes for the birthing and dying in particular. In one survey of physicians in high-risk specialties, 93 percent of respondents admitted to practicing defensive medicine. The most common practices were unnecessary use of imaging equipment and referring patients to other doctors.[12] More troubling practices included avoiding high-risk procedures altogether or avoiding complex patients or those who seem litigious.[13] Studies that focus on physician self-reports are the primary evidence advocates provide for the existence of a crisis of malpractice litigation that increases costs and harms patients.

Critics contend that the evidence is actually more nuanced and that relying on survey self-reports is an unreliable way to gage physician behavior. It is difficult to tease out the causes of unnecessary treatments, since defensive medicine may be mingled with the desire to keep patients happy, profit motives, and pressure from other doctors. Physicians may highlight fear of liability to explain overtreatment since it deflects blame away from them and onto broader impersonal causes. Because many surveys on the topic specifically ask about defensive medicine and the malpractice environment, critics argue that availability bias leads physicians to substantially overestimate how much of their treatment is due to liability fears.[14]

While the impact of the liability environment on physician behavior is still somewhat unclear, a broader concern with the tort system is that it fails to do what it is meant to do: compensate victims of existing malpractice and prevent medical malpractice in the first place. Recent analyses of the tort system demonstrate both the strengths and weaknesses of litigating medical errors. An article in the *New England Journal of Medicine* (*NEJM*) found that the tort system does a reasonable job of tracking the merits of claims.[15] Claims with merit are generally compensated, while claims without merit generally are not. Around 75 percent of claims decisions matched the merit of the claims, though that means that around 25 percent did not. Of those that did not, it was actually more likely for a meritorious claim to not be compensated than it was for an unmerited claim to be compensated.

On the more negative side, because the vast majority of victims of medical injuries do not report and do not sue, the tort system fails to compensate even a small minority of victims of medical malpractice. For those who do successfully sue, the process is both long and costly. The average claim in the *NEJM* study took five years to complete, and 54 percent of compensation went to administrative costs, including lawyers and expert witnesses. Trials cost three times more than those cases that were settled out of court, and plaintiffs are less likely to win in court, probably owing to the fact that clear-cut cases are more likely to be settled before a trial.[16] The unevenness of the tort system—the fact that most victims of medical malpractice receive no compensation at all—is one major criticism of the current system, with some advocates arguing for a system more like workplace injury compensation or administrative processes that compensate more patients with medical injuries while reducing the cost of the process itself.[17]

Overall, the tort system seems to be reasonably helpful at sifting merited from unmerited claims but quite unhelpful at compensating victims of malpractice and possibly also unhelpful at actually improving standards of practice. Yet medical errors themselves are a serious problem in the US healthcare system, with a recent report estimating medical errors to be the third leading cause of death in the United States.[18] Limiting patients' ability to sue is unlikely to have much effect on the overall cost of care in the United States and in fact may even drive costs by reducing incentives to improve care. One report estimated that tort reform would save around 0.1 percent of overall healthcare costs.[19] Conversely, some estimates suggest that as much as 35 percent of Medicare spending at the end of life is the result of physician behavior that is not supported by clinical evidence.[20] Yet tort reform, rather than poor medical practices, has been targeted by both the media and legislators at the state and federal levels as a major way to reduce healthcare costs.[21]

Tort reform is particularly difficult to defend given how the traditional model of self-policing in medicine has broken down over time. Ideally, licensing boards would play a role in limiting medical malpractice by sanctioning doctors who cause avoidable harm or even removing them from practice. In reality, however, such actions are rare.[22] While state licensing boards do create a barrier to entry for new practitioners, they often do very little to ensure good standards of practice once physicians are licensed. Around 1 percent of doctors are responsible for around 30 percent of all malpractice claims, which indicates at least the need for more investigation, though explanations other than malpractice exist.[23] One report found that it is not uncommon for a physician to lose clinical privileges at a hospital and be deemed an "immediate danger to health and safety" and yet still maintain a license to practice and continue seeing patients.[24] If licensing boards are not sanctioning physicians adequately, tort reform merely adds to patient risk by making it more difficult to sue rogue doctors. Any reforms to the tort system must account for the background context of a healthcare system beset by frequent medical errors and a lack of accountability provided by other institutions. In the absence of more comprehensive reforms, the tort system may be the best system for compensating victims, as imperfect as it is.

Risk, Liability, and Bias in Birth

The liability issue is especially complex in birth because birth itself presents a major challenge for accurately assessing risk. Risks to mothers and infants are not the same, and different interventions can lower risks to one while increasing them for the other. A low-risk pregnancy can become a high-risk pregnancy very quickly and sometimes with little warning. Complications from medical decisions, whether intervention or nonintervention, may not be immediately clear, such as placenta accreta after a cesarean section or pelvic floor damage after a vaginal birth, both of which can manifest years later. Because risks to the infant such as brain damage or death are so serious, physicians prioritize mitigating infant risk, which increases risks to the mother. Finally, the economic costs of infant birth injuries such as brain damage or paralysis are catastrophic, and many families with disabled infants feel that their only financial option is to sue, regardless of whether an injury could have been prevented. As a result, birth providers are juggling a complicated and sometimes contradictory set of risks, including preventing physical harm to both the mother and the child, respecting maternal autonomy, and protecting themselves and their staff from a variety of economic, reputational, and legal risks.

Birth and Malpractice

Malpractice concerns rank high for obstetrics providers. Doctors, nurses, and midwives all describe fear and anxiety about the liability environment, and professional workshops and conferences focus on the importance of removing liability. These concerns are not unfounded. Theresa Morris's recent study on the cesarean crisis found that the average obstetrician will be sued around three times in the course of his or her career.[25] These suits take on average four years to resolve. While most (65%) are decided in favor of the physician, the toll of ongoing litigation in terms of reputation, stress, and time away from practice is considerable. Moreover, while the actual number of claims has decreased over the past 25 years, award amounts continue to rise, with one 2011 cerebral palsy claim in Connecticut setting records at $58.6 million. Many of these suits, including many of those decided against the doctor, demonstrate no actual malpractice, unlike other kinds of medical malpractice cases where awards more closely track fault. Most suits are for stillbirth, shoulder dystocia, or cerebral palsy, none of which can be conclusively linked to practitioner quality or competence in most cases. In fact, as Morris points out, unlike in other areas of medical malpractice, "most malpractice payments [in obstetrics] are awarded for injuries that are not the result of medical error."[26] Cerebral palsy, which often results in the costliest suits for doctors and insurers, is still not well understood, but researchers believe that most cases result from prenatal or genetic causes, not from practitioner error.[27] In other words, the majority of obstetrics liability suits are cases that no competent medical provider could have prevented.

What is less clear is how much these patterns influence practitioner behavior and healthcare costs. Obstetricians argue that malpractice fears lead them to pursue unnecessary testing and interventions, including cesarean section, which drive up costs. Analyses at the macro level fail to turn up evidence that physicians use cesarean sections to avoid liability. States with relatively high malpractice insurance premiums had somewhat higher rates of caesarean section and lower rates of delivery by VBAC than did states with lower premiums, but the differences were relatively small.[28] States that have passed various reforms, such as caps on awards or limiting noneconomic damages, do not have significantly lower levels of cesarean sections or other "defensive" interventions than states that have not passed such reforms, indicating that the situation is not as simple as physicians responding to perceived risk with overtreatment. Interviews with doctors and midwives and other micro-level data suggest that practitioners at least believe that their risk aversion is linked to malpractice concerns.[29] The macro-level data also suggest at least one way in which doctors practice defensively, which is that obstetricians who have already been sued have higher cesarean rates than they did prelitigation.[30] Overall, the effect of malpractice concerns on practitioner behavior seems to be fairly small in the aggregate.

One possible explanation for the differences between the macro- and micro-level data is that doctors are indeed practicing medicine defensively but are not responding to reforms because they view such changes as marginal enough that they are unlikely to change the outcome of future suits, unstable because legislatures and courts could overturn them, or simply irrelevant given the environment of fear in which they operate. It would be no surprise to psychologists that individuals often respond not to the actual level of threat in their environment but to the perceived level of threat.[31] Surveys of obstetricians and midwives demonstrate that practitioners believe that this threat level is high.[32]

While the patterns of obstetrics suits might seem to support calls for tort reform, the narrative is further complicated when one looks at risk from the perspective of the patient, in this case at the rate of preventable birth injuries. A 2013 report found that negligent injuries to mothers and infants are relatively common, making up around 1 percent of births, or as many as 40,000 women a year.[33] Yet most of the victims of negligent injuries do not sue. Of those who sue, most do not win, and of those who win, around half of the money goes to court and legal costs. As is the case for general malpractice, the system does not do a good job of actually compensating people for negligent injuries, nor does it work to lessen rates of injuries themselves.[34] Moreover, evidence does not support claims by clinicians that liability costs threaten their livelihood as providers. Obstetricians have successfully increased revenue through procedure and test-intensive practice style and now have the second-highest salaries of any major specialty.[35] Nevertheless, liability concerns are a serious cause of stress and dissatisfaction among obstetrics providers, even if the financial impact of such concerns is relatively low.[36]

Even while meta-analyses of claims of defensive medicine among obstetricians do not generally support claims of doctors themselves that liability fears influence their practice, tort reforms do not seem effective, however that effectiveness is measured. When compared across states and across liability frameworks, medical interventions seem largely independent of either the cost or availability of liability insurance. Similarly, tort reforms and administrative compensation programs have little effect on the cesarean section rate, often touted as a major defensive procedure used by obstetricians.[37] The research suggests two possible explanations for this gap between physician self-reports and actual practice patterns: it could be that physicians are using liability as an excuse for high-intensity treatments, or they may believe the risks of lawsuits to be much higher than they in fact are.

So-called mega-awards heighten practitioner perception of risk. Despite an overall lower rate of suits filed in recent years, the number of awards at the extremes has increased, including awards like the one in Connecticut. The size of such awards places doctors at greater risk of exceeding their malpractice insurance cap, thus putting their personal assets at risk.[38] Mega-awards are also more likely to result in the cancellation of policies after the suit, resulting in doctors who either are unable to get any insurance at all, thus ending their careers, or are forced to pay for high-risk insurance, which prices them out of practice. In such a climate, where suits seem random but inevitable, payouts seem high, and the professional stakes seem soaring, practitioners would be highly sensitive to risks on the side of not doing enough and much less sensitive to the risks of doing too much. This sensitivity is heightened by an environment, as many doctors in Morris's sample argue, in which they are told by courts, by lawyers, and by their own professional organizations that the way to avoid liability is to perform surgeries early and often.[39]

Moreover, nothing about tort reform changes the nature of maternity practice itself, which is riddled with unknowns and a host of potential unseen complications. The reality of maternity care is that birth is an unpredictable and sometimes tragic event. When infants are injured before or during even the most competently assisted births, the results can be devastating. Neurological problems and severe disabilities swamp unsuspecting parents in medical bills they will struggle to pay for the rest of the child's life. Many parents see no option other than to sue as a way to provide care for a severely disabled child. Juries are often sympathetic and believe that having an insurer pay, even in cases where no malpractice was found, is morally superior to bankrupting the parents of a disabled infant. Juries usually know little about the long-term impacts of their decisions, such as the rising scarcity of ob stetricians and the impact on doctors themselves. Obstetrics thus poses unique challenges for the tort system. Injuries, when they occur, may be catastrophic, such injuries are statistically relatively common, and many (though not all) of the injuries are unavoidable by even the most competent obstetrician, barring one with second sight. Yet the harms of overtreatment and unnecessary interventions are not easily measured or accounted for by the tort system.

Risk Perception in Birth

The perceived risk of malpractice influences the way practitioners understand and balance other kinds of risks, including risks to patients. One concern critics have noted is that obstetrics research and guidelines from professional associations often underestimate the risks of high-intensity interventions while overestimating the risks associated with demedicalized interventions. VBAC is a well-studied example. VBAC rates are extremely low in the United States. By some estimates, less than 10 percent of women who attempt a VBAC will succeed.[40] The decline in successful VBAC was largely the result of fears of uterine rupture, since a uterus that has been compromised by an initial cesarean scar is somewhat more likely to split in a subsequent pregnancy. This rupture rate, however, is and has always been low, with ruptures occurring in less than 1 percent of all VBACs. Most uterine ruptures that occur during VBAC (in and of themselves very rare) are in fact minor tears that can be easily repaired.[41] Catastrophic uterine rupture is very rare.

Tellingly, for many years providers did not believe that the risk of rupture outweighed the benefits of vaginal birth, as evidenced by rates of attempted VBAC as high as 50 percent in the 1990s. What changed was not the medical risk of a VBAC itself but the salience of malpractice concerns in the late 1990s. As a result, VBAC rates fell dramatically in the late 1990s and never recovered.[42] The most recent research on VBAC shows not only that is it very safe but also that it is actually safer than repeat cesarean, particularly for women who go on to have subsequent pregnancies. Maternal deaths during both procedures are very rare, but the rate for repeat cesarean is 9.6 deaths per 100,000 births, while the rate for VBAC is 1.9 deaths per 100,000 births.[43] The disparity between theoretical risk and actual practice patterns is explained in part by who is held responsible for the risks of medicalized births. If a patient attempting a VBAC experiences a uterine rupture, the physician supervising the VBAC will be sued rather than the physician who did the original cesarean. A practitioner who performs an unnecessary cesarean section will, in turn, be unlikely to experience liability or other risk associated with complications because most life-threatening risks like placenta accreta and placenta previa do not show up until later pregnancies.[44] Moreover, juries themselves are biased and see more harm in undertreatment than overtreatment.

This pattern of prioritizing malpractice risk over other kinds of risks is not just found in VBAC attitudes. The emphasis on macrosomia (or large babies) discussed in chapter 1 is explained in part by the way providers balance risks of litigation against risks to infants. Obstetricians often recommend induction or cesarean section for large babies, even though the vast majority of large babies will be vaginally delivered without incident. Obstetrics providers also tend to focus on preventing excess weight gain throughout pregnancy, since weight gained during pregnancy is associated with the size of the infant at birth. Yet a mother gaining too little weight is more dangerous to the infant than gaining too much weight, and induction can increase the risk of low birth weight.[45] Low birth weight places infants at higher risk of breathing problems and other lifelong health risks and increases infant mortality. For providers, however, the liability risk of shoulder dystocia is greater than the medical risk of low birth weight. Dystocia is one of the major causes of malpractice lawsuits, since babies who get stuck in the vaginal canal sometimes require force to remove them, and it carries a risk of lifelong injuries to the infant, including permanent nerve damage.[46] None of the risks of low birth weight are compensable by a medical malpractice suit. The obstetric community's assessment of the directionality of risk in maternal and fetal weight tracks concerns about malpractice more closely than it tracks the real risks to mothers and infants.

A final piece in the puzzle comes from the economic incentives that accompany inflated perceptions of risk. Part of what changed the landscape for VBAC births were recommendations from the American College of Obstetricians and Gynecologists that VBAC deliveries require an operating room on site, constant physician attendance during labor, and blood banks on hand.[47] This guidance signaled to providers not only that VBAC is medically and legally risky but that handling these risks would lead to artificially inflated costs for both hospitals and providers. Many rural hospitals responded by refusing to provide VBAC at all because they could not afford such precautions, while many doctors refused to attend VBAC births because constant attendance during a VBAC labor made vaginal birth unprofitable. As a result of ACOG's recommendation, as many as 50 percent of hospitals in the United States have de facto VBAC bans, a major contributor to the rising cesarean section rate in the United States.[48] ACOG's recommendations were also not in fact responses to the real medical risk of VBACs to mothers or infants, but were instead responses to the perceived liability risk of VBAC among obstetrics providers. The VBAC case demonstrates how the liability tributary combines with the river of reimbursement to pull patients toward medicalized care. When medicalized management is associated with both lower liability risk and higher reimbursement rates, it is hardly surprising that physicians respond with higher rates of interventions.

Risk and Bias in Death

Concerns about risk in treating elderly and dying patients are also more complicated than those in other areas of medicine. Patients at the end of life have competing needs and values, including pain control, quality of life, and length of life. Patients who are unable to communicate, family conflicts, transfers of care, and shifting values all challenge the practicality of both informed consent and evidence-based decision making. The severity of patient symptoms at the end of life and the difficulty of managing the expectations of patients and their families in a politically charged area of medicine add further complexity.[49]

Legal Concerns at the End of Life

The legal environment of end-of-life care is complicated, since practitioners fear not just accusations of undertreatment, which is usually the case in lawsuits relating to birth, but also investigations of overtreatment, specifically with regard to the use of opiate pain medication. Additionally, legal and professional standards are still in flux. Political debates over the opioid epidemic, physician-assisted suicide, and "death panels" create significant fear in practitioners over how to ensure that they are providing the best patient care possible while avoiding entanglements with administrative, legal, or criminal bodies.[50]

The legal concerns of end-of-life care providers can trigger both under- and overtreatment. Palliative care doctors frequently use large doses of morphine and other drugs to control pain at the end of life, which can lead to scrutiny in light of political concerns about physician-assisted suicide and euthanasia. At the same time, physicians may be pressured into overtreatment as patients, families, and even other doctors protest against the withdrawal of treatments and procedures at the end of life, including artificial hydration and nutrition. These counterpressures place physicians and others who care for the dying in a medical-legal-ethical bind. They feel they cannot provide adequate pain relief to their patients without being accused of criminal behavior, but they also feel coerced into providing or supporting unnecessary treatments that actually increase pain at the end of life. End-of-life care is compromised in both directions. Undertreatment of pain is endemic, but unnecessary or harmful treatments are a major concern among patients and palliative care physicians as well.[51]

Both the media and contemporary political debates over end-of-life care have contributed to physician perception of risk. The combination of the media coverage of high-profile cases, such as that of Terri Schiavo, and the political and media frenzy over so-called death panels has led to changes in practice behavior, triggering undertreatment for pain and overtreatment in other areas like chemotherapy or artificial nutrition and hydration. Media and political attention both increase scrutiny of care at the end of life and heighten the perception of legal risk among practitioners. The current opioid epidemic further heightens fears, as physicians worry about being caught up in drug raids or being victimized by overzealous prosecutors, even if such risks are actually very low.

Risk and Undertreatment at the End of Life

Narcotic use is perhaps the primary area where physicians' legal fears influence their treatment of the dying. The widespread opioid epidemic and heightened political scrutiny have increased physicians' concerns about prescribing high doses of narcotics to patients at the end of life. Research from the 1990s, when the war on drugs was raging, found that more than half of physicians surveyed would "occasionally reduce drug dosage or quantity or limit refills because of fears of regulatory scrutiny."[52] Oncologists specifically reported that regulation of opioids created a serious challenge for effective pain management. Recent concerns over the escalation of the opioid epidemic and over how many addictions begin with legally prescribed opioids after injury have again heightened physicians' concerns about treating pain with narcotics.[53]

Complicating the picture is that most physicians who are investigated for narcotics use in end-of-life care are not initially targeted by law enforcement, but are instead reported by other staff. In fact, none of the available research supports a systematic targeting of palliative care or other end-of-life providers by enforcement agencies or prosecutors. One review of cases between 2000 and 2008 finds that most investigations "represent intercollegial discord and miscommunication or disagreements between providers and families, rather than suspicious or overzealous prosecutors."[54] Even without explicit targeting by prosecutors, criminal prosecutions of physicians increased from the 1990s onward, and the review noted some patterns. Prosecutions are more common in rural counties and more commonly aimed at doctors new to the area. Nurses were the most common informants. Many, though not all, of the cases show medical mismanagement at some point in the process. The more troubling cases are those that show no medical mismanagement and that are eventually thrown out, but not before they do substantial damage to the reputations and malpractice insurance costs of the accused. While convictions are rare, prosecutors sometimes use trials as a way to send messages to the medical community about opioid medications. Of those doctors who are formally investigated, "typical consequences for physicians included jail time, lost income, reduction in practice size and/or time, and emotional distress."[55] The costs, even of unsuccessful investigations, are high for physicians.

The result of these fears is an epidemic of a different sort, that of inadequate pain management. Around 60–70 percent of patients with severe pain are undertreated.[56] This epidemic is particularly troubling for those at the end of life whose pain is both severe and resistant to traditional nonmedical ways to manage pain. As one author notes, "A doctor, if he really wants to cover himself, is going to under-prescribe. There's no law against under-prescribing other than the law of compassion."[57] Just as there are very few lawsuits for unnecessary treatments in obstetrics, in pain management there are very few lawsuits for underuse of narcotics, even though patients are seriously harmed in both cases. Whether liability fears lead to undertreatment or overtreatment will depend in large part on which kind of treatment the legal standards are most sensitive to. The consequence is that patients and their families are forced to suffer because of fears about risks that are, in part, unrelated to evidence-based standards of care.

Part of the problem is that the pain management needs of terminally ill patients and the trade-offs involved are almost completely at odds with the needs and risks within the general population. Unlike the average patient, the risk of addiction in a terminal patient approaches zero, while the medical justification for increasing levels of strong pain medications increases over time. As one palliative care practitioner notes,

> The whole world of opiate treatment has gotten much more complex in the last ten years as a result of the opioid epidemic. There are tons of people who are not terminally ill but in a lot of pain who have been put on lots of opiates. Then they develop a tolerance to it and sometimes also addiction. There's a huge conundrum there. Then you take people at the end of life and there's much more of a clear indication and you're dying anyway and you care less about some of the risks. But applying the principles that hospice uses, for example, for terminally ill patients to the larger population for pain management has been seriously problematic.

Public policies cannot easily distinguish between the unique needs of terminal patients and those of the general population, which in turn affects practitioner prescribing habits. One hospice nurse noted, "When we call a community doctor [a doctor not directly affiliated with the hospice], generally they're ok prescribing things for hospice, but if [the patient is] not on hospice [i.e., not yet terminal] they won't prescribe. So that stuff is frustrating. It's not a law, but doctors are uncomfortable prescribing comfort medicines."

Pain medication is a crucial part of end-of-life care because terminal conditions like cancer are extremely painful and the pain is difficult to treat. Moreover, many pain medications have what is known as a "double effect," that is, they blunt or eliminate pain while also compromising or slowing various bodily functions, perhaps hastening death.[58] This double effect implicates not only debates over proper use of narcotics but also debates over physician-assisted suicide. Crucially and confusingly, the intent of the physician is the central determinant in what kinds of treatments cross the line from legal to illegal. A physician who prescribes a large amount of morphine to treat pain is objectively indistinguishable from a physician who prescribes a large amount of morphine to hasten death. Yet the legal system treats the first activity as legal and the second activity as illegal. The subjectivity of intent creates opportunities for miscommunication and disagreements within the care team and between family members and caregivers. Some palliative care physicians have criticized using double effect as a legal doctrine, since it can distort physician intentions and leads physicians to avoid care that they nevertheless believe to be in their patient's best interest.[59] It also supports the problematic legal standard that "what a physician says is more important than what he does."[60]

This subjectivity is magnified because the "standard of care," the usual way courts determine the appropriateness of a physician's actions, differs between different medical specialties. Palliative care physicians and nurses use opioids much differently and in much different doses than do other kinds of medical providers.[61] Pain medication doses are also patient specific, and terminally ill patients can develop high tolerances to opioids in the final weeks of life, while their pain is also escalating. In mixed-practice environments, doctors and nurses whose focus is on comfort at the end of life can find themselves in legally dangerous disagreement with medical or other practitioners whose goal is extending life. One study found that suspicion of hospice and palliative care providers among nursing home staff, particularly in terms of medication, was a serious barrier to quality of hospice care for patients in nursing homes.[62] A nurse interviewed in that study commented that nursing home providers "don't seem to worry that the patient's in pain. . . . They worry about drug addiction when the patients theoretically have less than 6 months to live."[63] The home environment prevents some of these conflicts because providers are more likely to be on the same page, with one home hospice nurse remarking, "We're so liberal with [narcotics] in home hospice that [the legality] doesn't bother us." The location of care and the mix of providers present have important implications for appropriate pain treatment. One palliative care physician expressed frustration that such fear also allows other physicians to shift responsibility for opioid management to already-overburdened palliative care teams or to fail to treat patient pain at all: "[Legal fear] makes it easier for other docs to just say 'I'm not going to prescribe any pain meds' because they're afraid of the DEA [Drug Enforcement Administration] looking into their life."

Risk and Overtreatment at the End of Life

Concerns about physician-assisted suicide contribute to overtreatment as well. The Terri Schiavo case and others like it were not about hastening death with drugs, but about the ethics and legality of withholding or withdrawing life-sustaining treatment at the end of life. The characterization of conversations about end-of-life goals as so-called death panels by vice presidential candidate Sarah Palin during the 2008 election shifted the debate around end-of-life conversations, not least by heightening the risks practitioners felt in even talking about end-of-life care.[64] Physicians, especially those without training in palliative techniques, may feel uncomfortable initiating conversations about withdrawing or withholding treatments with patients and their families and even more hesitant about withdrawing care, even when it is clearly futile.[65]

Legal precedent has clarified only one part of the puzzle. While the Supreme Court's decision in *Cruzan* (1990) that competent individuals have the right to refuse medical treatment clarified some end-of-life decision making, it left open what to do about patients whose wishes are not clear.[66] Even those with Do Not Resuscitate orders may end up being resuscitated as a result of poor communication or legal fears.[67]

Complicating things, advance directives and other legal documents out-lining care goals may be unclear, be irrelevant for the specific condition a patient is being treated for, or become moot in the moment as patient goals change when actually confronted with death. Clear communica-tion and informed consent can be difficult to obtain in the emotionally fraught circumstances of a dying loved one. Family members are fre-quently torn among trying to control pain, wanting their loved one to remain alert for quality time with family and friends, and balancing fears of or desires for death itself. Both sides try to shield the other from uncomfortable truths by not talking about it. In the confusion, physi-cians may unintentionally substitute their wishes for those of their pa-tient. While most physicians believe they know what individual patients want, most actually do not.[68] Physicians also confront the difficulty of making sure that all relevant decision makers are accounted for. A major concern physicians reference when refusing to withdraw treatments is the specter of family conflict, including unknown relatives arriving on the scene.[69] The result is miscommunication or conflicts of interest that make medical decisions morally and legally fraught.

End-of-life practitioners' perception of the risk of withdrawing care is inflated not only by the theoretical risk of administrative, civil, or criminal action triggered by confusion about care goals but also by actual comments made by patients, their families, and other healthcare providers. In one recent survey, over half of palliative care doctors had their work characterized as "murder" or "euthanasia" by friends, pa-tients, or other doctors.[70] Four percent of doctors in the study had been formally investigated by their institution, by their medical board, or by a district attorney. None were found guilty, though the costs of investi-gation ranged from losing DEA registration to suspension of a medical license to reputational damage, as well as fear, anxiety, and anger during the investigation itself. Perhaps surprisingly, doctors were most often reported by other doctors or medical professionals.[71]

High-profile cases add to the environment of fear and uncertainty. Dr. Naramore of Kansas was convicted in 1996 of attempted first-degree murder for trying to give a large dose of morphine to a dying cancer patient and then convicted again for second-degree murder for removing a patient who had suffered a stroke from respiratory support. He served more than two years in jail before the court reversed his convictions on appeal.[72] Dr. Anna Pou was charged in 2006 with euthanizing patients, both by withdrawing care from the patients least likely to survive and via overdose with morphine, in the chaos surrounding Hurricane Katrina. Though a grand jury declined to indict, the case continued to make national media headlines, including a front-page story in the *New York Times Magazine* in 2009.[73] Such cases, while rare, gain national attention and heighten practitioners' feeling of risk. While the actual risk of criminal prosecution is small, the fear of prosecution is a major reason given by the 40 percent of physicians who report acting against their medical conscience.[74]

As with opioid use, risk and perception of risk increase the more practitioners from different backgrounds interact with one another, promoting overtreatment. Hospice nurses report hostility from nursing home staff not only about narcotics use but also about conflicting standards for withholding of artificial hydration and nutrition.[75] Liability fears directly impact patient care by prompting unnecessary transfers to hospitals, with fear of liability considered a major cause of unnecessary hospitalizations of nursing home residents. One study found that as many as 40 percent of nursing home residents transferred to hospitals would have been better off remaining in place, but poor communication between staff members, state laws that protect the nursing home itself but leave physicians vulnerable to lawsuits, and perceived liability threats all contribute to high transfer rates and escalation of care.[76] Transfers to hospitals increase the risk of stress-related illnesses, social isolation, unnecessary treatments, and overall physical decline.[77]

Even before patients are transferred to hospitals from nursing homes, liability concerns can impact patient care in the form of "defensive on-site medicine," including overuse of medications alongside the underuse of pain medications like narcotics.[78] One palliative care doctor noted that "most meds for chronic illnesses in the last year of life are not indicated and yet most people refuse to stop them," which creates a cascade of other issues, including increased confusion, falls, and compromised quality of life.[79] Some state laws make the situation worse by holding medical directors of nursing homes liable for incidents involving patients, when in fact the medical director has little control over the main contributors to medical mistakes, such as poor staffing levels. Medical directors of nursing homes in those states may lean toward higher treatment levels as a way to balance out fears that stem from entirely differ-ent administrative causes.[80]

Risk Perception at the End of Life

The finality of death and the ever-growing number of interventions to combat it influence risk perception in more subtle ways. The medical anthropologist Sharon Kaufman has described how the very presence of medical options skews practitioner thinking about risk toward treat-ment. In one case she discusses, a physician who wanted to place an implantable cardioverter defibrillator (ICD) to restart the heart of an elderly man with chronic heart failure argued that the man, Mr. Jones, was risking death by not having an ICD placed. Kaufman argues, "Med-icine emphasizes that refusing an ICD puts one at risk for death—as if one (and certainly Mr. Jones) were not already at risk for death simply by having advanced heart failure in old age."[81] As Kaufman notes, tech-nology itself has changed physicians' attitudes toward risk. Since there is always one more tool to use, inaction is now seen as a risk in and of itself. She argues, "The changing means and ends of technology have enabled today's dominant cultural tendency: to think, to act as if most deaths are premature."[82]

Crucially, many of the intensive and invasive interventions that hos-pitals provide at the end of life do not increase function, improve qual-ity of life, or ease suffering. What they do accomplish is to prolong life, albeit for a very brief period. Too much attention to the risk that death itself poses diverts attention from other risks like uncontrolled pain, poor quality of life, and inability to communicate with loved ones. Which risks a physician perceives as most relevant will be strongly linked to the tools a physician has at her disposal, the setting of care and its risk bi-ases, and whether a patient's wishes can be clearly known. These vari-ables, in turn, influence how care options are framed for patients, with important implications for how "informed" patients can actually be in such a complex framework. Physicians may guide patients toward less legally risky care without even being fully conscious they are doing so. While legal concerns are by no means the only concerns that heighten practitioner attention to death as the primary risk to be avoided, legal fears contribute to an environment in which overtreatment is seen as less risky than more conservative kinds of care.

Hospitals and the Riptide of Risk

As in a real watershed, the tributaries of the healthcare watershed combine in unexpected ways. Regulations and reimbursement policies that centralize care in hospitals inadvertently contribute to the liability crisis by centralizing care in hospitals, the care location that is the most sensitive to both liability and risk. Regulations and reimbursement policies that wash away demedicalized providers or those who operate outside of hospitals shift patients from care settings with relatively low levels of liability anxiety into care settings with relatively high levels of such anxiety. In this way and others, the various tributaries in the watershed interact, each adding water volume that increases the speed of the current, pushing patients toward the rapids of medicalization.

Owing to their size, patient population, provider profile, and other characteristics, hospitals have both a heightened level of various kinds of risks and a heightened perception of those risks. Hospital-based care actually increases some medical risks, including unnecessary care, medical errors, hospital-borne infections, and heightened levels of infirmity post-hospitalization.[83] But hospitals also support medicalization by heightening *perceptions* of risk, particularly the risks of nonmedical alternatives, even when such alternatives are the most appropriate form of care. Hospitals also underestimate the risks of medical treatments themselves. The combination of a highly specialized staff, a complex patient profile, high patient volume, time-constrained decision making, and the need to standardize patient care escalates medicalization in hospitals compared to community-based care settings like birth centers, hospices, and nursing homes.

Hospital staffing is the most obvious way the hospital environment heightens perception of risk—both legal and medical—among practitioners. Most practitioners in hospitals are trained medical professionals, and medical training understandably emphasizes the benefits of medical interventions and underestimates the benefits of nonmedical care. Owing to time and curricular constraints, most new doctors do not experience either physiological birth or death in medical school. Medical providers are biased toward medical options simply because they have never seen a safe version of the alternative. And because medical practitioners are trained in using medical tools, they feel legally vulnerable (and may in fact be vulnerable) if they do not use all the tools at their disposal, particularly in borderline cases.[84] Midwives and hospice workers, familiar with physiological birth and death, are generally more comfortable with the risks inherent in demedicalized alternatives to birth and death and much less comfortable with the risks inherent in medical interventions.

Hospitals also heighten perception of risk by concentrating large numbers of providers together in one place. The sociologist Theresa Morris argued in her study of the cesarean section epidemic in the United States that "collaboration leads to more c-sections because it is a mechanism that allows the spread of liability fear."[85] A single lawsuit or rare complication can, in the presence of many providers, take on great weight via the rapid dissemination of hospital gossip in hallways and break rooms. Like everyone, nurses and doctors are more heavily influenced by negative experiences than by positive ones, compounding the bias toward intervention as a hedge against risk.[86] These factors create a kind of confirmation bias about risk; practitioners feel that high levels of treatment intensity are always appropriate precisely because they believe that risk levels, whether the risk of liability or the risk of medical catastrophe, are always high. Adding to the complexity, multiple teams of physicians often consult on a single patient. As one hospital palliative care specialist notes, "If you have someone with cancer, you have a whole cancer team on top of a whole palliative care team. And there might be a whole radiation team. It ends up being a lot of people. There are good things from all that expertise, but one of the downsides is that no one is really running the ship. No one is looking at the big picture." In team environments, each provider contributes her own perception of risk, with no one putting the entire picture together or comparing it to a more objective assessment.

Moreover, the patient population of hospitals heightens perception of risk and normalizes medicalized care because most patients in the hospital (with the exception of labor and delivery wards) are in fact sick, often with complex illnesses. In both birth and death, crises hit unexpectedly, making it more likely that providers will fall back on treatments they are familiar with and competent in providing. One of the benefits of both palliative care and midwifery philosophies in hospital settings is that both try to keep the big picture in view, referring back to patient goals of treatment, while other doctors and nurses are focused on the necessary minutiae of individual treatments. Demedicalized providers operate in some sense like the navigator whose job it is to keep the boat headed in the right direction, while the rest of the crew provides the tools to get it there.

The large volume of patients in hospitals also influences perception of risk by encouraging practitioners to think about the aggregate risk of an outcome, rather than the risk for any individual patient. As Morris notes, "The doctor's risk of overseeing a VBAC in which a uterine rupture occurs is not the same as a woman's risk that she will have a uterine rupture in a VBAC attempt. In other words, a physician experiences a different 'lifetime' risk of uterine rupture over his or her career than does a woman in her one-time risk of having a uterine rupture in a VBAC attempt."[87] The fear a physician has of uterine rupture in VBAC is therefore not actually related to the statistical likelihood of uterine rupture for an individual patient, which is extremely low. Uterine rupture, while extremely rare statistically, may be experienced once or even twice by a provider in the hospital environment over the course of a career. In turn, the hospital environment will ensure that many more physicians and nurses will hear about an individual case of uterine rupture, spreading the perception that such incidents are not only possible but common.

Of course, volume and risk perception work both ways. Community-based providers may underestimate risk because they have fewer overall patients and are less familiar with potential negative outcomes. One hospital-based nurse midwife acknowledged this difficulty, arguing that "a lot of the [direct-entry midwives] are not evidence-based, they base their practice on the 85% [of easy deliveries]. Most of them do maybe 20 deliveries a year. I do 20 deliveries a week. So I see the abnormal cases." At the same time, the same midwife acknowledged the tension of appropriate risk assessment in the hospital, saying that "the whole [hospital] mindset is 'everything is wrong and we need to fix it' instead of 'it's probably fine, so let's try to keep it that way.'" She believed that a central part of her job as hospital midwife is to "keep reminding [doctors] that this is normal, this is normal, this is normal."

The population of patients admitted to hospitals is also skewed in ways that elevate the risk practitioners feel about demedicalized birth and death. A common refrain from hospital providers is that home birth is incredibly risky, which is understandable since the home birth patients who are transferred to hospitals require medical care. Hospital staff do not see the much more common home births with positive outcomes, and they may resent that home birth complications become their "problem" and their liability risk when a patient is transferred. One maternal-fetal specialist lamented that this lack of experience with positive home births skews practitioner attitudes not just toward home birth itself but also toward patients who are transferred and the providers who transfer them, leading to mutual distrust and sometimes outright animosity. He remarked, "There's no reason [midwives] would want to take unnecessary risks. They want the patient to have a good experience. We only see the times they don't. I think that colors the interactions." He believes that obstetrics residents would benefit from rounding at home births as well as in hospitals to allow more positive experiences with home birth and improve interactions when transfers become necessary.

For all these reasons, hospitals are characterized by high perception of risk and ever-present liability fears. Hospital administrators respond to these heightened levels of real and perceived risk with protocols to mitigate liability risk but not medical risk itself. A hospital-based midwife described how liability fears play into daily conversations about best practices: "In a hospital there's a huge amount of pressure to practice by guidelines because you hear it 30 times a week—if you go to court, you can say 'I practice by guidelines.'" Such frequent references to legal liability affect the relationships between patients and their providers over time. One family practice physician said she has personally seen a breakdown of trust over the past 20 years of her practice: "Providers are worried about getting sued and it's really from both sides. Parents distrust the medical people and medical providers distrust their patients and it causes people to separate into sides. It's not like we're in this together." Such distrust is exacerbated by the protocols in hospitals that limit liability risk by compromising evidence-based care, such as prohibitions against laboring women moving or walking during labor or requirements for continuous fetal monitoring. ACOG and other professional organizations contribute to the problem by emphasizing liability avoidance over medical best practices. By one estimate, only around one-third of ACOG recommendations are based on the best-quality medical evidence, with many instead aimed at provider convenience or limiting liability.[88] At least some protocols to limit liability make medical errors or poor outcomes more likely, as in the case of routine continuous fetal monitoring.

Liability fears also create their own vicious cycle, influencing the standard of care, which in turn influences the liability environment. Breech vaginal deliveries, for example, once common, are now exceedingly rare. A maternal-fetal specialist argued that in order to understand why demedicalized options become less common, "we can't ignore the medical-legal context. If you look at the risks of [vaginal] breech deliveries, they're actually very low, but they're a little higher than a cesarean. So now since the standard is cesarean and if something happened [during a vaginal breech delivery] you would be in a bit of legal bind. How well could you justify doing the opposite of what everyone else is doing?" Because the standard for breech delivery is now cesarean section, few medical students receive any training in how to deliver a vaginal breech baby, even though, according to the maternal-fetal specialist, "the maneuvers to flip a breech baby are fairly similar between cesarean and vaginal. If you can do it in a cesarean incision you can do it vaginally." The risks of delivering a vaginal breech baby are higher now than they were 30 years ago, not because of anything inherent to breech deliveries themselves, but because the knowledge of how to appropriately manage such deliveries is gone. Not only does the current legal-medical standard of care affect practice in the moment, but it also eliminates options in the future as providers lose familiarity with demedicalized options, pulling patients and providers along toward greater levels of medicalization.

Risk in Community-Based Care

Community-based care, whether located in homes, birth centers, or hospices, changes the environment of risk because factors such as the character of the practitioners, the populations of patients, and the care setting itself lower levels of real and perceived risk, allowing providers to individualize care, which lowers risk even further. Unlike the vicious cycle of hospital liability fears, community-based providers benefit from a virtuous cycle of low risk perception and high levels of trust, which lowers medical and legal risks even further by increasing both communication and patient satisfaction. Birth centers and hospices cannot treat very complex patients precisely because their medical tools are limited by the very goals of supporting demedicalized birth and death. They also tend to attract providers who are drawn to demedicalized care and who, by both instinct and training, are less likely to resort to medicalized care. Because of the intensive one-on-one care each patient receives, both birth centers and hospices will necessarily treat a much lower volume of patients and many fewer complex patients. Finally, community-based providers are much less likely to experience lawsuits and prosecutions, owing again to the combination of closer relationships with patients, lower-risk patient populations, and less interaction with healthcare providers with different standards of care. The overall perception of how risky demedicalized birth and death are will be significantly different among community-based providers compared to their hospital-based counterparts.

This virtuous cycle protects providers in crucial ways that provide lessons for limiting liability even in other contexts. Anecdotal evidence, for example, suggests that midwives are sued much less frequently than obstetricians, owing at least in part to their more extensive relationships with the women they treat, honed over long prenatal appointments and hands-on human care during delivery. A nurse midwife who attends home births hypothesized that the nature of the relationship in decentralized care settings protects both providers and patients: "Honestly, very few midwives get sued because of the nature of the relationship we have with people. It's also nice to not have to follow the insurance company's requirement of 15-minute appointments. The hospital treats people like they don't trust them and so patients don't trust them either. When I get to know people, I can see their labs, I know their families, I can see how they're living at home, I can get a sense of their nutritional habits, etc., so it's that model of care that limits lawsuits." Research suggests that practitioners who communicate openly, who apologize for mistakes, and who ask for patient input and informed consent are less likely to be sued than practitioners who emphasize protocol and documentation.[89] Ironically, physicians and hospitals could immediately reduce their liability risk by being more forthcoming about explaining or apologizing for adverse events, such as informed consent violations, before patients feel forced to sue. Such a reform is, however, still at stark odds with the traditional advice of hospital legal teams and professional associations to avoid admitting fault.[90]

The insulation of community-based providers from liability fears improves outcomes as well. While community-based providers may be less aware of the aggregate risks of, say, an out-of-hospital VBAC, their perception more accurately reflects the actual risks each individual patient confronts. This lower standard of risk is also likely to be a more accurate assessment of both the real medical risks to patients and the real legal risks to providers. It is also a major reason why community-based care settings are better able to resist medicalizing birth and death than hospitals. The attitude toward care and the relationship providers have with their patients set up a mutually reinforcing cycle of trust where low perceived risk actually helps reduce liability risk by allowing practitioners to provide high-quality and individualized care. Hospital providers do not have this same freedom. Ironically, by downplaying both medical risk and liability risk, demedicalized providers reduce their vulnerability to both.

None of this means that liability concerns do not affect community-based care providers. Community-based care settings are limited by liability concerns not least because small-scale providers are increasingly overwhelmed by the rising cost of liability insurance. Insurance companies frequently fail to distinguish between the low-risk populations served by these settings and the more medically complex and legally riskier patients served by hospitals. Otherwise successful birth centers in many states face closure as a result of the current created by skyrocketing malpractice rates and low reimbursement rates from insurers. Malpractice insurance costs were the primary reason for the closure of the first US birthing center in Manhattan, despite excellent outcomes and low rate of lawsuits.[91] Some liability insurance policies privilege medicalized providers directly by excluding demedicalized options like VBAC from coverage.[92] Small providers are also threatened by the consolidation of insurance providers, as independent insurance companies that once provided malpractice coverage to birth centers, for example, are replaced by companies with links to a particular hospital or hospital center, creating potential conflicts of interest.[93]

Finally, liability concerns may prevent medical providers from collaborating with demedicalized providers, compromising patient care and encouraging medicalization. One direct-entry midwife noted in an interview, "It would be extremely helpful if I could have an OB who would monitor a minor risk; it would be wonderful to call a collaborating physician because this [issue during labor] could go either way, but it's really hard to do that because OBs don't want to work with midwives because it's a liability issue for them." Liability fears therefore prevent the collaboration between low-risk and high-risk providers that could keep many patients out of hospitals, furthering fragmentation of care.

While hospices face fewer of these concerns, malpractice concerns may be growing. The interdisciplinary nature of hospice and palliative care teams itself can create barriers in terms of malpractice coverage, which increases costs and creates barriers to finding medical directors. Doctors who serve as medical directors for hospices are sometimes only covered by hospice malpractice coverage for their administrative activities, leaving them vulnerable in the clinical sphere.[94] Contracting physicians must also be covered, and those who leave must be covered up to the statute of limitations, which ranges from 1 to 10 years depending on the state and when the harm was discovered. Recent attention to issues at some hospices, including cutting corners on care for complex patients, indicates an area of legal vulnerability for hospices that could escalate malpractice fears and increase costs.[95] For both birth centers and hospices, the combination of reimbursement rates that do not reflect the cost of care and malpractice insurance rates that do not reflect the actual level of legal risk makes it extremely difficult for community-based options to enter and stay in the market, even when the demand for them clearly exists. Hospitals, which tend to be favored both by Medicare and Medicaid policies and by agreements with malpractice insurance companies, are better able to absorb the costs associated with malpractice liability for this reason, another way in which patients end up in centralized care.

Conclusion

The tributary of risk, like the other policy tributaries, creates an undertow in the river of treatment options that pulls providers and patients toward centralized and therefore medicalized care. This tributary's force is even more powerful since the regulatory and reimbursement tributaries have washed away demedicalized alternatives along the shoreline. Once patients are channeled into hospitals, this risk undertow becomes a riptide. Hospitals, whose attempts to lessen legal risk heighten liability fears, inadvertently increase medical risk by prioritizing interventions and defensive documentation instead of evidence-based care and communication. Meanwhile, the tort system itself creates another powerful current as a result of biases in the trial process that make it easier to sue for undertreatment while failing to address the harms of overtreatment. Community-based providers' inability to absorb the costs of malpractice insurance owing to artificially low reimbursement rates completes the cycle of centralization. The combined effect of these three tributaries is a whirlpool of Charybdis proportions, inexorably pulling patients toward the highest intensity and most medicalized care.

Troublingly, traditional approaches to tort reform do not adequately address any of these concerns. Capping awards does little to curb defensive medical practices. State medical boards do little to provide accountability for overtreatment or medical errors. Neither addresses the incentives for overtreatment built into the hospital environment or the way in which that environment shapes the doctor-patient relationship. More foundationally, most tort reform proposals fail to address the harms caused by medical errors or the power imbalance between hospitals and patients that leaves trials as the only way for patients to find out what happened during treatment and why. And none of the most popular suggestions for malpractice reform take aim at the more subtle ways in which medicalization harms individuals at their most vulnerable, like laboring women and terminally ill patients. While traditional approaches to tort reform assume that the patients are the problem and that legal fixes like capping awards are the solution, any true reform must take into account the entirety of the healthcare watershed and the way in which centralization of care in hospitals increases the risks of errors and opens physicians and hospitals up to liability in the first place. I discuss potential reforms in the conclusion, but first, let's take a closer look at how medicalization harms the most vulnerable among us.

CHAPTER 7

Black Birth and Death in the Medicalized Rapids

You know why the blacks avoided the white doctors? Because, honey, they avoided the whites period. . . . And then they was treated so bad and so cold by the doctors. The doctors thought the black person was mostly too filthy for him to put his hands on. They talk to them just like they was a dog that didn't have human sense. They did not want that kinda treatment. They didn't deserve that kinda treatement. They didn't deserve that kinda treatment cause they were human beins.—*Onnie Lee Logan, granny midwife*

I think we all know that many doctors don't treat everybody the same. I think it is especially with African American people, it's like we don't know any better, so the doctor just thinks they can do whatever they think is best and don't give you all the options.
—Black caretaker of a terminally ill patient, from an ethnography of black experiences with hospice

THE SHAPE of the American healthcare watershed has particularly profound effects on the most vulnerable patients in the healthcare river, those with the fewest options and the most need for individualized care. Racial and ethnic minorities and low-income, disabled, and LGBTQ (lesbian, gay, bisexual, transgender, and queer) individuals are more likely to experience the paradox of medicalization than white individuals, suffering from high levels of intervention and a variety of harms. Many of these harms are due to the way poor communication, distrust of the medical system, and provider bias combine with centralized care in hospitals to standardize treatment and prevent preference-sensitive care. These disparities can be seen most clearly in the black community, as black Americans give birth and die in peculiarly medicalized ways. Black women have much higher rates of surgical birth and maternal and infant mortality than white women, even when controlling for poverty and other confounding factors. Black Americans are much more likely to die with high rates of intervention and have lower rates of hospice and palliative care use than white Americans. They are also more likely to die with uncontrolled pain and higher levels of disability. Not coincidentally, black Americans are also more likely to give birth and die in hospitals than white Americans.

The experiences of black Americans in the healthcare system are therefore illustrative of broader concerns about how the shape of the healthcare watershed prevents individualized care. They also demonstrate how the shape of the healthcare watershed contributes to unequal access and a variety of health disparities that challenge the bioethical commitment to justice. Not only is there a bias in the watershed toward those who can pay out of pocket for care, but it also biases treatment in peculiarly unequal ways, ways that harm those most vulnerable to that harm. The principle of justice does not require absolutely equal outcomes of medical care, which would be impossible for a variety of practical reasons, but it does require that harms and benefits of medical treatment are relatively equally dispersed and that some populations, particularly historically vulnerable populations, are not forced to absorb harms in the process of benefiting others.[1] As we shall see, the US medical system fails on those grounds alone. While this chapter focuses on the black American experience, the lessons of the chapter apply more broadly to the way the watershed creates harms for all birthing and dying Americans, escalates costs, and undermines our most foundational bioethical commitments.

Racial Disparities in Birth and Death

While the research on racial health disparities is both complicated and ongoing, recent research provides some clues for why medicalization disproportionately affects black Americans. Most obviously, black Americans are more likely to suffer from chronic illnesses like heart disease and diabetes than white Americans, which can cause complications during pregnancy and at the end of life that make interventions more likely.[2] The causes of those illnesses are, in turn, complex because they cannot be entirely explained by socioeconomic status, education, health behaviors, or genetic markers. Recent work suggests that heightened stress contributes to a "weathering" effect on minorities that makes them more vulnerable to chronic health problems, particularly high blood pressure and heart disease.[3] This stress is linked to what is known in the literature as "perceived racism," or the everyday experiences with what black individuals believe to be discriminatory or racist behavior and attitudes.[4] In addition to raising levels of chronic stress, the belief that one must navigate a constantly antagonistic world may contribute to distrust of the medical community, creating another barrier to care.

Heightened stress is also linked to socioeconomic differences, which explain part, but not all, of the health disparities black Americans face. Higher rates of poverty and greater use of Medicaid make it harder for minority Americans to find providers, particularly providers who are familiar with relevant cultural and religious variables that play an important role in medical decision making. Poverty, in turn, increases stress levels, which exacerbates a variety of conditions and increases the risk for complications that require intensive interventions. Yet disparities exist even while controlling for education level and socioeconomic status, suggesting that poverty alone cannot explain the heightened levels of stress black Americans face. The universality of daily experiences with racism and discriminatory practices may help explain why black Americans of all socioeconomic and education levels face greater health risks than similarly situated white Americans.[5]

While black Americans face unique health risks, their trust in medical providers has been undermined by the history of medical practice itself. As medicine marketed itself in the nineteenth and twentieth centuries as grounded in an objective and reductionist understanding of the world, this same scientific method of medicine was inextricably linked to and bound up with the scientific racism that held sway at the time. As physicians claimed superiority over folk healers as a consequence of their objective and scientific approach to the study of medicine, the very same physicians were using this "scientific" approach to justify racist and white supremacist beliefs, ostensibly supported by "objective" measures like skull size and shape and intelligence testing.[6] These same physicians and their professional associations lobbied for policies, including segregation and forced sterilization, that not only entailed horrific violations of individuals but also left a legacy of distrust of the motivations of physicians and medical providers in its wake. This distrust continues today, as poor communication and cultural differences stymie interactions between white providers and nonwhite patients.[7] While physicians interpret distrust of the medical system as a lack of medical literacy, evidence suggests that provider bias contributes to this continued distrust.[8] Distrust of medical providers may prevent black Americans from seeking care early in a pregnancy or illness. It may also affect their use of demedicalized providers, which patients with a background of discrimination are more likely to see as cost-cutting efforts than real initiatives to improve care.

The hospital environment aggravates this distrust. The isolation of maternity wards and intensive care units is especially damaging for individuals who rely heavily on strong social networks and religious communities for support. The lack of consistent caregivers in hospitals can make communication more difficult, resulting in both higher levels of stress and care less likely to be aligned with patient wishes.[9] The cultural and individual import of birth and death makes cultural expectations particularly relevant, yet such factors are more likely to be misunderstood or neglected in the hospital environment.[10] One study found that black Americans are more likely to report a lack of respect for their preferences in hospitals than white patients, which can have profound impacts on birth and end-of-life decisions.[11]

Evidence suggests that this distrust is rooted in more than mere perception. Research across healthcare contexts suggests that provider bias is common and manifests itself in a variety of ways. Black Americans in the ER are triaged differently than white patients with the same complaint, resulting in longer wait times.[12] Black stroke patients had longer waiting times in the ER than white patients, increasing their risk for serious complications later.[13] Providers consistently underestimate the pain levels of black patients.[14] Overall, research suggests that black patients are less likely to be taken seriously and their preferences more likely to be overlooked or overridden by hospital staff than white patients.

In birth and death, these patterns of distrust and bias generate seemingly contradictory patterns in care, with black Americans more likely to get medically unnecessary interventions in the hospital and more likely to have poor outcomes than their white counterparts. Hospital-based care produces the paradoxical outcomes of overtreatment and worse outcomes for minority patients because of the mismatch between a population with unique social, cultural, religious, and medical needs and the standardized care hospitals must provide. This mismatch limits communication, creates distrust between patients and providers, and can even drive minority patients out of the healthcare system altogether.

While centralized care serves minority patients less well than other kinds of care, minority patients are even more likely to end up in hospitals at the beginning and end of life than white patients are. Black Americans are more likely to give birth and die in hospitals than white Americans, and they have fewer decentralized options available to them. The dearth of nonhospital options has its roots in historical events that shaped the healthcare watershed itself and is compounded by current regulatory pressures and demographic realities. In particular, the elimination of traditional caregivers like granny midwives and black physicians in the early twentieth century led to lower access to high-quality primary care and a lack of black providers. Higher poverty rates, themselves the result of discriminatory policies over the past century, mean that black Americans tend to rely more heavily on public insurance like Medicaid than white Americans, insurance that is less likely to cover out-of-hospital care. All these factors, combined with geographic and transportation limitations, increase the likelihood that black Americans will be cared for in hospitals.[15]

Race and Birth

Racial disparities in health begin at birth. Black Americans have the worst maternal and infant outcomes in the United States. Black women are three to four times more likely than white women to die or have serious complications after birth.[16] In New York City, black mothers die at 12 times the rate of white mothers. Black infants nationwide die at almost twice the rate of the United States as a whole. Black women have the highest rate of preterm birth of any group in the United States (11.1 percent of all births compared to 6.9 among white women). Black mothers also experience the highest rate of cesarean section in low-risk births (29.9%) of any racial or ethnic group, which places both mothers and infants at greater risk for complications and poor health outcomes, particularly in later births.[17] Black mothers have some of the most medically intensive care, at least in terms of surgical or induced births, and the worst outcomes.

Black mothers are also more likely to die from complications that black mothers and white mothers are equally likely to face, like hemorrhage. In fact, many of the major causes of maternal mortality are experienced by white women and black women at the same rate, but black women are two to three times more likely to die from them.[18] Explanations for this higher rate of mortality include lower rates of prenatal care, higher rates of other complicating conditions, lower access to medical care, and lower quality of medical care when accessed.[19] Some conditions like preeclampsia can have lifelong effects, including increased risk of heart disease later in life.[20] Complications during pregnancy do not end with delivery, sometimes compromising health for years and even lowering life expectancy.

Some of these disparities are explained by the fact that black mothers are, on average, less healthy than white mothers. Some have attributed this to the effects of greater rates of poverty among black Americans, though the same patterns are not found in Hispanic mothers with the same poverty level. The weathering effect of stress on the body is particularly relevant during pregnancy, when the body is both under stress and more sensitive to stress. Black mothers report high levels of stress associated with workplace discrimination and fears for their children in what they perceive to be a racist society.[21] Whether such discrimination actually exists matters less than the fact that the perception alone has powerful effects on stress levels and health. Perceived racism has also been linked to hypertension, with researchers concluding that perceived discrimination increases stress levels and also deters black women from seeking medical care.[22] Maternal stress impacts infants as well, with research linking stress to both high blood pressure and preterm birth, all of which are also associated with lower birth weight in black babies. Low birth weight puts infants at risk for a variety of health problems, including increased risk of death in the first year.[23] Education and high income reduce, but do not eliminate, these various risks. Black college graduates still die during childbirth at rates comparable to white women who have never graduated high school.

The link between preterm birth and stress is compelling but not yet wholly accepted. The causal story is complex, since many of the variables at play overlap. Black women have higher levels of complex health issues than white women. Moreover, stress is linked to education level and workplace stability, so it is difficult to untangle discrimination, for example, from other stressors. At the same time, commonly cited risk factors for preterm birth such as drug use, smoking, and some other stressors are actually more common among white women than black women.[24] Black women may, however, be exposed to environmental toxins like lead at greater levels than white women, which can increase the risk of preterm birth.[25] While some research has shown genetic links to preterm birth, the research is still unclear. According to one analysis, race alone explains only about 4 percent of the difference between white and black rates of preterm birth, while other factors such as income level, education, and access to prenatal care explain more.[26]

Aside from risk factors, black women may be more vulnerable to over-treatment and unnecessary treatment during birth. Black women are somewhat more likely to receive cesarean sections than white women, and racial disparities were the greatest among the lowest-risk women, indicating that medical need is not driving the increase.[27] One analysis found evidence that black women were less likely to have medically necessary cesareans and more likely to have medically unnecessary cesareans than their white counterparts.[28] Some have argued that these patterns come from a lack of trust between minority patients and white providers and an overall lack of power within the system. Black patients, who are more likely to rely on Medicaid to pay for pregnancy and birth than white women, are less likely to have a choice of providers and less able to "fire" providers who are not providing quality care.[29]

Patients of color are also more likely to experience coercive treatments and disrespectful behavior than white patients. While the case of Angela Carder—a white, terminally ill woman forced to undergo a court-ordered cesarean section—made headlines in 1987, a *New England Journal of Medicine* article published the same year found that 86 percent of patients who underwent court-ordered cesarean sections were black, Hispanic, or Asian.[30] Hospital environment played an important role in that all the patients in the sample were treated at teaching hospitals or were on public assistance, making them much more vulnerable to coercive interventions. At the same time, black women are more likely to be tested for drugs during pregnancy and are, by some estimates, as much as 10 times more likely to be reported to Child Protective Services than white women, even though the rate of drug use among both populations is similar.[31]

Hospital providers, who often lack previous relationships with patients, may rely on heuristics about patient populations, contributing to health disparities by stereotyping black patients or those on public assistance. Qualitative research on the experiences of women of color found that disrespectful and discriminatory experiences were common and added to the stress pregnant women are already under.[32] One black home birth midwife recalled in an interview that when she brought a black mother in labor into a local hospital for pain relief, the physician on call asked the laboring mother twice about her plans for birth control, before she had even given birth. The midwife finally told the doctor, "She doesn't need to talk about birth control; she hasn't pushed out the baby she has." The midwife believed that the physician's questions were a stereotyped response because the laboring woman was black, looked young, and was on Medicaid (but was in fact a graduate student). She also argued that "those little microaggressions weighing on you consistently is just a lot" for pregnant women to handle.

Such experiences fuel distrust of providers that, in turn, can prevent black women from seeking prenatal or postpartum care. In general, black women access prenatal care later than their white counterparts. In addition to fears of biased care, reasons include difficulty finding providers who take Medicaid in their area, less flexible schedules due to juggling multiple jobs, less access to reliable transportation, and significant stressors related to work, finances, and partners. Black women are also less likely to continue prenatal care regularly, with some evidence suggesting that black women respond to perceived discrimination in their prenatal visits by refusing to return.[33] Some reforms have helped, including managed care models, home visits, group-based prenatal care, and other community-based approaches. It is no accident that the approaches that have the most impact are those that individualize care, focusing on individual women and adapting care to the unique variables in their daily lives. In contrast, simply expanding the number of practitioners in a given area does not seem to have a significant effect on either outcomes or the number of women who access care.[34]

While black women, owing to higher rates of poverty and discrimination, face unique stressors when accessing care, hospitals inadvertently increase these difficulties. Maternity wards are impersonal, often staffed largely by white providers, and limit the number of visitors or support people, isolating patients during vulnerable times. The social isolation and patterns of bias in hospitals may increase distrust of providers and lead to higher levels of stress in patients. Black women also give birth at a relatively small number of hospitals, which have a high concentration of black patients. Research has shown that hospitals that primarily serve black patients have higher levels of mortality and morbidity than hospitals that primarily serve white women. Black women who give birth at majority white hospitals have better outcomes than black women who give birth at majority black hospitals, and white women who give birth at majority black hospitals have higher mortality and morbidity than white women who give birth at majority white hospitals.[35]

While it is not yet clear precisely what causes these disparities, some suggestions are a combination of provider-, system-, and patient-level errors. Some kinds of standardization of care, including checklists and team trainings for serious health emergencies like hemorrhage and blood clots, can help women at risk.[36] Addressing structural characteristics such as the presence of specialists who treat complex patients and high-quality neonatal units for premature infants can also help. Many of these reforms, however, do little to address the reasons black women and their infants are at higher risk for complications in the first place. Training in better communication with diverse patient populations, diversifying support staff, and addressing implicit bias can help improve both patient experience and outcomes.[37] As one black home birth midwife put it, "I love being a black woman. . . . It brings a richness and a knowing to your experience that you're just not going to get from another care provider." This experiential knowledge can be particularly important during the emotionally and physically vulnerable time of pregnancy and birth.

Race and Decentralized Birth

Black American birth was not always centralized in hospitals. In the eighteenth and nineteenth centuries, black Americans were excluded almost entirely from mainstream medical care, so informal traditional midwifery was the main mode of giving birth. Black women gave birth with "granny" midwives, women who had learned their craft through an apprenticeship model that began with the first importation of black midwives on slave ships in 1619. Granny midwives had impressive safety records, rarely losing a mother or a baby. Because they served a population with little money or resources, granny midwives were largely ignored during the initial wave of professionalization of medicine. As a result, black birth remained decentralized well into the twentieth century.[38]

This benign neglect changed in the 1920s. The Sheppard-Towner Act of 1921 established prenatal and children's health centers while also increasing the training available to traditional midwives, training most midwives welcomed enthusiastically.[39] Initially, the policy focused on providing basic training in hygiene and emergency techniques to traditional black midwives, who used their training not only to safely deliver babies but also to provide comprehensive care to low-income rural black families.[40] While the early stages of the policy emphasized and supported the traditional self-help networks within black communities, over time the policy focus shifted to emphasize nurse midwives with formal medical training. As professionalization of medicine spread even to rural areas and standardization of care became a major policy goal, escalating restrictions on granny midwives throughout the 1930s all but destroyed traditional black midwifery in the South.[41] Despite efforts to train black nurse midwives, the structural racism that prevailed during Jim Crow excluded most black women from accessing formal education, and those who did succeed in becoming nurse midwives faced official discrimination that excluded them from membership in professional midwifery organizations and limited their access to hospitals, patients, and even housing.[42]

As a result, in 1920 there were as many as 5,000 black midwives in Georgia alone, but by 2002 there were just 15.[43] Today just 8 percent of black women use midwives for labor and delivery today, a sharp contrast to the 50 percent of black births still attended by midwives in the 1950s.[44] Black midwives continue to be an anomaly, with over 90 percent of nurse midwives self-reporting their race as white.[45] One direct-entry black midwife pointed out the way this disparity operates today: "There's also racism in midwifery. Midwifery care is better than obstetrical care in my opinion, but midwifery is also a ridiculously white profession. So a lot of the issues you deal with in obstetrics you also deal with in midwifery. We had a whole midwifery conference on health disparities and it was the lowest attended conference we had ever had." White midwives, just like white physicians, may be unaware of the needs of black patients, may harbor their own damaging biases about black mothers, or may simply not have adequate training in dealing with the effects of perceived racism and discrimination on pregnant women. That ignorance can compromise care.

Perhaps unsurprisingly, the shift toward formal medical care did not and has not resulted in better outcomes for black mothers and their babies. Even in the 1930s, as physicians were working to limit access to midwives, disparities between physician and midwife births were clear. In Alabama, for example, one historian found that "doctors attended three-fourths of the women who died in childbirth in 1933."[46] While these deaths were frequently blamed on the mothers themselves in official paperwork, state medical boards recognized that these deaths were likely caused by poor physician training, indifference, or both.

The disappearance of the black midwife represented not just a loss of competent providers but also the loss of individualized culturally competent care that addressed every part of a black woman's life. Granny midwives provided prenatal care in the home, helped with other children, did laundry while mothers were on bed rest, and helped organize other modes of social support for pregnant women and new mothers.[47] They saw midwifery as a religious calling, and the traditions of black midwifery were heavily rooted in the black community's focus on faith and family. Granny midwives emphasized care for the mother, inadvertently treating the very stress that evidence suggests is a danger to black mothers today.[48] Midwives also provided care physicians wouldn't, care that was crucial to helping new mothers navigate motherhood in an impoverished environment. Onnie Lee Logan, an Alabama granny midwife whose career spanned decades, described the activities her mother engaged in as a midwife when out on calls: "Mother would do whatever needs to be done. Sometime she would get the house all cleaned up. Mother all settled and baby all settled. See the doctor's not go'n bathe that baby, not go'n dress that baby or nothin like that. That's go'n be the midwife."[49] Midwives were known to make clothing for new babies while the mother was in labor, provide care in their own homes for premature babies for weeks or months at a time, and even adopt babies they delivered when maternal death or homelessness left infants vulnerable.[50] Black midwives were also some of the only trained providers at the time who rejected the prevailing racist stereotypes of black women as little better than animals, stereotypes that had profound effects on the kind of medical care providers offered, as we shall see.[51]

Midwives also had enormous influence in their communities and played a crucial role in educating families about hygiene and childcare, including teaching pregnant women how to sterilize clothing and cloth pads for labor and how to arrange safe sleeping locations for new babies.

They also guided black families toward more formal medical care as local governments embraced community-based clinics for prenatal and maternity care throughout the 1920s.[52] The care they provided was individualized, community based, rooted in the culture and traditions of black Americans, and comprehensive, a powerful counter to the racist and reductionist view of rural black Americans that prevailed at the time.[53] Ironically, as midwifery came under increasing scrutiny from professional medical associations, its very strength became seen as a weakness. According to one historian, "the attention to the personal, individual needs of a woman was interpreted as a sign of primitive care. Rigid order and procedure were valued more highly than flexibility and adaptability to specific needs."[54] As formal medical control over birth gained traction, standardization became the norm, and the unique needs of black women were deemphasized in favor of procedural rigor.

Standardization became more problematic as black women moved to hospitals to give birth. As the midwife and historian Jenny Luke points out, black wards and hospitals were actively dangerous places for patients. She quotes one survey in the 1930s that found some hospitals "so filthy and inadequately equipped and managed that one would hesitate to take a drink of water in them, much less submit to even the most minor surgical procedure."[55] Intervention rates were high and maternal mortality staggering.[56] The care was typically "impersonal and mechanized," but even the standardization of hospitals did not apply equally to black patients, with black mothers routinely denied privacy, pain relief, and other care standard for white patients.[57] Even more disturbing, the move to formalized medical care left black women vulnerable to medical tools wielded by racist physicians. In one county in Mississippi, physicians performed postpartum hysterectomies on 60 percent of the black women who delivered there without their knowledge, a procedure common enough to have the nickname "Mississippi Appendectomy."[58]

The limits of hospital-based care continue to challenge black women's health and autonomy today, and recent interest in racial disparities in birth has provoked black women to share their experiences giving birth in hospitals. In 2018 tennis champion Serena Williams detailed her experience directing her own treatment for life-threatening blood clots after medical staff failed to take her breathing concerns seriously.[59] Her account inspired widespread social media commentary by black women sharing their own stories of hospital-based care. On various social media forums, black women described hospital-based birth as traumatic and dehumanizing. Many reported believing that their access to adequate pain control and other medications was restricted based on their race, and many reported struggling to convince staff to take their medical needs seriously. Some described life-threatening complications that resulted from delays in care. In 2019 in *Time*, academic and author Tressie McMillan Cottom described the avoidable death of her premature daughter, recounting how despite seeking medical care over multiple days for bleeding and rectal pain and being told that her symptoms were normal, a nurse nevertheless blamed Cottom for her baby's death after she went into premature labor. She attributed the rejection of her concerns to widespread views of black women as incompetent. As a married black professor, she notes that "all of my status characteristics screamed 'competent,' but nothing could shut down what my blackness screams when I walk into the room."[60] One consistent theme in all these accounts is that black women do not trust hospital-based care but also feel trapped by limited options and the lack of alternatives.

As a response to these failures and the corresponding crisis of maternal and infant mortality facing black families, grassroots interest in community-based birthing care, particularly midwifery, for black women is growing.[61] The number of black-owned birth centers in urban areas is increasing, and a number of formal and informal initiatives are working to increase the number of black healthcare and birth workers, including groups like the Black Mamas Matter Alliance, Black Women Birthing Justice, SisterSong, and the Black Doulas Association, among many others.[62] The growth of social media has made it easier to connect with like-minded birth workers across the United States, allowing black birth workers to connect and share strategies for growth.

Black birth workers differ from white birth workers in seeing their profession as dual pronged: to save lives while also addressing racial health disparities in birth. One study found that many black birth providers linked their interest in birth care to a broader interest in recreating the tradition of granny midwives that had been destroyed by state regulations. Many in the study also argued that individualized care had positively impacted their own birth experiences and that they wanted to engage in birth work to share that experience with other women.[63] A strong strain of activism exists among black birth workers, many of whom see themselves not just as providing care for individual women but as confronting what they see as systemic biases and entrenched racism within the American healthcare system.[64] Many black birth workers view midwifery and birth care as both an act of resistance and an alternative mode of healthcare delivery, much like the holistic and comprehensive role of granny midwives in the past.

The very structure of midwifery individualizes care, addressing both holistic needs and complex health concerns.[65] Midwives center their practice around longer prenatal appointments—up to an hour long—that can uncover and address lifestyle and environmental issues that affect pregnancy outcomes, including stress, domestic violence, nutrition, and chronic illness. In these appointments, in addition to addressing medical needs, midwives emphasize relaxation practices to reduce stress during pregnancy and help manage labor pains, which may help women handle stress in other areas of life, including the stress associated with perceived racism and discrimination. A focus on individual empowerment within these meetings encourages women to ask questions of providers and play a partnering role in their care, which research has shown improves outcomes.[66] Perhaps most crucially, evidence suggests that midwifery care and the close relationships midwives have with patients foster higher levels of trust between patients and providers than exists in obstetrics.[67] In an article on black midwives in Los Angeles, one black woman described midwifery care after a traumatic hospital birth: "'At my first appointment, they just wanted to get to know me. That was such a shock, to just put the paperwork aside,' she says. 'That's not what you get at the hospital. It's procedure. It's routine. They stick you. They poke you. You don't feel like a person.'"[68] Evidence suggests that midwifery care produces better outcomes and experiences for minority patients than traditional obstetrics and hospital-based care precisely because it allows providers to individualize care and fosters trust. As a black midwife noted in an interview, "We get to know the person, we hear their experiences, and a lot of it is what's happening in their lives, not just fetal heart tones and blood pressure. We treat all parts of a person's life. We work with women on every part of their lives. . . . Just being heard and being seen eliminates a lot of the stressors."

Other community-based approaches include doulas aimed at black mothers, such as the Birthing Beautiful Communities initiative in Cleveland, Ohio, which works to address high rates of infant mortality in urban Cleveland communities. The group provides extensive prenatal care, support, and parenting classes.[69] One requirement of the program is that doulas live in the communities in which they work, in order to enhance understanding of the lives of the women they are assisting.[70] Other programs, such as CenteringPregnancy, a national initiative, provide prenatal care to vulnerable populations in a group format so that women can address issues in their lives in a supportive environment. Prenatal visits are over an hour long, meaning that women have a longer window in which to ask questions and discuss concerns with providers than they would in an individual format. Other options include "maternal homes," community-based clinics that aim to address the constellation of issues pregnant women face with trained case managers who are usually from the community. Many of these programs also focus on postpartum care, providing breastfeeding and parenting classes, as well as links to other services like housing and continuing education. Early research on such initiatives is positive, suggesting that a comprehensive approach to care can reduce the number of preterm births, increase breastfeeding initiation and continuation, reduce risk of postpartum depression, reduce HIV transmission to infants, and help control gestational diabetes.[71]

Interest in birth centers specifically is growing as a way to improve outcomes for black mothers and their babies by providing a holistic and preference-oriented approach to prenatal, birth, and postpartum care. The number of birth centers in urban areas is slowly growing, including some targeted at providing black women with black providers who are trained to meet the needs of expecting black mothers.[72] Midwifery care in a birth center is associated with lower rates of interventions, lower rates of preterm births, and higher birth weights for low-income and black women and their babies.[73] Scholars studying the benefits of midwifery care for minority patients hypothesize that outcomes, particularly those related to stress, are better for minority patients in birth centers because birth center care allows for "highly individualized prenatal care delivered in a culturally relevant and comfortable environment."[74] For black mothers in particular, birth center care results in fewer cesarean sections, lower likelihood of preterm birth, and higher infant birth weight, all while lowering costs compared to hospital birth.[75]

Despite these benefits, community-based and midwifery care is even less accessible to black women than it is to the general population. Medicaid limitations on midwifery and birth center care and low reimbursement rates for care limit many birth centers to suburbs where a wealthier clientele can pay out of pocket. Black women are also more likely to be uninsured than their white counterparts and more likely to live in urban environments. Even seemingly minor policies such as the Medicare requirement that ambulances only deliver patients to hospitals contribute to centralization of care since women living in urban areas are less likely to have access to reliable transportation and rely more heavily on ambulances when in labor.[76] The combination of these variables makes it more likely that black women will give birth in hospitals with high rates of interventions, poor outcomes, and coercive experiences. Improving access will require reshaping the tributaries that limit black women's options, including reimbursement limitations and legal and liability barriers.

Race and Death

Racial disparities also affect patient experiences and outcomes at the end of life. Despite higher rates of cancer and chronic illnesses, black Americans are less likely to have access to palliative care or hospice and less likely to use them when they have access to them. Black patients are more likely than white patients to die in hospital ICUs, and their pain tends to be less controlled at the end of life.[77] In one study of ICU use, nonwhite patients were less likely to have a Do Not Resuscitate order or living will, more likely to die on life support, and more likely to have conflicts between family members or between the patient and clinicians about end-of-life goals.[78] Another study found "strikingly greater use of life-sustaining interventions" in Hispanic and black patients dying in ICUs compared to white patients.[79] Higher levels of interventions are one major reason for higher healthcare costs among minority patients at the end of life. Despite high rates of interventions, black patients with pain are less likely to receive adequate pain control compared to white patients, even those with painful conditions like cancer.[80] The same combination of overtreatment and undertreatment found at birth is also found at death.

Explanations for these patterns are various and complex. Some of these differences stem from the way the black experience with the medical system has shaped current attitudes. Distrust of the medical profession is high in black communities, a legacy of both the infamous Tuskegee experiment and segregated medical care. Structural racism in healthcare spanned much of the twentieth century and helped shape the black experience with medical care as one in which black Americans' well-being was firmly secondary to other goals. One study found that the Tuskegee experiment alone lowered life expectancy among black males by as much as 1.5 years, presumably owing to avoidance of medical professionals after the experiment was disclosed.[81] Distrust, combined with higher rates of poverty, limits black Americans' access to primary care, which disrupts doctor-patient relationships, preventing early discussions about end-of-life options. Lack of a relationship with a trusted medical professional may make black Americans much less comfortable discussing end-of-life options, especially those involving withholding treatment. The black experience of being consistently denied access to lifesaving medical innovations by white gatekeepers also explains why black Americans indicate high levels of trust in medical innovations alongside high levels of distrust of medical providers and policy makers. Black Americans are also more likely than white Americans to hold religious beliefs about death, including the prevalence of miracles, that support high-intensity care at the end of life.[82] These factors have real-world consequences for the way black Americans think about disease and treatments. As an example, one study found that black cancer patients are much more likely than white cancer patients to misunderstand their prognosis and to believe that chemotherapy would cure their disease, when in fact it would only extend life for a few months.[83]

Provider bias also influences the care that black Americans receive at the end of life and, as such, reinforces the distrust black Americans feel toward providers. One study found that about half of white medical students and residents in an experiment espoused incorrect beliefs about biological differences between black people and white people, such as the belief that black people feel less pain than white people. These beliefs in turn affected the recommendations residents were likely to make for treating pain.[84] Other research finds that providers consistently underestimate the pain severity of minority patients.[85] Some bias is subtle but has important implications for end-of-life care. One study found that physicians have fewer positive nonverbal encounters with dying black patients than with white patients. While the content of communication was similar in conversations with patients of different races, nonverbal interactions such as touch and facial expression were less positive with black patients. The researchers posited that such nonverbal cues could encourage families to choose more aggressive care because they distrust the recommendations providers offer.[86] Other forms of bias stem from ignorance. Since most physicians are white, they may not understand the unique way in which religion, community, and family interact in decision making about end-of-life decisions for many black patients. Failure to understand the full context in which decisions are made limits the ways doctors communicate with black Americans about treatment options.[87]

The combination of provider bias and patient distrust is likely to be higher in hospitals owing to the limits on communication and less familiarity with patients. At the same time, black Americans are more likely to receive care in hospitals than white Americans and, interestingly, are more likely to rate that care positively, perhaps because they see interventions as a sign of high-quality care.[88] Black Americans are also almost twice as likely as white Americans to be hospitalized at the end of life.[89] One study of nursing home patients found that black patients were less likely to have DNR orders and advance directives than white patients and were also more likely to end up with feeding tubes than white patients. These findings are consistent both with black American preferences for life-sustaining care and with institutional factors that contribute to overtreatment. While the study did not find differences in hospitalization at the end of life among blacks and whites in the same facility, researchers did find dramatic differences in hospitalization rates among patients across facilities. In particular, patients in majority black nursing homes were far more likely to die in hospitals and far less likely to use hospice than patients of any race in majority white nursing homes. The authors hypothesize that these patterns can be explained in part by the incentives nursing homes have under Medicare and Medicaid policies to hospitalize patients and prevent them from moving to the lower-reimbursed hospice rate and in part by the lower quality of end-of-life care in nursing homes where black patients are more likely to end up.[90] Majority black nursing homes are also more likely to serve a large Medicaid population, which may influence end-of-life care, particularly in the way incentives for dual-eligible patients —those who receive both Medicare and the Medicaid nursing home benefit—align. Whatever the complex causes, black Americans are more likely to receive intensive hospital care and less likely to receive hospice care at the end of life.[91]

As in birth, the centralization of care for black Americans at the end of life began with a series of policy decisions in the early 1900s and was solidified by the desegregation of hospitals in the 1960s. One response to segregation was to build hospitals in black communities where black practitioners could practice, and in the early days of Jim Crow, dying black patients (those who made it to hospitals at all) were cared for in segregated hospitals or wards.[92] Black practitioners, meanwhile, were limited to practicing in their own communities by state law and American Medical Association policies.[93] Both black patients and black providers were carefully segregated from mainstream white hospitals. While these hospitals were admittedly severely under-resourced, they offered care by culturally competent providers in the communities in which black patients lived.[94]

As in the case of midwifery, the growth of grassroots black-oriented medical care was halted by public policies that aimed to standardize and professionalize medicine. The Flexner Report of 1910, whose goal was to standardize medical practice and make the profession more scientifically grounded, recommended the closure of many minority-run medical schools and increased barriers to medical education, which dramatically reduced the numbers of minority doctors in practice. As older black physicians retired and died, there were no trained physicians to replace them. While Abraham Flexner discussed the importance of improving care for black patients, his emphasis was on the threat black Americans posed as "a potential source of infection and contagion."[95] Improving black healthcare was secondary to protecting white health. As a result of the changes spurred by the Flexner Report, there were proportionally fewer black physicians in the 1970s than in the 1940s.[96]

Counterintuitively, desegregation made this situation worse. The closing of black hospitals and integration with white hospitals harmed black communities by removing black doctors from practice, since the AMA did not require hospitals and medical schools to desegregate staff until a decade after *Brown v. Board of Education* was decided in 1954. Black doctors could not practice in many hospitals, even the newly desegregated ones, and fewer black doctors overall were trained as a result of discriminatory policies in medical schools and professional associations.[97] The closure of black hospitals meant fewer hospital-based practitioners with the cultural competence to treat black patients, as well as fewer physicians overall in black communities. According to an Institute of Medicine report, the closure of these hospitals "meant a loss of geographic convenience and accessibility to care, a sense of safety with known institutions, and a loss of a major source of employment within the community."[98] As a result of all these changes, black Americans were more likely to receive routine care in relatively anonymous desegregated hospitals and clinics, rather than in private offices with a primary care provider, because black physicians could no longer rely on attending patients in hospitals to support their community practices.[99]

Today, black patients receive peculiarly centralized care in that not only do they receive more care from hospitals but they also tend to receive more care from a small number of hospitals. In one study, just 5 percent of hospitals treated 45 percent of elderly black patients.[100] While the study found only minor differences in the quality of care provided by these high-minority-serving hospitals (unlike in maternity care, where the disparities were larger), more research needs to be done on end-of-life care, including whether high-minority-serving hospitals are more or less likely to have palliative care teams and how staff at these hospitals communicate with seriously ill patients about end-of-life options. Some evidence shows that black Americans receive better care from more diverse hospitals, perhaps reflecting greater staff awareness of the needs of minority patients, though that research did not touch on end-of-life options.[101] Broadly speaking, black Americans are more likely to die in hospitals but are less satisfied with the quality of care and quality of communication at the end of life.[102] Troublingly, some research suggests that conversations between black patients and their providers are less likely to result in care that is aligned with their wishes than similar conversations with whites.[103] Black patients are more likely to get unnecessary interventions, less likely to receive adequate pain management, and more likely to express distrust in the quality of their care. At the same time, they express greater trust in the role of medical interventions at the end of life. Black Americans are, whatever the causes, more likely to experience medicalized death than their white counterparts.

Many of the same cultural and social pressures that lead to aggressive care at the end of life serve to turn black patients and their families away from hospice and palliative care. Black patients are much less likely to use hospice than their white counterparts, despite being more likely to suffer from cancer, heart disease, and stroke, the most common illnesses among hospice patients.[104] Black patients may not have a trusting relationship with a primary care doctor who can adequately explain what hospice care is and what its benefits are. A strong orientation toward family and community and misunderstandings about who provides hospice care can lead black families to see hospice as a rejection of the community duty to care for one's own.[105] The strength of extended family connections can, counterintuitively, complicate conversations about care. As one palliative care nurse practitioner explained, "[With black patients] you are much more likely to walk into a room with siblings and cousins and aunts and second cousins," all of whom feel an obligation to participate in medical decision making for their loved one. Providers may acquiesce to the desires of the family member who wants the most aggressive interventions simply because consensus on limiting or withdrawing treatment is difficult to achieve with so many stakeholders.

Ethnographic reports from black American hospice patients highlight how informal communication within the community limits access to hospice. Word of mouth plays an important role in black patients' willingness to follow physician suggestions. These interviews also highlight many of the structural barriers black Americans believe they face in healthcare, such as lack of early diagnosis, physicians who fail to discuss the full range of options, and a general unfamiliarity with the healthcare system as a result of previous lack of access. As one black hospice patient in the study pointed out, "I think you have a lot of Black folks who wouldn't have a doctor they trusted enough to allow that person to put them in hospice."[106] The current generation of elderly black Americans may be particularly resistant to hospice owing to the combination of memories of segregated medical facilities, belief that they cannot afford hospice care, distrust of physicians' intentions, and the habit, entrenched in many older minority communities, of taking care of themselves rather than seeking out care in what can be seen as "white" healthcare environments.[107] One participant summed up her thoughts by saying, "Well, I'm gonna tell you what I'd always been told about hospice. Hospice doesn't care about the patient; they are only there for the patient to just let them die and not take care of them."[108]

The structure of the Medicare Hospice Benefit compounds these concerns, particularly its requirement that patients not seek curative treatment. Some black Americans report being concerned that they are forgoing treatment as a cost-cutting measure rather than seeing hospice as legitimate and high-quality care.[109] This requirement also conflicts with the views of some black Americans that medical interventions themselves constitute high-quality care. As a result, the MHB may disproportionately harm black patients by increasing distrust and inadvertently encouraging unnecessary and harmful care among a population that is already poorly served by the medical community. A hospice patient in one study made this concern explicit, arguing, "One of the things I never understood is why does a person have to choose if they can go to a hospice or keeping getting better. I think one thing you'll see is among Black folks that there is a strong will, I mean a real strong feeling that you can't be giving up the fight."[110] Palliative care providers are particularly likely to be viewed with suspicion in this framework, with many reporting that black patients often view referrals to palliative care as physicians simply giving up on black patients.

Suspicion of the motives of providers and the incentives within the healthcare system therefore directly influence black Americans' decisions about end-of-life care. Black Americans interviewed by the *New York Times*, for example, expressed concern that advance directives are a way to limit insurance coverage for interventions. They seemed to view these documents as another way that their care can be limited and conscribed rather than as a way for their preferences to be recorded and respected.[111] In an interview, a palliative care nurse practitioner recalled one black family with whom she was discussing end-of-life options: "They were very polite, but they made it clear that they thought I was trying to save the hospital money by taking their relative off the ventilator." Perhaps as a result of the combination of poorly structured policies, patient distrust, and poor provider communication, that nurse practitioner said that "the most challenging family meetings we have [as palliative care teams] are with African American families."

A variety of initiatives may help break down some of these barriers. Some involve changing hospital protocol, while others involve decentralizing care altogether. Many hospices have focused on marketing that aligns more closely with black American values, including emphasizing the role family members play in caregiving in the hospice model, the ability to stay at home close to family and spiritual centers, and the role of chaplains and religious figures in the interdisciplinary hospice care team.[112] Role models and stories from black American hospice patients about their experiences can also change attitudes.[113] Training healthcare providers to have conversations that emphasize how hospice and palliative care can help meet the unique needs of minority patients may also reduce resistance.[114] Other initiatives have emphasized the importance of home-based palliative care teams that both help families navigate end-of-life decision making and ensure that goals of care are consistent across care locations.[115] One study found that an emphasis on patient education and support to keep patients at home and avoid hospitalizations increased hospice rates among black Americans specifically.[116] Finally, in-hospital practices such as providing palliative care consults to all seriously ill patients can increase the chances that minority patients fill out advance directives, which can help limit conflict where large extended families are concerned, a common problem in minority end-of-life care.[117]

Movement has been slower at the grassroots level, perhaps because, unlike midwifery, hospice does not have strong traditional roots in the black community. Some of the resistance may be because black Americans still see hospice as a service created by and offered by whites, rather than coming from the black community itself.[118] The resistance is even greater to relatively new supports like death doulas. A black death doula and end-of-life planner said in an interview that black Americans still see "death doula" as a "fancy white lady term." She also noted that reimbursement limitations mean that she cannot bill insurance, a serious barrier for low-income families. Still, there are some areas of growth. Black families that have had good experiences with hospice are now speaking out in their churches to counter the fears many members of their community have. In some limited cases, pastors and other religious leaders have tried to clarify the religious teachings at stake in refusing aggressive care at the end of life and to encourage conversations about goals of care between family members. The *New York Times* described how one family's positive experience with hospice inspired the wives of black pastors in Upstate New York to encourage discussions of advanced care planning among their congregations.[119] The death doula noted that she is now seeing more black clients seeking end-of-life planning services as well. Word of mouth may be the most powerful driver of change in the community.

As with birth, however, the healthcare watershed creates powerful currents that make hospice access difficult for black patients. The MHB limitation on curative treatment may be the most direct barrier to accessing hospice care. Medicare and Medicaid reimbursement policies prioritize interventions over high-quality communication, which harms minority patients even more than whites precisely because such communication is needed to overcome cultural differences and trust issues. Lack of consistent relationships with providers and provider bias in the hospital frustrate conversations about end-of-life care. All these forces combine to form a forceful current that hinders black patients' ability to navigate the rapids of interventions, particularly at the end of life.

Decentralized Care and the Failure of Political Will

Despite ample evidence suggesting that individualized and decentralized care at the beginning and end of life improves outcomes for all, but especially minority, patients, such options continue to be the exception rather than the norm. The shape of the healthcare watershed plays an important role in limiting access for everyone, but these barriers are particularly high for underserved populations. The struggle faced by Ruth Lubic and her Family Health and Birth Center in Washington, DC, is one case study among many that illustrates how powerful currents in the healthcare watershed can wash away alternatives to hospital-based care in minority communities. Lubic, a major figure in the midwifery community for the past 50 years and winner of a MacArthur Foundation "genius" grant, spent decades working to increase access to birth center care as a way to lower disparities in pregnancy and birth outcomes for low-income mothers. In 2000, she used her MacArthur grant of $375,000 to open the Family Health and Birth Center in northeast Washington, DC, as a way to target that city's high racial disparities in birth. Most of the patients at the birth center are low-income black women.

Care at the clinic offers precisely the individualized care that medicalized options lack. Mothers have the option of in-depth group prenatal care, births attended by midwives either at the birth center or at a local hospital, breastfeeding support, and referrals to other services such as housing, wellness courses, medical, dental, and parenting classes. The center also provides doula services, postpartum support, and pediatric care for newborns. The comprehensive approach allows the center to individualize care to the needs of specific mothers and provides an interdisciplinary net of care that supports women and their babies from early pregnancy through the first year of life and beyond, emphasizing culturally competent care with a range of providers.

Medical outcomes at the birth center are excellent. Mothers giving birth at the center have much lower rates of preterm birth than similar populations at area hospitals, and the cesarean section rate for first-time black mothers at the center was 15.3 percent, compared to 29 percent in the rest of the city.[120] Evidence also suggests that the birth center has lower rates of newborns with low birth weight as well. In addition to providing excellent outcomes for mothers and their infants, these benefits save money as well. According to Lubic's analysis, care at the center saved the healthcare system more than it cost to run the facility in many years, largely because the costs of preterm births are so high. Independent research demonstrates significantly improved outcomes for mothers using the center, compared with Washington, DC, averages.[121]

Lowering the rates of preterm birth, primary cesarean section, and low birth weight represents significant cost savings in both the short term and the long term, especially when taking into account the challenges mothers and infants face over the life span as a result of pregnancy and birth complications. Individualized care improves outcomes by encouraging mothers, particularly those with previous negative interactions with care providers, to return for follow-up appointments. In a *Washington Post* article about the center, expectant mothers said that the care they received at the center made them feel empowered. One teenage mother living in a group home spoke of the care she received: "'They explain stuff to you,' Smith says. 'They don't get irritated.'"[122] Empowerment, emerging from trust and communication, has significant effects on medical outcomes by encouraging patients to work with providers to identify risk factors and complications early on in a pregnancy.

Despite excellent outcomes, lower-cost care, and cost savings for the healthcare system as a whole, the Family Health and Birth Center must rely on donations and assistance from the District of Columbia Council to support its operations. The same pressures discussed in earlier chapters weigh heavily on the center. Until a recent reorganization, the clinic was reimbursed for less than half of what most births cost in personnel and upkeep of facilities owing to artificially low Medicaid reimbursement rates for midwifery and birth center care. Regulations and bureaucratic tangles with the city increased costs and delayed the clinic's opening. Even more seriously, skyrocketing malpractice premiums threatened an otherwise successful model. Premiums at the clinic increased from $90,000 to $300,000 between 2005 and 2008 and continue to rise, despite the clinic's excellent safety record.[123] While malpractice premiums threaten both hospital maternity wards and birth centers nationwide, birth centers are particularly vulnerable since they explicitly do not offer the more lucrative interventions that can help offset expensive premiums.[124]

While the Family Health and Birth Center remains an example of high-quality and individualized maternity care provided to vulnerable women at relatively low cost, it is not clear whether such a model can be transferred to other areas. Even now, the clinic is under pressure to find a new location given escalating real estate prices, another common problem in urban areas. More broadly, the center's success relies on Lubic's personality and reputation, including powerful friends like Supreme Court justice Ruth Bader Ginsburg. As a sign of the vulnerability of the birth center model, the center was recently forced to move under the umbrella of another "federally qualified health center," a designation that protects it from rising malpractice insurance costs and increases Medicaid reimbursements.[125] Such a move comes with greater oversight and requirements to standardize care in line with federal standards. Lubic initially resisted this move, and her concerns reflect broader concerns individualized and community-based providers face as they struggle against corporatization and bureaucratization. Providers who offer the most individualized care have the fewest resources available. Access to greater levels of funding such as Medicare and Medicaid dollars requires layers of bureaucracy and standardized procedures that threaten the very individualization that makes such care beneficial in the first place.[126] Access to the tributary of reimbursement brings with it powerful currents from the regulatory tributary, both of which threaten the very power of community-based providers to offer low-cost, evidence-based care that respects individual preferences.

Conclusion

The causes of racial disparities in birth and death are complex, but solutions that address a constellation of these causes are relatively straightforward. All Americans, but particularly Americans with unique needs, benefit from individualized care at the beginning and end of life, care that can be provided in the community at relatively low cost. The black American experience in the healthcare watershed is but one example of how a greater understanding of individual-level variation can illuminate the damaging way medicalization, centralization of care in hospitals, and the accompanying standardization of care harm patients. It also casts light on some of the most underappreciated causes of medicalization and provides lessons for the future.

One of the most important lessons gleaned from the black experience is how the standardizing currents of regulations and reimbursement policies eliminated many of the traditional community-oriented solutions that black Americans created as both hedges against white control and alternatives to the health systems they were intentionally excluded from. As one group of black scholars pointed out about birth, "There is no answer to solving this crisis that Black women do not already know."[127] The importance of traditional self-help institutions is reflected in the modern grassroots initiatives growing out of black communities across the nation, including the slow but steady growth of black birth workers and black death workers in a variety of fields. Solutions coming directly from black communities have the advantage of being both more flexible and more immediate than waiting for mostly white policy makers to decide what black communities need, an approach that has consistently failed to improve black lives over the years and has in many cases caused real harm.[128] Reducing restrictions on community-based options would allow black Americans the flexibility to develop the kinds of care structures they know they need rather than relying on the largely white policy makers whose predecessors destroyed uniquely black healthcare options in the first place. As one black midwife argued in an interview, "I actually think that health care, policing, all of that is [moving to] looking at it more from a community perspective. You live in the community you serve, you understand the community you serve, you're going to be more aware of the needs of the people there. Community care, I think it's super super important." Unfortunately, serious barriers to self-organizing solutions to community challenges are built into our policy framework.

Providing black communities the freedom to innovate and experiment with community-oriented care is just one way to undo the decades of government policies that intentionally or unintentionally centralized care. The eradication of the granny midwife and the destruction of black medical schools many decades ago generated powerful ripple effects that denied culturally competent care to generations of black Americans, and these policies still affect the options available today. Medicare and Medicaid policies perpetuate these harms by standardizing care for those who need individualized care the most. Low Medicaid and Medicare reimbursement and an overwhelmingly fee-for-service model prevent high-touch, low-tech options like birth centers and residential hospices from being economically viable, particularly in urban and low-income areas. These policies, combined with restrictive licensing laws, create almost constant pressure on culturally competent grassroots providers, pressure that ultimately undermines innovation and exacerbates injustices.

Another broad theme that extends beyond the black American case is that decentralization itself improves care for vulnerable populations. By individualizing care and providing care in a comfortable environment with culturally competent caregivers, many of the dangers of medicalization, such as mechanization and overtreatment, can be avoided. Decentralized care is uniquely poised to address the challenges minority patients face, such as unstable relationships with providers, lack of access to primary care, and distrust of the medical profession. Hospitals, as beneficial as they are in other contexts, are likely to exacerbate precisely the barriers that minority patients face in the quest for a "good" birth or death. Decentralized care is also a way for groups like black Americans to rediscover the rich tradition of self-help and community assistance that was destroyed by standardized and bureaucratic policies. Black Americans want care that originates in their community with roots in their own traditions, but such care is simply not viable under current regulatory and reimbursement limitations.

Additionally, the black American experience illuminates how to individualize care for other populations that are just now entering the mainstream. Growing immigrant populations will require birth and palliative care teams that are able to work with non-English speakers. Persons with nontypical intellectual or physical abilities also require individualized care that is flexible enough to accommodate specific and unique needs.[129] Victims of emotional and physical trauma—including refugee populations, sexual abuse survivors, and victims of violent crimes —need much more emotional, psychological, and spiritual support during birth and death than patients without traumatic pasts. The growth in the population of transgender individuals will challenge birth and death workers to provide sensitive and medically appropriate care at a time when an individual's identity is both peculiarly relevant and particularly vulnerable.[130]

Individualizing care cannot be solved by one-off solutions like cultural competency training modules because patient preferences and needs are irreducibly complex and because birth and death are uniquely preference sensitive. Race, ethnicity, gender, income, religion, sexual orientation, sexual identity, and a myriad of other variables combine to produce irreducible individuals who may or may not hold the values one expects from their visible background.[131] Because of this complexity, helping people give birth and die in respectful and supportive ways requires high-quality communication that includes attention to communication content and style. This kind of care is not specific to a particular racial or ethnic group, but instead, as one physician's guide to end-of-life care makes explicit, these are skills "needed to serve any patient or family who is facing death."[132] The best practices for providing high-quality care at birth and the end of life start with the time and space to access and respect individual preferences and frequent examination of biases and assumptions about patients of all kinds. Such communication requires addressing issues like patient distrust of the medical profession openly, assessing and reassessing comprehension on both sides (including working with trained translators when necessary), and working directly with patients and their families when cultural, ethical, and medical conflicts arise.[133] Unfortunately, most of the financial and legal incentives in the US healthcare system work against physicians having the time and space for this kind of contact, often explicitly.

The way black Americans give birth and die is, while an extreme case in some ways, also fundamentally an *American* experience. The shape of the American healthcare watershed actively prevents individuals of all backgrounds from giving birth and dying the way they desire. Because birth and death are where individual differences matter the most, they are also where standardization and centralization do the most harm. Moving away from standardized and centralized care in hospitals and individualizing care for every American will require a fundamental shift in how Americans pay for, regulate, and legislate on healthcare at all levels of government. Until those reforms are in place, options for truly individualized care at birth and death will remain few and far between.

Reshaping the Watershed

The sovereign extends its arms over society as a whole; it covers its surface with a network of small, complicated, painstaking, uniform rules through which those most original minds and the most vigorous souls cannot clear a way to surpass the crowd; it does not break wills, but it softens them, bends them, and directs them; it rarely forces one to act, but it constantly opposes itself to one's acting; it does not destroy, it prevents things from being born.
—Tocqueville, *Democracy in America*

T HE SHAPE of the US healthcare watershed has far-reaching consequences for the way in which Americans give birth and die. Powerful currents in the watershed push laboring women and terminally ill patients into centralized hospitals, where their experiences are reduced to their medical parts. These currents challenge deeply held principles of medical practice, including commitments to respect patient autonomy, minimize harm, and ensure just access. One of the most ironic trade-offs of medicalization is that as the number of available interventions has expanded, patient autonomy has become increasingly circumscribed. The watershed prevents informed consent by eliminating options that provide individualized, low-cost, and evidence-based care, instead incentivizing standardized, high-cost, medically intensive options that facilitate overtreatment and ignore patient wishes.

What is striking about the American system is, given the American commitment to freedom, how little control Americans have over their most profound life events and how little they even understand this fact. American birth and death are structured and limited by a tangle of regulations, legal structures, and financial policies that have very little to do with medical evidence or patient choice. In the best case, these limitations lead to expensive and sometimes inappropriate care. In the worst case, they lead to avoidable emotional trauma and serious physical harm. The reality of American birth and death is that interest groups, insurance companies, regulators, and legislators have far more influence on how someone gives birth or dies than individuals or their healthcare providers. The options patients have at the beginning and end of life are like a sheer wall built by regulators, insurers, medical coders, lawyers, hospital administrators, and professional associations. The individuals who matter most—whom the system is ostensibly set up to serve—are swept away.

Reshaping the Watershed for Autonomy, Quality, Cost, and Access

In contrast to the American healthcare watershed, characterized by steep walls, raging rapids, and strong currents that centralize care, the ideal watershed is a slow-moving river of healthcare options, with diverse places to land on the shore, trained navigators to assist individuals in both deciding where they want to go and how to get there, and a logic to the currents that guides high-need patients toward acute hospital care while preserving the ability of all patients, when possible given the vicissitudes of disease, to plot their own course. The ideal healthcare watershed is full of people as well as machines: trained navigators certainly, but also family, friends, children, and caregivers of all kinds, pulling together, joining in the paddling when appropriate, and creating a culture of care that protects individuals when they are at their most vulnerable.[1]

The best reforms not only individualize and resocialize medical care but also increase access for the most vulnerable patients in the watershed, providing them with boats and navigation teams to help them find care that fits their unique needs. As part of this access, demedicalized providers must be granted independence from the medical establishment. Such independence would support a flourishing ecosystem of diverse and innovative providers with different philosophies of care: some rooted in religious motivations, others in profit, and still others in activism. It would free entrepreneurial midwives and compassionate comfort care homes and sprawling medical research centers and small rural hospitals from the tangle of bureaucracy, allowing each to provide the best medical care they know how for the unique and irreducible individuals they treat. The Miriams and Josephs of the world, who had so few options in our introduction, would not find their desires strangled by a system that prioritizes bureaucratic rules over the humans those rules purportedly protect.

Reforms to the watershed to allow patient-centered, evidence-based care will require a combination of reshaping the main tributaries to slow currents of centralization and medicalization, providing navigators and support staff to help patients identify their preferences and how those preferences map onto the watershed itself, as well as emergency equipment in the boats themselves to protect patients from the sometimes unavoidable rapids of medicalized care. The most important of the reforms are those that limit the power of the tributaries themselves, but these are, predictably, the most difficult to achieve.

Perhaps most frustrating is that changing how Americans give birth and die seems relatively easy at first glance. Decentralizing and individualizing care is, on average, less expensive and results in better outcomes than hospital-based care. Yet the reality of the US healthcare system is that reform is rendered exceedingly difficult by the complexity of the system itself, the perverse incentives built into its structure, and the disjunct between patient preferences and who pays for and organizes care. That complexity has led entrenched players like hospitals, large insurers, and other interested parties to pour considerable resources into lobbying to prevent reforms that would return power and control to patients and their providers.

These lobbying forces are themselves made possible by a healthcare system that is structured in a peculiarly poor way, one that separates cause and effect, patient and payments, and whose complexity makes it difficult for patients and providers to pinpoint any one specific area of blame.[2] These causes are well known to healthcare policy analysts. The complexity of the system makes locating responsible parties difficult and creates a kind of internal logic that defies reform. It also makes it easier for interested parties to stay in control. Local hospital lobbies use state certificate-of-need laws and federal Medicare policies to limit the options available in ways that most patients and physicians do not understand. When a patient asks for a palliative care consult or a pregnant woman asks for a trial of labor after a cesarean, she and her doctor might have no idea why those options are unavailable.

Hampering reform, centralization of care is increasingly moving toward outright consolidation of care, as small numbers of large insurers and hospital systems increasingly control the payment for and provision of healthcare and traditionally independent, community-based providers are swallowed up by corporate providers. According to one recent analysis, consolidation of care results in "anticompetitive behavior, increasing prices, and exploitation of and less choice for consumers."[3] Meanwhile, federal and state policies encourage such consolidation through protectionist regulations and reimbursement policies that privilege institutionalized and high-intensity care. Consolidation of care does not just reduce the overall options available; it also fractures the relationship between patient and provider, a relationship that is already hindered by the limits put in place by the third-party payment system.

Both consolidation and third-party payers put increasing distance between patients, providers, and treatment options, which shifts medical decision making away from the patient-provider dyad and toward centralized decision makers. Decisions about provision of care are increasingly being made on the basis of population-level trends, rather than individual needs. Put another way, the individual is becoming less and less important in medical care. A recent analysis by the *Journal of the American Medical Association* of the American healthcare system described what it calls the "ascendancy of the public health and social policy perspective over that of traditional, individually focused medicine."[4] The emphasis on aggregate data, population averages, and standardization of care driven by large-scale payers actively prevents personalized and individually appropriate kinds of care. Physicians are limited by the protocols of their affiliated institutions, and patients are limited by the policies of their insurance carriers. Consolidation also means that the same organization may control a variety of inpatient and outpatient treatment centers, further standardizing care and crowding out more innovative or flexible alternatives. A final effect of consolidation is that the physician-patient relationship is increasingly being replaced by a relationship to a broader institution with a wide range of providers, each of whom has only a piece of an individual's specific story.[5] All these forces deepen the chasm between the individual and decisions about his or her own care.

Reform becomes even more difficult because it needs to occur at every level of governance, and each reform is likely to have ripple effects on other levels. Owing to the diversity in the number and kinds of actors involved and the levels of governance at which policies are made, serious efforts at reform in one area are stymied by resistance at another level by actors who have no idea that the initial reform is even taking place. Organizations lobbying for better care have limited resources and often have to choose battles carefully, resulting in incremental change, if change happens at all. Hard-fought but uncoordinated incremental changes are vulnerable to being destroyed by larger, more substantive changes in higher-level policies. Is the lack of birth centers a result of state regulations or Medicaid reimbursement policies? Both, but knowing which reform must come first can be difficult, given limited funding and lobbying resources.

Reforming the Regulatory Tributary

Regulatory reform of state laws is in one sense the most direct kind of reform because it involves simply eliminating laws that prevent evidence-based and preference-based options from proliferating. In another sense it is difficult to achieve uniformly because it requires that reforms be carried out in all 50 states, each of which has its own unique set of entrenched interests and players. State policies may also involve a combination of legislation, administrative court decisions, health codes, and other policies that are difficult to access and reform, as in the case of corporate practice of medicine regulations. Still, regulatory reform at the state level has the potential to move more quickly than national reforms of large-scale policies like Medicare, precisely because the scope of change is smaller, because community-based providers are themselves job creators and patients are direct constituents, and because many states face pressing financial considerations that make reforms more palatable. Lobbying efforts can be more closely targeted to local needs and are less likely to be diluted among a more diverse group of legislators than they are on the national level.

The most direct regulatory reforms that relate to birth and death are those that dampen the strength of the currents leading toward centralized care. Eliminating CON laws for birth centers and hospices would prevent both the centralization of care in hospitals and the centralization of care in corporatized for-profit alternatives that benefit from a highly regulated environment, such as the exploding for-profit hospice sector. Eliminating corporate practice of medicine laws would allow hospices and birth centers to hire physicians directly and would reduce some of the political jockeying over scope-of-practice discussions for nurse practitioners, as in California.

The other obvious area for reform is to expand the scope of practice for lower-cost, highly trained providers like nurse practitioners and certified nurse midwives, who are more likely to practice in community-based clinics and agencies. Many reform advocates view nurse practitioners and nurse midwives as a primary hedge against the plummeting numbers of both primary care and maternity workers, both of whom provide important protections against escalation of care into hospitals.[6] Bills to allow advanced practice nurses full independence within the scope of their training have made progress in some states, but they continue to be limited in the most populous states, such as California, Texas, and those on the Atlantic Coast.[7] It is probably no accident that the states mostly likely to allow advanced practice nurses to practice independently are rural states that have a difficult time retaining physicians and where physician lobbying has been balanced by pressing public health needs.

Competition among providers and care settings, often hailed primarily as a cost-cutting measure, matters for informed consent as well. A lack of alternative providers not only limits patient choice but also may influence the behavior of existing providers. Practitioners who believe they are the only available option for patients have little incentive to respect or protect patient wishes when such wishes conflict with their financial or legal interests. One analysis of obstetric violence, or the abuse and violation of informed consent during childbirth, argued that such violence is made possible in part by a dearth of maternity providers, the consolidation of independent practitioners into large medical groups that standardize care, and the reimbursement incentives that make interventions more lucrative than demedicalized options.[8] This explanation is supported by correlational data that find that states with fewer limitations on nonphysician maternity providers like midwives have lower rates of induction and cesarean section, suggesting that medicalized birth is at least partially driven by a lack of competition.[9] The same is likely to be true of demedicalized death. One study found that competition improved the quality of services hospices offered, except in the most competitive markets, where some quality markers went down.[10] Interestingly, quality drops were clearest in states with CON laws in place. What the study does not address, which would be more difficult, is how increases in the number of hospice providers affect patient care within hospitals themselves.

In general, patients, providers, and insurers should question the motivations of a variety of regulatory initiatives. Too often, regulations in the healthcare context serve protectionist goals of a few special interests and fail to provide quality, cost savings, or choice. While a considerable amount of academic work has investigated the perverse incentives created by a variety of healthcare regulations, the lay narrative that healthcare regulations exist primarily to protect the quality of healthcare or to reduce costs persists. More public education on the complex outcomes of the regulatory framework, including how that framework seriously limits patient choice and the range of alternatives available, could help state reform efforts move forward. Unfortunately, without more public awareness, both politicians and industry benefit from a system in which regulations serve protectionist motives while individuals and their communities bear the costs of that protectionism.

Reforming the Reimbursement Headwater

Perhaps the most important area of reform is also the most difficult to achieve. The reimbursement tributary pumps water into the system, and its powerful current determines what kinds of care systems succeed and which dry up or are washed away. This tributary creates perverse incentives in the first and most obvious way because patients do not control what kind of care their insurance premiums pay for. The indirect way patients pay for medical care interferes with autonomy directly by limiting the options insurers will cover but also indirectly by preventing alternatives from entering the market in the first place. If patients had greater control over their insurance premiums or had a more flexible system such as that provided by health savings accounts, they could choose to support medical care that more closely aligns with their goals and values. Patients would have more control in the moment and more options available to choose from over the long term.

In part because of the separation between patient and payer, but also because of the incentives within federal insurance programs, resources end up being poured into the most centralized and high-intensity care. Changing the payment structure of fee-for-service care in Medicare would incentivize more investment in less intensive options, while also correcting the imbalance between procedure-heavy specialists and the physicians who provide more holistic kinds of care.[11] Currently, the United States has the largest proportion of specialists (especially those who do procedures) in the developed world, alongside a dearth of primary care providers. Incentives, particularly in Medicare but also in other insurance payment structures broadly, privilege interventions over more appropriate and less intensive forms of care. Predictably, medical school students respond to these incentives by choosing the most lucrative fields.

While Medicare and Medicaid are politically entrenched and unlikely to go anywhere, there has been a growth of interest in developing alternatives to the fee-for-service model these programs rely on. Initiatives emphasizing "value-based care" are growing, with Medicare and Medicaid both floating a variety of experiments to incorporate patient outcomes into the reimbursement structure. While this chapter is not the place for an extensive discussion of healthcare reform, a few important initiatives could hold promise for demedicalizing birth and death. Perhaps the most obvious is something like a capitated payment system, which became popular in health management organizations in the 1990s but came under fire for requiring red tape, including third-party authorization. Newer capitation models would eliminate insurance gatekeepers and allow physicians to keep some of the cost savings while still controlling for quality care. On this model, physicians or hospitals would receive risk-adjusted monthly payments to provide all care for a patient, limited only by quality control reporting.[12]

While most reforms, including what is broadly known as "value-based care," involve linking reimbursement to outcomes as a way to challenge the incentives for overtreatment found in fee-for-service models, birth and death challenge such models because outcomes are difficult to both determine and assess.[13] Patients with diverse needs require a careful and individualized balancing of different outcomes, and too much of an emphasis by insurers on some outcomes may come at the cost of others. Birth and death themselves, because of their unique nature as only quasi-medical events, have outcomes that are different in degree and kind from other kinds of medical outcomes.[14] Birth outcomes are heterogeneous because intervention rates have to be balanced against both maternal and infant mortality, and maternal health outcomes must be balanced against infant health outcomes as well. Other important variables will not show up in the medical data at all. A woman who is disrespected and violated during birth may very well have a "successful" birth on paper if both she and the baby survive with minimal permanent physical damage. Death and dying, where patients typically have a mix of needs, including primary and secondary diagnoses, as well as the expectation of both medical crisis and eventual death, lead to outcomes that will necessarily be different from standard health measures.[15] As with birth, other important outcomes, such as a dying patient who does not receive adequate pain medication or enough time with his family, will not show up in data on health outcomes at all unless a medical provider somehow charts them. Because both birth and death are so preference sensitive, any measurement of outcomes must account for how patient preferences might contribute to particular outcomes, even if those outcomes are not considered "ideal."

Moreover, disagreement within the medical community about how to determine and assess outcomes, such as the current uncertainty over what the ideal rate of cesarean section should be or the ideal length of a hospice stay, further complicates the picture. As long as internal medical disagreements between obstetricians and midwives or between palliative care and critical care practitioners exist, external reviewers and payers and policy makers will struggle to make decisions about what kind of care to prioritize and how to measure and assess outcomes. Complicating the picture is that the movement toward a public health perspective that standardizes care leaves unique patients more vulnerable and fails to address crucial but difficult-to-measure individual needs. Unless outcomes are carefully determined, some scholars fear that "physicians and patients will be driven apart when they should be allies."[16] A final concern is that an emphasis on outcomes could push providers away from the most complex patients or those most in need, further exacerbating disparities in care.[17]

Some quality outcome measures, such as avoiding hospital readmission or reducing medical errors, apply to both birth and death and are worth pursuing.[18] And in both birth and death there exists widespread use of interventions with dubious benefits to patients, such as continuous fetal monitoring, routine episiotomy, and tube-feeding. Insurers could use evidence-based assessments to determine which interventions are most overused and target those interventions for further investigation.

Medicare's value modifier program, which reimburses physicians in part based on outcomes, will provide important data for future research.[19]

Other recommendations call for moving away from a hospital-centered approach and toward a more integrated patient- and condition-centered approach. Calls to create "integrated practice units" that operate together across care locations would assist the birthing and dying by providing access to nonclinical providers such as doulas, social workers, and other support staff who work directly with medical providers to provide care across a variety of contexts.[20] Though many of the experiments currently in practice do not deal with birth and death specifically, both could benefit from this approach because care locations are diverse and communication between providers can be challenging. An integrated care approach improves outcomes by improving communication among providers, managing risks, and keeping low-risk or low-need individuals in low medical intensity environments, including providing care at home where appropriate. Measuring outcomes and integrated care go hand in hand, since it is not possible to measure and track outcomes unless all members of the team are on the same page about what those outcomes should be. If a primary care provider is unaware of a hospital admission or a social worker is unaware of a recent serious diagnosis that changes the care plan trajectory, measurement of outcomes becomes impossible.[21]

One example of something like an integrated practice unit that takes advantage of a bundled care payment approach is the experiment at the Minnesota Birth Center, where a group of practitioners have what they call a BirthBundle, where midwives and obstetricians partner together to provide comprehensive maternal and newborn care. The midwifery practice is fully integrated into the hospital system, and the medical director is a maternal-fetal specialist who is able to handle complications when they arise. In this program, the outpatient birth center essentially bundles together all the fee-for-service payments each member receives and spreads those across the providers, reducing the incentives for high-intensity treatment and supporting collaboration since midwives and physicians are part of the same bundled payment system, rather than competing with each other for payments.

Outcomes are excellent, with high maternal satisfaction, low intervention rates, and low rates of maternal and infant mortality and morbidity. Care is provided via a natural triage system where low-risk mothers give birth in the birth center outside the hospital, but if com-plications arise, they can be quickly and easily transferred to the hospital to be attended by their midwife or an obstetrician when medically necessary. Because risks are spread out across a variety of providers and because decisions about how to manage risk are made between the mother and her providers, the payment system is both flexible and personalized. As the birth center itself reports, however, financial limitations in state Medicaid reimbursement models prevent the expansion of this model. If successful experiments like these in both birth and death are to spread, states must change the incentives within their Medicaid models and the federal government must overhaul Medicare payment structures to ensure that collaborative, high-value, low-volume care can flourish.[22]

Similar kinds of programs in end-of-life care also hold promise. One 2003 study investigated four models, including managed care plans and hospices that provide fully integrated and comprehensive palliative care to patients in some states. They share in common a capitated payment model and an interdisciplinary team that coordinates care and follows patients across care locations. All four are also somewhat unique in that they provide comprehensive palliative care services to all patients, even those who opt out of the Medicare Hospice Benefit and its attendant restrictions. They differ somewhat in their target population, with the managed care plans aimed primarily at nursing home residents, with palliative care bundled into the primary care framework. The hospice in the group accepted a wide range of patients, including terminally ill children and adults both under and over 65. In addition to the capitated payments it negotiates with Medicaid for hospice coverage for low-income Americans, the hospice also relies on fundraising to cover expenses not covered by the low hospice rate. Despite success in offering integrated high-quality care for patients at the end of life, all four providers faced significant barriers related to the structure of Medicare and Medicaid hospice reimbursement that limited expansion of these programs across states lines.[23] Importantly, many of the positive outcomes of these initiatives were associated with the provision of concurrent care, which allows patients to receive both palliative care and medical treatments at the same time. Some hospice providers offer concurrent care to some patients via Medicare's Home Health Benefit, but the services provided are limited and Medicare's reimbursement rates frequently fail to cover the actual cost of care. Expanding opportunities for concurrent care could prevent the binary choice many seriously ill patients face between giving up all treatment and pursuing hospice care at home.

Better integration of care, particularly for nonmedical providers, is particularly important for fulfilling our bioethical commitment to justice. Low-income patients frequently lack transportation, support networks, and the medical literacy to understand complex and sometimes conflicting information. Low-cost integrated options for maternity care, including prenatal support groups, social workers, and other nonmedical providers, have shown benefits in improving the health of mothers and their infants and reducing interventions during labor and delivery.[24] Similar kinds of support for the elderly and dying individuals help improve medical outcomes by increasing patient awareness of the costs and benefits of interventions, reducing resistance to options like palliative care and hospice, and reducing medical errors and unnecessary hospitalizations.[25] Expanding reimbursement to provide a variety of integrated support throughout the care process would improve outcomes in birth and death specifically, since in both cases involvement with the medical community may span many months and many of the needs involved are nonmedical in nature.

Another possible alternative to even these capitated payment models removes the middleman of insurers altogether and places payment for care directly with the patient. The rise of so-called concierge medicine provides patients direct access to a doctor on retainer. Once reserved for the wealthy, it has become an increasingly affordable alternative to more fragmented relationships with primary care providers.[26] The concept is common in birth center or home births, where women pay a flat rate out of pocket for comprehensive prenatal and newborn care, though limitations on the model due to poor relationships with hospitals have already been discussed. Concierge medicine offers a way to rediscover the traditional physician-patient relationship and cut out the middlemen of managed care, but this model still suffers from the same perverse incentives and heavy regulations that make consolidation of care attractive and more likely.[27] The costs of concierge medicine have dropped dramatically over just the past decade, suggesting that patient demand for high-quality individualized care exists and that, provided that the regulatory framework moves aside to make room, patients are willing to forgo insurance covering standardized care to allow for more individualized options. Some physicians providing concierge medicine specifically advertise geriatric and end-of-life care among their services, with one concierge physician emphasizing that he provides "continuity and coordination of care" for elderly patients.[28] Benefits for patients and providers include better communication and better coordinated care since providers spend less time on paperwork and more time with patients. The growth of such practices is likely to increase in the coming years as both patients and providers seek alternatives to the bureaucratic and consolidated model that constrains both patients and providers.

Unsurprisingly, many reforms focus on decentralizing care, since centralization plays a major role in poor outcomes and escalating costs. Increasing interest in moving many patients out of hospitals by providing comprehensive support at home could help challenge the hegemony of hospitals in both birth and death. Programs like Hospital at Home provide comprehensive care for patients recovering from a variety of conditions, while at the same time lowering costs and improving outcomes and patient satisfaction.[29] Physicians are better able to individualize care in a home environment and tend to do less reflexive testing and procedures since they are farther away from the technology that fuels interventions. Other reforms will be necessary to make such a model work, including changes to wage scales for home healthcare workers, who typically make much less than those with similar jobs in an inpatient setting.[30] Lower wages result in more turnover, which can compromise patient care. As with other kinds of decentralized reforms, however, burdensome regulations must be shifted, and payers need to either directly support such initiatives or provide more flexibility in how patients use their healthcare dollars. Individual-centered approaches like health savings accounts could be helpful in this area.

Whether any of these changes will happen on a large scale is unclear. Hospitals are a powerful lobbying force, and given the amount of money already poured into hospital infrastructure, it is difficult politically to make the argument to withdraw funds that would move resources elsewhere. Localities where hospitals are major employers may be particularly resistant to changing protectionist policies. One explanation for why states were slow to enforce changes requiring Medicaid coverage for midwives and birth centers laid out in the Affordable Care Act is that most lobbying from hospital groups occurs at the state level, where the power of hospitals as regional employers is considerable. Physicians also hold powerful sway at the state and federal levels, impeding the progress of reforms that would allow licensure for nonphysician providers, who are increasingly important in community-based care.[31]

Finally, the American experience of birth and death provides a powerful lesson for healthcare reform as a whole. Recent research has shifted away from patient demand as a primary explanation of the growth of healthcare costs, instead looking at the role of unusually high prices in the US healthcare marketplace.[32] While suggestions like price control, rationing, managed care, and a variety of other top-down policies are suggested as a way to limit that growth, these fixes ignore part of the reason prices are so high in the first place, which is that competition from low-cost providers is intentionally limited by a tangle of regulations and agreements with insurers. Home healthcare, hospice, and birth centers are limited in their ability to provide low-cost, low-tech options by a variety of state and federal policies that intentionally or unintentionally funnel patients toward high-cost, high-tech providers. Medicare has begun to recognize this trend and has initiated a series of experiments to encourage home healthcare, including its Home Health Value-Based Purchasing Model, which provides incentives to home healthcare agencies to provide more high-quality and more efficient care.[33] This program was implemented in nine states in 2016, and results are forthcoming.[34] Expanding the reimbursable scope of practice for nurses, midwives, and physician assistants and creating space for community-based options like residential hospice and birth centers can provide the starting point for demedicalized, decentralized, and individualized birth and death. Listening to patient demand, loosening restrictions on de-medicalized and community-based providers, and supporting innovative efforts for community-based care can lower costs and improve care without the need for price controls or rationing, both of which can have damaging unintended side effects and further constrain individual control over healthcare options.

Calming the Riptide of Risk

Perhaps the most hopeful area of reform is in calming the riptide of risk that funnels patients and providers into centralized care. Despite the popular narrative to the contrary, research suggests that some reforms work well to reduce the risk of liability and make it less likely that suits will reach the expensive trial phase. The first are quality assurance programs. The California Maternal Quality Care Collaborative program, for example, has reduced maternal mortality in California by 55 percent, while rates are increasing elsewhere across the nation. The program rigorously tracks preventable deaths and creates tool kits and protocols for how to respond in the future. The program also works to disincentivize medicalized practices that are not based in evidence, such as unnecessary cesarean sections (which increase the risk of maternal mortality in subsequent pregnancies) and nonmedically indicated early inductions (which increase risks to infants).[35] While the benefits to mothers and infants in terms of improved outcomes have been striking, an additional benefit is lowered malpractice rates. It makes intuitive sense that reducing medical errors and violations of informed consent would reduce malpractice litigation, but these are rarely the focus of the tort reforms discussed in the media. Given how uneven the US medical system is, how common medical errors and violations of consent are, and how poor outcomes are for the birthing and dying, instituting stricter quality assurance reforms seems necessary not only on the practical side of reducing liability risk but also as a basic requirement of medical ethics.[36]

Medical organizations can also play an important role in more aggressively defending less medicalized evidence-based practices in the media, at the policy level, to malpractice insurers, and in court when necessary. The American College of Obstetricians and Gynecologists has finally begun issuing recommendations for how to support physiological birth, how to reduce the incidence of primary cesarean sections, and the best way to support vaginal birth after cesarean and other less medicalized alternatives.[37] Hospitals and providers have been relatively slow to follow suit, perhaps because they still feel sufficiently fearful about liability and because the new recommendations are, in some cases, directly contradictory to previous recommendations about appropriate standards of care. Maternity care providers and end-of-life care providers are both vulnerable to public perceptions about the safety or efficacy of medicine, which can color patients' (and juries') attitudes toward the quality and quantity of medical care. Professional associations can work to resist the further medicalization of standards of care in the courtroom, providing clear and peer-reviewed guidance on the risks of medical care and the reasonableness of expectations.

One type of reform that directly affects the medicalization of birth and death are what the American Medical Association call "liability safe harbors for the practice of evidence-based medicine." These safe harbors would limit physician liability in cases where following evidence-based medicine resulted in an unavoidable patient injury. A variety of limitations and protections of various sorts are built into the proposal, but the overall goal would be to protect physicians who provide evidence-based care and to limit the heightened risk perception that follows from less medicalized options.[38] These safe harbors would be particularly helpful for maternity care, where evidence suggests that liability fears contribute to overtreatment, including the use of technology that provides little to no benefits to patients.

Perhaps even more importantly, research demonstrates that better communication between doctors, staff, and patients reduces liability exposure, more so after an adverse event has taken place. Encouraging informed consent, spending the time to understand patient wishes, and then apologizing for adverse events are all ways to reduce liability exposure, but they are rarely emphasized by reform advocates.[39] Rather than discussing adverse events with patients directly, hospitals tend to circle the wagons, shutting down communication with patients as a way to stave off lawsuits. Evidence suggests that this is the worst approach since it leaves patients with no option other than filing a suit to access records and staff accounts to determine what actually occurred.[40] One recent suit in which the patient was awarded $16.5 million as a result of permanent nerve damage during birth was triggered largely because the hospital did not respond to the woman's requests for information about what occurred during her care.[41] Despite the research supporting a relationship between better communication and reduced liability risk, a recent Joint Commission publication noted that "beyond distributing advice for patients, little was being done to support systems change or encourage health care professionals to facilitate greater or more effective involvement of patients in their own care—for the sake of safety or otherwise."[42] Despite the alignment between best medical practices and the best practices to limit malpractice risk, many physicians and hospital systems are not instituting changes that would improve outcomes, enhance communication, or reduce legal risk in meaningful ways.

There are, however, innovative experiments that demonstrate that change is both possible and beneficial. Communication-and-resolution programs (CRPs) are perhaps the most commonsense solution to the problem. In this model, providers and care settings like hospitals communicate with patients about adverse events immediately after detection, apologize, and provide adequate compensation. Such programs also allow for tracking of errors and injuries, potentially leading to higher-quality care. The evidence on existing CRPs is positive, with lower payouts and many fewer claims making it to litigation, supporting the hypothesis that many patients sue as a way to find out information that providers and institutions withhold out of fear.[43] The success of such programs relies on the ability of providers and institutions to feel secure in admitting fault without fear of expensive litigation later and on patients feeling comfortable with the explanations and compensation provided. The evidence so far supports the idea that better communication about adverse events helps lower the psychological burden of such events on both patients and providers, helps support the patient-provider relationship, and protects institutions from the expense of unnecessary litigation that serves only to unearth facts that could be provided much earlier in the process at much lower cost.[44]

The importance of communication in lowering liability risk has important implications for the way reimbursement and regulatory structures interact with liability fear to impact patient care. The emphasis on standardization and documentation in hospitals as a way to protect themselves against both lawsuits and government audits compromises quality of care by reducing the time spent with patients, especially the less lucrative time communicating with patients. Research finds that residents spend more time on documentation than they do with patients.[45] Hospital protocols then emphasize preparing for an inevitable lawsuit rather than avoiding the lawsuit in the first place with high-quality communication and time spent with patients. Regulators and insurers, particularly Medicare and Medicaid, must also recognize how documentation burdens contribute to poor patient outcomes, putting providers and institutions at risk of lawsuits.[46] Since poor communication is a major barrier to high-quality care at the beginning and end of life, regulators, physicians, and hospitals must work together to reduce the documentation burden on practitioners and make time for the activities that actually improve patient outcomes.[47] These bureaucratic barriers to communication are another reason that community-based providers are somewhat more immune to liability fears, since communication about goals of care is a hallmark of both midwifery and hospice.

Poor communication hampers quality of care in other ways as well, especially when it comes to transitions between care locations. For both birth and death, failure to communicate between members of the care team (including poor communication between community-based providers and hospital staff) is a significant contributor to poor patient outcomes that can result in a lawsuit.[48] In death, where members of the medical team or the family are the most likely informants to administrators or police, careful, consistent, and continual communication is necessary to prevent miscommunication and to reorient care when goals change. One author notes the importance of institutional guidelines for end-of-life care, not only to guide the practitioners involved but also to educate nurses and other members of the care team on controversial practices, such as when high doses of opioids might be used.[49] Such guidelines, in conjunction with frequent team meetings and conversations with the patient and his or her family, can help alleviate concerns and ensure that members of the team are on the same page. Similar guidelines for birth, as well as policies making home birth and birth center transfers smoother for expecting mothers, would reduce miscommunication and stress on patients involved in transfers from community-based to hospital-based care. Perhaps most importantly, eliciting informed consent early and often, particularly when treatment goals change, is central to clarifying the course of treatment and justifying decisions about treatment options.

Holding practitioners accountable for medical malpractice, including unnecessary treatments, remains an important role of the tort system, and one that is probably underused given how common medical errors and overtreatment actually are. There is no one simple path to reform, since the causes of overtreatment are so complex and what constitutes overtreatment varies dramatically by condition and by patient. But better guidelines and better communication protocols are two proven ways to increase the quality of care while decreasing liability risk. Both are also central to the ethical commitments of medicine to do no harm and respect patient autonomy. Both, incidentally, require more time spent with patients, which will in turn require changes to the reimbursement structures of American healthcare.

One final problem is cultural rather than systemic, and that is that despite an imperfect medical system and the intrinsic fallibility of all medicine and of all providers, Americans have unrealistic expectations about the care and outcomes medicine can provide. Every parent expects a perfect child, and every loved one expects a death with dignity. The reality is that both birth and death are unpredictable, painful, and sometimes tragic. Understanding the limitations of the medical field and protecting competent and well-intentioned providers from unrealistic expectations are important steps in demedicalizing these uniquely human experiences. As one palliative care practitioner pointed out, medicalization itself has changed the culture in important ways: "The big thing is how hard it is to help people to understand the limits of medical treatment. The 6:30 news every night has a new drug or new treatment. It's very hard to know when you get sicker that there isn't something that could fix this. There's a real seduction to aggressive medical intervention that's very hard to stand up to unless you've really thought these things through." Attitudes toward the acceptable level of risk in medical care will be highly dependent on what treatments and interventions are available. Medicalization itself—both its successes and its failures—may be a primary driver of liability concerns. Better communication between patients and providers, unrestricted by liability fears, reimbursement incentives, and regulatory limitations, is one straightforward way to protect providers while providing high-quality medical care that reduces harms to patients and respects patient autonomy.

Emergency Equipment for the Medicalized Rapids

While systemic reform will involve shaping the tributaries themselves to control the direction and power of currents in the river, there are also more minor reforms, what might be considered the emergency equipment on the boat itself, that can help patients and providers better navigate the existing watershed. These include reforms to the medical school curriculum that emphasize the importance of birth plans or end-of-life counseling and training in how to communicate with patients about goals of care. Institutional reforms include standardized protocols to address complications when they arise (as opposed to standardizing care in anticipation of a complication arising) and protocols on the best practices for de-escalating interventions. Incorporating standardized communication points into care plans is one way to ensure that conversations about care happen at least somewhat frequently. One way to think about this is as standardizing the individualization of care. The "pause points" discussed in chapter 2 are one way in which hospitals and practitioners can attempt to standardize assessing patient preferences. Another might be a specific prenatal appointment devoted to crafting a birth plan at around 20 weeks. Other ways of making individualization a standard part of medical care include short debriefing sessions after an intervention or event so that providers and patients can share their experiences and discuss how to proceed. Of course, such "standardizing to individualize" requires that incentives point in the right direction, that providers have the time to discuss options with patients early and often, and that practitioners are reassured that communication will not have adverse liability outcomes.

As part of these conversations, standard emergency equipment in the river of healthcare options should be documents that explain patient preferences and goals of care. While there are practical limitations of healthcare planning documents such as advance directives, living wills, and birth plans, having written records of patient desires can help patients and their caregivers find a focal point for conversations with their providers. These documents should, ideally, come from conversations between patients and their providers over the course of treatment and should be updated frequently to reflect changes in medical reality. But such plans can serve an important centering purpose, whatever their legal status, in reminding the patient and her provider that, at least in birth and death, patient preferences are central to achieving good outcomes and that the treatment is for the person, and not the other way around. Unless and until insurers reimburse providers adequately for these conversations over the course of treatment, the efficacy of these documents will be limited.

Doulas: Navigating toward Individualized Care

Just as every boat needs someone with a map, all pregnant women, terminally ill patients, and elderly people should have trained support persons who can help individualize and rehumanize care no matter what the care location or goals of care. Unlike physicians or nurses, who help navigate the explicitly medical parts of birth and death, doulas can help patients navigate the nonmedical aspects, providing social, emotional, and psychological support and putting patients in touch with nonmedical resources that can help them avoid hospitalization and the rapids of medicalization. In both birth and death, doulas provide social support and institutional and generational knowledge about physiological birth and death to help individuals navigate vulnerable and precarious transitions.[50] They also, crucially, help access and assess patient preferences to facilitate and coordinate individualized care.

At their most powerful, doulas are like trained navigators, helping patients negotiate the complicated healthcare watershed. Because they have experience within the local healthcare environment and are familiar with the culture at various hospitals and other institutions, they can help patients make informed choices about where to seek care and which providers might be most in line with their treatment goals. Because birth and death are not frequent occurrences in any one person's life, patients rarely have the institutional knowledge themselves to make informed decisions about settings of care or providers. Doulas also provide some of the lost knowledge of physiological birth and death, providing comfort to patients and families and normalizing some of the more concerning realities of how people give birth and die, such as the loss of appetite in terminal patients or the escalation of pain at the end of labor that signals transition and that birth is near. They can help family members moisten the lips of a dying patient or teach a husband how to provide counterpressure during labor contractions. They can help set up postpartum care for mothers or help patients and their families plan funerals and memorial services when death seems near.

Crucially, doulas are not limited to demedicalized births and deaths. They can, and should, stay in the boat with their client even if the boat ends up in the rapids of medicalized care, helping patients navigate those rapids and, if possible, return to safer waters as soon as they are able. Birth doulas have been found to be helpful in the hospital context, where women have the least institutional knowledge and the most constraints on their choices. While women with doulas are overall less likely to have surgical births, women who had doulas present during their cesarean sections reported less emotional stress and better physical recovery than those who did not.[51] Similarly, death doulas are perhaps most helpful for patients who end up transitioning between multiple locations of care. Doulas represent a strong and consistent force in the river of healthcare options that tethers providers to patient preferences across care locations. As navigators on the healthcare watershed, doulas, as well as social workers and other nonmedical providers, keep their maps of the watershed at the ready and help patients identify currents leading to the rapids of medicalization before they get there. And they can pick up a paddle and support patients even when a medicalized birth or death becomes inevitable, providing support and guidance until everyone is safely on the other side.

While reforms like increasing access to doulas, expanding the role of communication in medical school curricula, and standardizing individualized care are all important parts of the "emergency equipment" in the boat, these reforms are limited in their efficacy by the political and legal structures that shape a watershed that both harms patients and reduces alternatives for care. The institutionalization of care for the birthing and dying creates its own momentum. Reforms must focus on changing the shape of the watershed from one of steep cliffs that channel patients into centralized care toward one that meanders and provides a wealth of community-based and centralized options to accommodate patients with a wide range of medical and social needs. But these reforms are political and legal reforms, not reforms that the medical community can make on its own. Moreover, without the proper political and legal reforms in place, the medical community simply does not have the incentives to provide consistently high-quality and low-cost care. The first step in reform requires the political will to care about how individuals giving birth and dying are treated and to reemphasize individual choice and control in healthcare, especially during our most vulnerable and our most human moments.

Principles and Politics in the Healthcare Watershed

As this book has argued, the outcomes of the US healthcare watershed create moral quandaries that go beyond the usual discussions of healthcare policy because they challenge every principle on which the US medical and political systems are ostensibly based. Despite the promise to "do no harm," new mothers and the elderly undergo unnecessary and harmful interventions, resulting in physical and emotional trauma. Despite the commitment to freedom and informed consent, hospitals and providers systematically reject individual values and beliefs in favor of standardized protocols. Despite a commitment to democratic governance, special interests influence policy, overriding medical evidence about best practices, involving both providers and patients in harmful cycles of intervention. Despite a commitment to equality and justice, policies encourage disparities in care across socioeconomic and racial lines, harming the most vulnerable. When our ideological commitments mean so little during our most profound and meaningful life events—when getting it right arguably matters the most—one wonders whether these commitments mean anything at all.

There are, however, alternatives. There are ways to create a watershed that results in outcomes consistent with our most closely held political and medical values. There are ways for individuals to choose inexpensive, high-quality, and medically appropriate options at the beginning and end of life. It will require more than emergency equipment. It will require rethinking the way Americans pay for and provision healthcare, the kinds of regulations policymakers and legislators deem necessary, and the way patients and providers think about and manage risk. But the resulting watershed would be compatible with the human needs of the individuals whom both medicine and politics claim to serve. It can be a healthcare system that provides medically appropriate, individually focused care that does not bankrupt either individuals or the society those individuals depend on. It can be one where floating down the river of healthcare options need not be disorienting or traumatic, but might instead be characterized by hope and trust. But the political world must provide a way for medicine to reach its full lifegiving and lifesaving potential. It will require Herculean political will to reshape a watershed. For all those who will be born and who will die—for us all—we must find it.

Methods

While most of this book is the result of straightforward research and policy analysis, I also conducted interviews with a series of practitioners to find out how they viewed birth and death in the hospital context and what kind of care they believe patients receive. Having experienced the deaths of relatives and the births of my three children, I had some experience from the patient side of things, but I felt that it was important to find out from providers about their experiences with birth and death inside and outside hospitals. As a result, I conducted in-person and phone interviews with a range of providers, including critical care nurses, hospice administrators, palliative care physicians, midwives, maternal-fetal specialists, and death doulas. These interviews are not meant to be scientific, nor is this meant to be an in-depth ethnographic study, which I am unqualified to attempt. Instead, these interviews provided me with background on hospital and out-of-hospital practices for birth and death, providing a range of experiences and attitudes. I also used quotes from these interviews to highlight or clarify parts of my argument. The sample is not meant to be exhaustive of the stakeholders in birth and death, and I do not claim any particular objectivity, either of my sample or of the people I interviewed.

In all, I interviewed 18 practitioners, whose titles are listed below. All of the interviewees agreed to the use of their words in the book and to the use of their real names, but for a variety of reasons I use their titles alone throughout. I found providers through a combination of referrals, snowball sampling, and outreach via social media. Practitioner interviews ranged from one to four hours in length, with follow-up emails where necessary. In addition to these providers, I also surveyed more than 400 individuals about their experiences with birth and death, both in and out of hospitals, to get both a broader and more individual understanding of different attitudes and experiences with American birth and death. The surveys were conducted using SurveyMonkey, and participants were recruited via social media. All responses were anonymous, and the survey instruments were approved by the institutional review board approval process of the Rochester Institute of Technology. The survey data were used as background information to clarify areas for further research, but I also used selected quotes from survey respondents who agreed to have their words used in the final book, particularly in the chapter on reimbursement barriers, an area where patients have the most direct experience with and knowledge of the policies that affect their care.

In-Depth Practitioner Interviews

Two palliative care physicians: one a faculty member at a large medical
    school, and one the supervising physician in a large urban palliative care
    practice
Hospice administrator
Hospice nurse
Palliative care nurse practitioner
Critical care nurse
Director of a "home for the dying"
Family practice doctor
Two hospital-based nurse midwives, practicing in different urban hospitals
Home birth nurse midwife
Home birth direct-entry midwife
Three obstetricians: one birth center owner and obstetrician, one private
    practice obstetrician, and one maternal-fetal specialist on the faculty of
    a medical school
Two birth center owners: both nurse midwives
Death doula and end-of-life planner

advance directive—A legal document that provides information to medical providers about a person's medical wishes, particularly at the end of life. May include living wills or, in some states, documents called medical or physician orders for life-sustaining treatment (MOLST or POLST, depending on the state) that provide immunity to medical staff who forgo lifesaving interventions in accordance with patient wishes.

advanced practice nurse—An umbrella term for a nurse who has a master's or post-master's level of education and is a specialist in a particular area such as midwifery or anesthesiology; an advanced practice nurse has scope-of-practice limitations that set boundaries for what she is and is not allowed to practice (see also "certified nurse midwife" and "nurse practitioner").

Affordable Care Act (commonly known as "Obamacare")—Comprehensive health reform legislation signed into law by President Barack Obama in March 2010 that expands Medicaid for low-income people, provides subsidies for middle-income families, and makes it easier for small businesses to offer health insurance.

American Association of Birth Centers—A nonprofit membership organization that supports research, education, and policy initiatives that promote the birth center model of care.

American College of Obstetricians and Gynecologists—The main national professional association for obstetricians and gynecologists in the United States.

American Medical Association—A professional organization created in the mid-1880s to standardize medical education.

autonomy—The right of an individual to make decisions relating to their own healthcare needs and body (see also "informed consent" and "relational autonomy").

beneficence—The principle of acting for the benefit and welfare of others; physicians are obligated to not only avoid doing harm but also act for the benefit of their patients (see also "bioethical principles").

bioethical principles—Four basic ethical guidelines physicians must follow when making decisions about procedures or treatment: autonomy, justice, beneficence, and nonmaleficence (see also "autonomy," "beneficence," "justice," and "nonmaleficence").

birth activism—Action taken to effect political or social change relating to birth issues, such as efforts to increase access to community-based birthing options. For example, birth activist groups such as the Black Mamas Matter Alliance, Black Women Birthing Justice, SisterSong, and the Black Doulas Association were formed by black healthcare and birth workers to provide community-based birthing care, particularly midwifery, to black women.

birth center (accredited)—A freestanding, home-like healthcare facility for childbirth that is separate from hospitals and staffed by midwives, nurse midwives, and/or obstetricians.

birth plan—A document in which a woman outlines her goals and desires for her labor and birthing experience; this document has no legal or clinical status.

#breakthesilence campaign—An initiative to collect and publicize, usually through social media, incidents of obstetric violence and violations of consent during birth.

capitated payment system—A system of reimbursement in which physicians or hospitals receive payment according to the number of patients they serve in a given period of time, regardless of the number of times the patients seek care. Newer capitation models provide hospitals with risk-adjusted monthly payments to provide all care for a patient, limited only by quality control reporting.

"cascade of interventions"—The tendency for one intervention to trigger further interventions either due to complications and side effects or practitioner proximity to interventions (see also "healthcare watershed").

centralization of care—The concentration of caregiving and medical resources in one place, such as in urban hospitals (see also "Hill-Burton Act").

certificate-of-need laws—Legislation instituted in many states and some federal jurisdictions in the 1970s to control the building or expansion of hospitals and other healthcare facilities based on community need. Because these laws allow existing providers to protest or even veto the entrance of potential competitors, hospitals use them to prevent competition from community-based care facilities.

certification—An official document verifying that an individual has achieved a certain level of skill or status.

certification of terminal illness—A document signed by a physician that declares the life expectancy of a patient to be six months or less if the terminal illness follows its normal course.

certified nurse midwife—An advanced practice nurse with a master's degree in midwifery who is trained to provide pre- and postnatal care, to provide support to women in labor, and to deliver babies (see also "advanced practice nurse"). Referred to in the text as "nurse midwife."

code—A slang term used by physicians in hospitals or clinics to refer to an emergency, such as a patient who has had a cardiopulmonary arrest; terms such as "code red" or "code blue" correspond with particular medical emergencies.

collaborative agreement—An agreement between a physician and another provider, often a midwife or nurse practitioner, that allows the physician to provide prescriptions or medical backup to patients seen by the other provider; often required by state health boards.

comfort care homes (also called homes for the dying)—Small facilities that provide care for dying patients. They fit within state regulations for end-of-life care by limiting themselves to two beds and avoid Medicare regulations by relying solely on donations.

Commission for the Accreditation of Birth Centers—The accrediting body for birth centers in the United States.

communication-and-resolution programs—A model in which providers and hospitals communicate with patients about adverse events immediately after detection, investigate what went wrong, offer an explanation, and, when warranted, apologize and provide compensation to the patient.

community-based care—Healthcare provided in either homes or outpatient facilities that tends to be low cost, evidence based, and patient centered; the provision of comprehensive healthcare, including social and emotional support in a nonmechanized setting, can help limit the need for medical intervention, particularly in birth and death situations. Examples of community-based care options include independent birth centers, residential hospice, home birth, and home hospice.

concierge medicine—A payment structure in which a patient pays a fee as a retainer in order to have direct access to a physician.

consolidation of care—A move toward smaller numbers of large insurers and hospital systems controlling payment for and provision of healthcare.

continuous fetal monitoring—The use of electronic monitors for constant monitoring of the activity and distress levels of the fetus during labor. This standard practice tends to be a gateway medical intervention that leads to other interventions during labor and birth. While medical evidence does not support its use for low-risk women, it is commonly used for liability reasons.

"conveyor belt" of care—A phrase coined by physician Jessica Zitter in her book, *Extreme Measures*, that refers to the way one medical intervention makes another much more likely and to the lack of information given to patients regarding long-term risks of interventions.

corporate practice of medicine laws—Legislation that regulates medical care by prohibiting corporations from employing physicians or engaging in medicine. These laws may limit innovations in healthcare by limiting the places and conditions in which physicians and advanced practice nurses work.

CPR (cardiopulmonary resuscitation)—An emergency procedure used to restart the heart and/or lungs. Its use on elderly or terminally ill patients may result in serious harm.

C-section (cesarean section)—A surgical operation to deliver a baby through an incision in a pregnant woman's abdomen.

curative treatment—Treatment that aims to treat or cure a patient of an illness. This is contrasted with palliative treatment, which emphasizes symptom management, though physicians disagree on how useful the distinction is in practice. The Medicare Hospice Benefit requires that patients limit all curative treatment to qualify.

death doula (also referred to as a "death midwife")—Nonmedical provider who supports and guides a dying patient through the process of physiological death; may also make meals for families, do light cleaning, keep the dying person comfortable, run errands, and assist the family during and after death.

death midwife—See "death doula."

"death panels"—A phrase coined by Sarah Palin, former Republican governor of Alaska, to characterize physicians' conversations about end-of-life care as bureaucrats making decisions about whether or not the elderly and disabled are "worthy of healthcare." She used the phrase to generate opposition to the Democrats' proposed Affordable Care Act healthcare legislation in 2009 (see also "Affordable Care Act").

defensive medicine—The use of extra caution by physicians in their practice to prevent or defend themselves against legal action due to malpractice. Defensive medicine is frequently linked to overtreatment, since the legal risks of overtreatment are lower than those of undertreatment.

demechanization of care—A movement away from mechanized treatments and technological monitoring and toward human-provided care that includes social and emotional support alongside treatment.

demedicalization of birth and death—A movement away from treating birth and death as illnesses that necessarily require medical intervention and toward an understanding of birth and death as human processes with social, emotional, and psychological import.

destandardization of care—Care that is free from the protocols and standards of hospitals and allows for individual choices and preferences.

direct-entry midwife—A midwife with an apprenticeship-based education and no medical training who has completed a licensing process through the state and may also be accredited by a national midwifery organization. Also called a "licensed midwife" or "certified professional midwife."

Do Not Resuscitate order—A directive added to a patient's medical file informing medical staff that the patient does not wish to receive CPR if their heart fails or their breathing stops.

double effect—The effect of a medication treating pain while at the same time, or in different doses, hastening death.

doula—A trained attendant during birth or at the end of life who provides social and emotional support and helps clarify healthcare goals and values.

episiotomy—An incision made in the tissue at the opening of the vagina during the second stage of labor to help widen the opening and facilitate delivery of the baby.

evidence-based practice—The integration of individual clinical expertise, research-based evidence, and patient preferences and values in making decisions about a patient's care.

expectant management—A characteristic approach of midwifery care that involves waiting and watching rather than assuming full control of the labor and birthing process; this approach is more difficult in hospital environments.

fee-for-service—A system in which a doctor or other healthcare provider is paid separately for each service offered, thereby incentivizing procedures over other types of care.

"the feminine mystique"—Phrase from and title of a book written by Betty Friedan, published in 1963, in which Friedan challenges the assumption that women find fulfillment through their roles as housewives and mothers alone.

Flexner Report (1910)—A move to standardize medical practice in the United States and make the profession more scientifically grounded. This report recommended the closure of many minority-run medical schools, which dramatically reduced the number of minority doctors in practice.

Friedman's curve—A guideline from the 1950s used by many hospitals as a basis for the "normal" length of each stage of labor; many researchers now view this guideline as outdated.

granny midwife—A traditional black midwife in the South who used practical intelligence and "motherwit" in assisting women in labor and childbirth, delivering babies, and helping with household tasks (see also "motherwit").

healthcare watershed—A metaphor for the variety of federal, state, local, and hospital policies that structure and determine the outcome of care. Just as the geography of the landscape directs water into valleys and downhill, the structure of the landscape of healthcare policies directs care downstream toward more intensive options (see also "cascade of interventions").

health disparity—The inequality of health status of different groups, with certain racial, ethnic, and socioeconomic groups having higher rates of certain diseases than others.

Hill-Burton Act—A federal law passed in 1946 that prioritized spending on hospital construction. This act resulted in a 40 percent increase in the number of hospital beds and a $1.8 billion investment in hospital construction.

home birth—A birth that takes place in one's home rather than in a hospital or at a birthing center; these usually involve little or no medical intervention.

homes for the dying—See "comfort care homes."

hospice—A general term referring to any support for the terminally ill at the end of life that focuses on comfort and symptom management. Also, a specific term indicating federal regulation of end-of-life care for patients who have less than six months to live and choose hospice care over other Medicare-covered benefits.

hospice care—End-of-life care for a terminally ill patient where attempts to cure this person's illness have been stopped. Hospice care may take place in a person's home, a nursing home, or another hospice facility (see also "palliative care").

iatrogenic birth trauma—Trauma inadvertently caused by medicalized birth practices that have no medical indications (e.g., restricted movement and the use of a catheter for a woman in labor) (see also "obstetric violence").

iatrogenic harm—Unintended harm caused in the process of a medical treatment.

induction—The use of medicine or manual interventions to initiate the labor process, most commonly because of macrosomia (a larger-than-average baby) or prolonged pregnancy.

informed consent—The idea that a patient, in the course of agreeing to a particular treatment, understands the need for the treatment (is informed) and is in control of her actions (gives consent) (see also "autonomy").

justice (with respect to healthcare)—The principle of respect for individual human rights, respect for morally acceptable laws, and fairness in the distribution of resources.

Lewin Report—A report commissioned by the Federal Trade Commission in 1981 chronicling substantial physician opposition to the Manhattan Birth Center. The report outlined the resignations of 10 of the

18 members of the Medical Advisory Board, formal opposition by physicians to insurance reimbursement for the birth center, informal opposition in the form of rumors about quality, and pressure on residents at the admitting hospital to avoid cooperating with the birth center.

liability safe harbor—A provision in a law that protects physicians who provide evidence-based care from liability. This limits the heightened risk perception of physicians in choosing less medicalized options.

licensing—The granting of permission by a regulatory body to perform a service in a particular geographic area (e.g., a direct-entry midwife who has been licensed to practice in a particular state).

malpractice environment—A context in which the threat of liability for improper or negligent treatment prevents physicians from practicing medicine in a way that is consistent with best practices and patient preferences, driving medicalization (see also "malpractice litigation").

malpractice litigation—Legal action taken against a professional for negligence or mistreatment that causes injury. Often cited as a primary reason for defensive medicine or the use of medical treatments to limit liability (see also "malpractice environment" and "defensive medicine").

maternal-fetal specialist—An obstetrician who specializes in high-risk pregnancies.

mechanization of care—The use of machines for testing, monitoring, and/or replacing bodily functions to allow staff to be in many places at once, to reduce human error, and to increase hospital efficiency.

Medicaid—A health insurance program started in 1965 and coadministered by states and the federal government that provides health coverage for individuals and families with low income.

medical intervention—Measures taken to prevent harm or to treat a medical condition. In the case of childbirth, examples include forceps delivery, episiotomies, and labor augmentation.

medicalization—The process by which a human experience or condition comes to be treated as an illness or disease, as is the case with experiences of birth and death.

Medicare—A federal health insurance program started in 1965 that provides health coverage for those over 65 years old or the disabled. Its payment structure and rules privilege hospitals over less interventionist providers.

Medicare Home Health Benefit—Covers the cost of health services such as nursing care and therapy in the home. Does not cover most day-to-day tasks like cleaning, cooking, and personal care (see also "Medicare Hospice Benefit").

Medicare Hospice Benefit—Provides coverage for palliative care in the home or a hospice facility for patients with less than six months to live who also agree to refuse other curative treatments. Signed into law in 1982, it was a measure to promote the hospice model to limit out-of-control costs and to address overtreatment of dying patients.

MOLST (medical order for life-sustaining treatment)—A legal form that provides immunity to medical staff who forgo lifesaving interventions and protects patient wishes.

motherwit—A combination of common sense and intuition that has guided traditional midwives for thousands of years (see also "granny midwife").

nonmaleficence—The principle of avoiding morally wrongful behavior or actions that inflict harm (see also "bioethical principles").

nurse practitioner—A registered nurse with advanced education and experience; provides some of the medical care formerly provided by physicians (see also "advanced practice nurse").

nursing home—A care home for the elderly or disabled. Medicaid covers nursing home care for low-income Americans, but there is no coverage under Medicare.

obstetric violence—Actions taken by providers during birth that involve high rates of intervention and lack of informed consent, such as forced cesarean sections and abusive conduct by providers during birth (see also "iatrogenic birth trauma" and "informed consent").

overtreatment—A level of medical treatment that exceeds the correct level of treatment, whether determined by professional standards or patient preferences (see also "undertreatment").

palliative care—Comprehensive care of a seriously ill patient in a hospital, a nursing home, a palliative care clinic, or the home that may include both measures to cure a person's illness and end-of-life comfort measures (see also "hospice care").

perceived racism—The interpretation of a situation or experience as discriminatory on the basis of race. Perceived racism may contribute to heightened stress in black individuals, making them more vulnerable to chronic health problems (see also "weathering effect").

perceived risk—The belief in a level of risk that may not relate to the real level of risk as supported by evidence.

perinatal mortality rate—A measure of the number of stillbirths and early neonatal deaths.

physician-assisted suicide—The voluntary ending of one's own life with the aid of a physician.

prodromal labor—Early false labor that starts and stops before active labor begins and can last days or weeks before active labor begins.

provider bias—The often subtle and unconscious preferential treatment given to white patients over black patients by healthcare providers, such as shorter wait times for white patients in the ER than for black patients with the same complaint because of different triaging.

reductionism—The notion that by reducing diseases and illness to the sum of their parts, researchers can determine causes and isolate treatments.

relational autonomy—Shared decision making between a patient and their family or friends relating to the patient's healthcare needs (see also "autonomy").

respite care—Short-term care for elderly or disabled people to give their regular caregivers a break from their ongoing caregiving responsibilities. It is not available in many areas owing to limited providers.

scope of practice—The roles, processes, and procedures that a healthcare provider is allowed to undertake based on their professional designation, often defined by state licensing requirements.

Sheppard-Towner Act—A 1921 federal policy promoting maternal and infant healthcare through the establishment of prenatal and children's programs and health centers. This act led to a shift in favor of nurse midwives with formal medical training over traditional midwives, contributing to the near elimination of black midwifery in the South.

skilled nursing facility—An area of a hospital or a special facility that provides professional nursing services to patients; it is covered under Medicare for a limited amount of time after a hospitalization and cannot usually be used concurrently with the hospice benefit.

standardization of care—The requirement that healthcare providers follow strict protocols and standard care procedures to eliminate human error and use resources in the most efficient way.

standardizing to individualize care—The implementation of standard protocols to prevent and address complications in order to provide care that meets the particular health needs and preferences of an individual, such as pause points with those who are dying, as an attempt to standardize assessing patient preferences.

SUPPORT study—A study published in 1996 that outlined serious shortcomings in the way Americans die in hospitals, such as high levels of aggressive treatment and confusion over end-of-life wishes, and demonstrated the difficulty of reform.

terminal patient—A person expected to die in a relatively short period of time from an end-stage illness.

terminal weaning—The gradual reduction of oxygen and removal of a mechanical ventilator from a patient who, owing to illness or injury, is not expected to breathe independently again; also known as "extubation" or the removal of life support.

third-party payers—Groups such as insurance companies or government agencies that reimburse healthcare expenses of a patient.

tort law—An area of civil law that protects people from wrongful acts by others.

traditional midwife—A midwife with an apprenticeship-based education and no medical training who refuses any licensing or certification limits on her practice.

transfer agreement—A written agreement that contains relevant clinical information about a patient who is being transferred from one healthcare facility to another; this is particularly relevant in the case of birth when a laboring woman is transferred from home or a birth center to a hospital.

Tricare—A healthcare insurance program for military members, retirees, and their families.

undertreatment—Failure to diagnose a condition, treat an illness, or manage pain at the level needed according to professional standards or patient preferences.

value-based care—The incorporation of patient outcomes into the reimbursement structure; an alternative to the fee-for-service model, which provides incentives for overtreatment.

value modifier program—A Medicare program that reimburses physicians based on quality of care and cost of services.

VBAC (vaginal birth after cesarean)—A vaginal birth by a woman who previously gave birth by cesarean section.

weathering effect—The compounding effect of stress and perceived racism on black Americans that contributes to chronic illnesses (see also "perceived racism").

Introduction. The Watershed of Healthcare Decision Making

1. Miriam is a pseudonym.

2. Nina Bernstein, "Fighting to Honor a Father's Last Wish: To Die at Home," *New York Times*, September 25, 2014, www.nytimes.com/2014/09/26 /nyregion/family-fights-health-care-system-for-simple-request-to-die-at-home .html.

3. Bernstein, "Fighting."

4. Richard A. Deyo, "Cascade Effects of Medical Technology," *Annual Review of Public Health* 23, no. 1 (2002): 23–44; Courtenay R. Bruce, John E. Fetter, and J. S. Blumenthal-Barby, "Cascade Effects in Critical Care Medicine: A Call for Practice Changes," *American Journal of Respiratory and Critical Care Medicine* 188, no. 12 (December 15, 2013): 1384–85, https://doi.org/10.1164 /rccm.201309-1606ED.

5. The term "medicalization" originated in the sociological literature in the 1970s, and the current literature discusses everything from psychiatric disorders to sexual identities to male pattern baldness. See Peter Conrad, *The Medicalization of Society: On the Transformation of Human Conditions into Treatable Disorders* (Baltimore: Johns Hopkins University Press, 2007).

6. Jessica Nutik Zitter, "De-medicalizing Death," *Health Affairs* (blog), September 28, 2017, http://healthaffairs.org/blog/2017/09/28/de-medicalizing -death/; Ira Byock, *Best Care Possible: A Physician's Quest to Transform Care through the End of Life* (New York: Avery, 2013); Angelo E. Volandes, *The Conversation: A Revolutionary Plan for End-of-Life Care* (New York: Blooms-bury, 2016); Amy Michelle DeBaets, "From Birth Plan to Birth Partnership: Enhancing Communication in Childbirth," *American Journal of Obstetrics and Gynecology* 216, no. 1 (January 2017): 31.e1–31.e4, https://doi.org/10.1016/j .ajog.2016.09.087.

7. Attitudes toward medicalization vary in the sociological literature. While contemporary sociologists like Peter Conrad seek to understand the process of medicalization from a descriptive standpoint, earlier critics like Thomas

Szasz and Ivan Illich rebelled against a medical model that they saw broadening the field of medical control well past its legitimate boundaries, crowding out human elements, and challenging foundational principles like autonomy and self-determination. Ivan Illich, *Medical Nemesis: The Expropriation of Health* (New York: Pantheon Books, 1976); Conrad, *Medicalization of Society*; Thomas Szasz, *The Medicalization of Everyday Life: Selected Essays* (Syracuse, NY: Syracuse University Press, 2007); Roslyn Lindheim, "Birthing Centers and Hospices: Reclaiming Birth and Death," *Annual Review of Public Health* 2 (1981): 1–29, https://doi.org/10.1146/annurev.pu.02.050181.000245.

8. Centers for Disease Control and Prevention, "FastStats: Life Expectancy," www.cdc.gov/nchs/fastats/life-expectancy.htm; www.cdc.gov/nchs/data/hus /2010/022.pdf.

9. Carol Sakala, Maureen P. Corry, and Milbank Memorial Fund, *Evidence-Based Maternity Care: What It Is and What It Can Achieve* (New York: Milbank Memorial Fund, 2008).

10. Sakala, Corry, and Milbank Memorial Fund, *Evidence-Based Maternity Care*.

11. Haider Warraich, *Modern Death: How Medicine Changed the End of Life* (New York: St. Martin's, 2017).

12. Institute of Medicine (US) and Committee on Approaching Death: Addressing Key End-of-Life Issues, *Dying in America: Improving Quality and Honoring Individual Preferences near the End of Life* (Washington, DC: National Academies Press, 2015).

13. Institute of Medicine (US) and Committee on Approaching Death, *Dying in America*.

14. "End of Life Care," *Dartmouth Atlas of Health Care* (blog), www .dartmouthatlas.org/interactive-apps/end-of-life-care/.

15. Kei Ouchi et al., "Prognosis after Emergency Department Intubation to Inform Shared Decision-Making," *Journal of the American Geriatrics Society* 66, no. 7 (July 2018): 1377–81, https://doi.org/10.1111/jgs.15361; Van Gijn et al., "The Chance of Survival and the Functional Outcome after In-Hospital Cardiopulmonary Resuscitation in Older People: A Systematic Review," *Age and Ageing* 43, no. 4 (July 1, 2014): 456–63, https://doi.org/10.1093/ageing /afu035.

16. Henry J. Kaiser Family Foundation, "Medicaid Pocket Primer," June 2017, http://files.kff.org/attachment/Fact-Sheet-Medicaid-Pocket-Primer.

17. Amber E. Barnato et al., "Trends in Inpatient Treatment Intensity among Medicare Beneficiaries at the End of Life," *Health Services Research* 39, no. 2 (April 1, 2004): 363–76, http://dx.doi.org/10.1111/j.1475-6773.2004.00232.x.

18. Kenneth A. Fisher, Lindsay E. Rockwell, and Missy Scott, *In Defiance of Death: Exposing the Real Costs of End-of-Life Care* (Westport, CT: Praeger, 2008).

19. Harold Y. Vanderpool, *Palliative Care: The 400-Year Quest for a Good Death* (Jefferson, NC: McFarland, 2015), 94; Conrad, *Medicalization of Society*.

20. Conrad, *Medicalization of Society*.

21. Lindheim, "Birthing Centers and Hospices."

22. Barbara Ehrenreich and Deirdre English, *For Her Own Good: Two Centuries of the Experts' Advice to Women* (New York: Anchor Books, 2005), 103–11.

23. Roslyn Lindheim, *Birthing Centers and Hospices: Reclaiming Birth and Death* (Berkeley, CA: Center for Environmental Design Research, 1981), 5.

24. Paul Starr, *The Social Transformation of American Medicine: The Rise of a Sovereign Profession and the Making of a Vast Industry* (New York: Basic Books, 1984), 347.

25. Starr, *Social Transformation of American Medicine*, 349.

26. Lindheim, "Birthing Centers and Hospices," 2.

27. Starr, *Social Transformation of American Medicine*, 350.

28. Lindheim, "Birthing Centers and Hospices," 6.

29. Lindheim, "Birthing Centers and Hospices," 6.

30. Roslyn Lindheim, "An Architect's Perspective," in *Humanizing Health Care*, ed. Jan Howard and Anselm Strauss (New York: John Wiley, 1975), 299.

31. Starr, *Social Transformation of American Medicine*, 385.

32. Starr, *Social Transformation of American Medicine*, 376.

33. Margaret Bingley, *In Sickness and in Wealth* (London: Severn, 1987), 114.

34. According to Lindheim, "the goal of professional medical organizations is toward the closing of small hospitals and the location of birth in larger, more centralized units that have the immediate capability of handling high risk pregnancies and, to varying degrees, high risk infant care." Lindheim, "Birthing Centers and Hospices," 16.

35. Lindheim, "Birthing Centers and Hospices," 16.

36. Theresa Morris, *Cut It Out: The C-Section Epidemic in America* (New York: New York University Press, 2013).

37. Certificate-of-need laws are discussed at length in chap. 4.

38. Attitudes toward medicalization vary in the sociological literature. While contemporary sociologists like Peter Conrad seek to understand the process of medicalization from a descriptive standpoint, earlier critics like Thomas Szasz and Ivan Illich rebelled against a medical model that they saw broadening the field of medical control well past its legitimate boundaries, crowding out human elements, and challenging foundational principles like autonomy and self-determination. I try to use medicalization descriptively, reserving "overtreatment" for areas where I am making normative claims. See Illich, *Medical Nemesis*; Conrad, *Medicalization of Society*; Szasz, *Medicalization of Everyday Life*; Lindheim, "Birthing Centers and Hospices."

39. Conrad, *Medicalization of Society*.

40. "The APA Removes 'Gender Identity Disorder' from Updated Mental Health Guide," GLAAD, December 3, 2012, www.glaad.org/blog/apa-removes -gender-identity-disorder-updated-mental-health-guide.

41. Szasz, *Medicalization of Everyday Life*, 21.

42. Elisabeth Kübler-Ross, *On Death and Dying: What the Dying Have to Teach Doctors, Nurses, Clergy and Their Own Families* (New York: Scribner, 2014).

43. Fisher, Rockwell, and Scott, *In Defiance of Death*.

44. Tom L. Beauchamp and James F. Childress, *Principles of Biomedical Ethics* (New York: Oxford University Press, 2016). I follow Beauchamp and Childress here while also being aware that there are considerable debates within both the biomedical ethics community and the broader philosophic community on the meaning of these various terms and whether such a framework is either complete or consistent. I am approaching these questions not from a detailed analytic perspective, but from the perspective of a layperson who is interested in the basic harms and benefits different medical systems provide.

45. Ruth R. Faden, Tom L. Beauchamp, and Nancy M. P. King, *A History and Theory of Informed Consent*, 1st ed. (New York: Oxford University Press, 1986), 76–91.

46. Harriet A. Washington, *Medical Apartheid: The Dark History of Medical Experimentation on Black Americans from Colonial Times to the Present* (New York: Anchor Books, 2008).

47. As part of the research on this book, I interviewed 17 providers, including physicians, midwives, nurses, hospice administrators, and doulas. For a variety of reasons, I refer to the providers by generic titles rather than (what I felt would be) more distracting pseudonyms. More information on the interviews and the full list of providers are available in the appendix. I also interviewed patients and families about their experiences with medicalized birth and death, including two surveys. These survey results are used primarily to provide anecdotal support and narrative force for more traditional research.

Chapter 1. Medicalized Birth and the Current of Centralized Care

1. European countries, for example, have much higher use of midwives, home birth, and birth center births, alongside comparable rates of infant mortality and much lower maternal mortality. Jane Sandall, "Place of Birth in Europe," *Entre Nous* 81 (2015), www.euro.who.int/__data/assets/pdf_file/0010 /277741/Place-of-birth-in-Europe.pdf?ua=1. *Rinat Dray v. Staten Island University Hospital*, no. 500510/2014.

2. Kate Womersley, "Why Giving Birth Is Safer in Britain Than in the U.S.," *ProPublica*, August 31, 2017, www.propublica.org/article/why-giving-birth-is -safer-in-britain-than-in-the-u-s.

3. Ariadne Labs, *Designing Capacity of High Value Healthcare: The Impact of Design on Clinical Care in Childbirth* (Ariadne Labs, 2017), https://massdesign group.org/sites/default/files/file/2017/170223_Ariadne%20Report_Final.pdf.

4. Dorothy Shaw et al., "Drivers of Maternity Care in High-Income Countries: Can Health Systems Support Woman-Centred Care?," *Lancet* 388, no. 10057 (November 5, 2016): 2286, https://doi.org/10.1016/S0140-6736(16) 31527-6.

5. Jill Alliman and Julia C. Phillippi, "Maternal Outcomes in Birth Centers: An Integrative Review of the Literature," *Journal of Midwifery and Women's Health* 61, no. 1 (January 2016): 21–51, https://doi.org/10.1111/jmwh.12356.

6. Carol Sakala, Maureen P. Corry, and Milbank Memorial Fund, *Evidence-Based Maternity Care: What It Is and What It Can Achieve* (New York: Milbank Memorial Fund, 2008), 11.

7. François Laliberté et al., "Medicaid Spending on Contraceptive Coverage and Pregnancy-Related Care," *Reproductive Health* 11, no. 1 (2014): 20, https:// doi.org/10.1186/1742-4755-11-20; Susan Rutledge Stapleton, Cara Osborne, and Jessica Illuzzi, "Outcomes of Care in Birth Centers: Demonstration of a Durable Model," *Journal of Midwifery and Women's Health* 58, no. 1 (January 2013): 3–14, https://doi.org/10.1111/jmwh.12003.

8. Laliberté et al., "Medicaid Spending."

9. Truven Health Analytics, "The Cost of Having a Baby in the United States," January 2013, www.chqpr.org/downloads/CostofHavingaBaby.pdf.

10. Victoria G. Woo, Arnold Milstein, and Terry Platchek, "Hospital-Affiliated Outpatient Birth Centers," *Journal of the American Medical Association* 316, no. 14 (2016): 1441, https://doi.org/10.1001/jama.2016.11770.

11. Centers for Disease Control, "Severe Maternal Morbidity in the United States," November 27, 2017, www.cdc.gov/reproductivehealth/maternalinfant health/severematernalmorbidity.html.

12. Shiliang Liu et al., "Maternal Mortality and Severe Morbidity Associated with Low-Risk Planned Cesarean Delivery versus Planned Vaginal Delivery at Term," *Canadian Medical Association Journal* 176, no. 4 (February 13, 2007): 455–60, https://doi.org/10.1503/cmaj.060870.

13. Centers for Disease Control and Prevention, "FastStats: Births, Method of Delivery," www.cdc.gov/nchs/fastats/delivery.htm.

14. Giacomo Biasucci et al., "Cesarean Delivery May Affect the Early Biodiversity of Intestinal Bacteria," *Journal of Nutrition* 138, no. 9 (September 1, 2008): 1796S–1800S.

15. Liu et al., "Maternal Mortality."

16. Sakala, Corry, and Milbank Memorial Fund, *Evidence-Based Maternity Care*, 11.

17. Sakala, Corry, and Milbank Memorial Fund, *Evidence-Based Maternity Care*, 14.

18. American College of Obstetricians and Gynecologists, "Committee Opinion: Approaches to Limit Intervention during Labor and Birth," February 2017, www.acog.org/Clinical-Guidance-and-Publications/Committee-Opinions/Committee-on-Obstetric-Practice/Approaches-to-Limit-Intervention-During-Labor-and-Birth.

19. Richard Johanson, Mary Newburn, and Alison Macfarlane, "Has the Medicalisation of Childbirth Gone Too Far?," *BMJ* 324, no. 7342 (April 13, 2002): 892–95.

20. Neel Shah, "A NICE Delivery—the Cross-Atlantic Divide over Treatment Intensity in Childbirth," *New England Journal of Medicine* 372, no. 23 (June 3, 2015): 2181–83, https://doi.org/10.1056/NEJMp1501461.

21. Mandisa Singata, Joan Tranmer, and Gillian ML Gyte, "Restricting Oral Fluid and Food Intake during Labour," in *Cochrane Database of Systematic Reviews*, ed. The Cochrane Collaboration (Chichester, UK: John Wiley & Sons, 2010), http://doi.wiley.com/10.1002/14651858.CD003930.pub2.

22. Jane Sandall et al., "Midwife-Led Continuity Models versus Other Models of Care for Childbearing Women," in *Cochrane Database of Systematic Reviews*, ed. The Cochrane Collaboration (Chichester, UK: John Wiley & Sons, 2015), http://doi.wiley.com/10.1002/14651858.CD004667.pub4.

23. Giliane Fenech and Gill Thomson, "Tormented by Ghosts from Their Past': A Meta-Synthesis to Explore the Psychosocial Implications of a Traumatic Birth on Maternal Well-Being," *Midwifery* 30, no. 2 (February 2014): 185–93, https://doi.org/10.1016/j.midw.2013.12.004.

24. Henci Goer, "Cruelty in Maternity Wards: Fifty Years Later," *Journal of Perinatal Education* 19, no. 3 (2010): 33–42, https://doi.org/10.1624/105812410X514413; Elizabeth Kukura, "Obstetric Violence," *Georgetown Law Journal* 106 (May 2018): 721–801.

25. D. K. Creedy, I. M. Shochet, and J. Horsfall, "Childbirth and the Development of Acute Trauma Symptoms: Incidence and Contributing Factors," *Birth* 27, no. 2 (June 2000): 104–11.

26. See, e.g., stories relating to two recent cases: Beth Greenfield, "Mom Who Sued Hospital for Traumatic Birth Wins $16 Million," *Yahoo News*, August 8, 2016, www.yahoo.com/beauty/mom-who-sued-hospital-for-traumatic-birth-wins-16-million-173203800.html; Improving Birth, "'Kelly,' Who Had a Forced Episiotomy, Goes to Court," Crowdrise, www.crowdrise.com/kellygoestocourt. See also John Cooper, Samantha Burton v. State of Florida, no. 1D99-1958 (Circuit Court for Leon County, August 12, 2010).

27. Brandy Zadrozny, "New Mom Begged Doc: 'No, Don't Cut Me!,'" *Daily Beast*, June 5, 2015, www.thedailybeast.com/articles/2015/06/05/new-mom-begged-doc-no-don-t-cut-me.html. See also Fenech and Thomson, "Tormented by Ghosts."

28. Greenfield, "Mom Who Sued Hospital."

29. Phoebe Friesan, "Educational Pelvic Exams on Anesthetized Women: Why Consent Matters," *Bioethics* 32, no. 5 (April 23, 2018): 298–307, https://doi.org/10.1111/bioe.12441.

30. See, e.g., https://improvingbirth.org/2014/08/vid/.

31. Alan Levine, Robert Oshel, and Sidney Wolfe, "State Medical Boards Fail to Discipline Doctors with Hospital Actions against Them," *Public Citizen*, March 2011, www.citizen.org/sites/default/files/1937.pdf.

32. R. Hamowy, "The Early Development of Medical Licensing Laws in the United States, 1875–1900," *Journal of Libertarian Studies* 3, no. 1 (1979): 73–119.

33. Richard W. Wertz and Dorothy C. Wertz, *Lying-In: A History of Childbirth in America* (New York: Free Press, 1977).

34. Barbara Ehrenreich and Deirdre English, *For Her Own Good: Two Centuries of the Experts' Advice to Women* (New York: Anchor Books, 2005).

35. J. Whitridge Williams, "Medical Education and the Midwife Problem in the United States," *Journal of the American Medical Association* 58, no. 1 (January 6, 1912): 1, https://doi.org/10.1001/jama.1912.04260010003001.

36. Eugene R. Declercq, "The Trials of Hanna Porn: The Campaign to Abolish Midwifery in Massachusetts," *American Journal of Public Health* 84, no. 6 (1994): 1022–28.

37. Declercq, "Trials of Hanna Porn."

38. Roslyn Lindheim, "Birthing Centers and Hospices: Reclaiming Birth and Death," *Annual Review of Public Health* 2 (1981): 4, https://doi.org/10.1146/annurev.pu.02.050181.000245.

39. Wertz and Wertz, *Lying-In*, 140–42.

40. Wertz and Wertz, *Lying-In*, 143.

41. Wertz and Wertz, *Lying-In*, 126–28.

42. Wertz and Wertz, *Lying-In*, 153.

43. Wertz and Wertz, *Lying-In*, 167.

44. Lindheim, "Birthing Centers and Hospices," 5.

45. Wertz and Wertz, *Lying-In*, 167.

46. Quoted in Lindheim, "Birthing Centers and Hospices," 6.

47. Wertz and Wertz, *Lying-In*, 137; Anat Shmueli et al., "Episiotomy—Risk Factors and Outcomes," *Journal of Maternal-Fetal and Neonatal Medicine: The Official Journal of the European Association of Perinatal Medicine, the Federation of Asia and Oceania Perinatal Societies, the International Society of Perinatal Obstetricians* 30, no. 3 (February 2017): 251–56, https://doi.org/10.3109/14767058.2016.1169527; Vittorio Basevi and Tina Lavender, "Routine Perineal Shaving on Admission in Labour," in *Cochrane Database of Systematic Reviews*, ed. The Cochrane Collaboration (Chichester, UK: John Wiley & Sons, 2014), http://doi.wiley.com/10.1002/14651858.CD001236.pub2.

48. Wertz and Wertz, *Lying-In*, 168.

49. Ebony B. Carter et al., "Number of Prenatal Visits and Pregnancy Outcomes in Low-Risk Women," *Journal of Perinatology: Official Journal of the California Perinatal Association* 36, no. 3 (March 2016): 178–81, https://doi.org/10.1038/jp.2015.183.

50. Wertz and Wertz, *Lying-In*, 165.

51. Elizabeth Moore et al., "Early Skin-to-Skin Contact for Mothers and Their Healthy Newborn Infants," *Cochrane Database of Systematic Reviews* 2 (May 16, 2012): CD003519, doi:10.1002/14651858.CD003519.pub3; Debra S. Lefkowitz, Chiara Baxt, and Jacquelyn R. Evans, "Prevalence and Correlates of Posttraumatic Stress and Postpartum Depression in Parents of Infants in the Neonatal Intensive Care Unit (NICU)," *Journal of Clinical Psychology in Medical Settings* 17, no. 3 (September 1, 2010): 230–37, https://doi.org/10.1007/s10880-010-9202-7.

52. Theresa Morris, *Cut It Out: The C-Section Epidemic in America* (New York: New York University Press, 2013), 57.

53. "ACOG Refines Fetal Heart Rate Monitoring Guidelines—ACOG," June 22, 2009, http://obgyn.med.sc.edu/documents/antepartum_fetal_2.pdf.

54. Morris, *Cut It Out*, 129.

55. Howard Minkoff and Dmitry Fridman, "The Immediately Available Physician Standard," *Seminars in Perinatology* 34, no. 5 (October 1, 2010): 325–30, https://doi.org/10.1053/j.semperi.2010.05.005.

56. Lindheim, "Birthing Centers and Hospices."

57. Wertz and Wertz, *Lying-In*, 170–71.

58. Wertz and Wertz, *Lying-In*, 182–83.

59. Anna Seijmonsbergen-Schermers et al., "Variations in Childbirth Interventions in High-Income Countries: Protocol for a Multinational Cross-Sectional Study," *BMJ Open* 8, no. 1 (January 10, 2018), https://doi.org/10.1136/bmjopen-2017-017993.

60. Richard A. Deyo, "Cascade Effects of Medical Technology," *Annual Review of Public Health* 23, no. 1 (2002): 23–44.

61. Ros Goddard, "Electronic Fetal Monitoring," *BMJ* 322, no. 7300 (June 16, 2001): 1436–37.

62. Sakala, Corry, and Milbank Memorial Fund, *Evidence-Based Maternity Care*.

63. Jennifer L. Bailit et al., "Hospital Primary Cesarean Delivery Rates and the Risk of Poor Neonatal Outcomes," *American Journal of Obstetrics and Gynecology* 187, no. 3 (September 2002): 721–27, https://doi.org/10.1067/mob.2002.125886.

64. J. Christopher Glantz, "Obstetric Variation, Intervention, and Outcomes: Doing More but Accomplishing Less," *Birth* 39, no. 4 (December 1, 2012): 286–90, https://doi.org/10.1111/birt.12002; Katy Backes Kozhimannil, Michael R. Law, and Beth A. Virnig, "Cesarean Delivery Rates Vary Tenfold among US

Hospitals; Reducing Variation May Address Quality and Cost Issues," *Health Affairs* 32, no. 3 (March 2013): 527–35.

65. Deyo, "Cascade Effects," 35.

66. Shah, "NICE Delivery." Shah points out that "nearly all Americans are currently born in settings that are essentially intensive care units (ICUs): labor floors have multipaneled telemetry monitors, medications that require minute-by-minute titration, and some of the highest staffing ratios in the hospital. Most labor floors are actually more intensive than other ICUs in that they contain their own operating rooms. Surely every birth does not require an ICU."

67. Ariadne Labs, *Designing Capacity*, 4.

68. Ariadne Labs, *Designing Capacity*.

69. "ACOG Expands Recommendations to Treat Postpartum Hemorrhage—ACOG," www.acog.org/About-ACOG/News-Room/News-Releases/2017/ACOG-Expands-Recommendations-to-Treat-Postpartum-Hemorrhage?IsMobileSet=false.

70. Womersley, "Why Giving Birth Is Safer."

71. Sarah Blaffer Hrdy, *Mother Nature: A History of Mothers, Infants and Natural Selection* (New York: Pantheon Books, 1999), 137–39.

72. Ina May Gaskin, *Ina May's Guide to Childbirth* (New York: Bantam Books, 2003), 139, 144–49.

73. Annemarie Lawrence et al., "Maternal Positions and Mobility during First Stage Labour," *Cochrane Database of Systematic Reviews*, no. 8 (2013): CD003934, https://doi.org/10.1002/14651858.CD003934.pub3.

74. Jun Zhang et al., "Contemporary Patterns of Spontaneous Labor with Normal Neonatal Outcomes," *Obstetrics and Gynecology* 116, no. 6 (December 2010): 1281–87, https://doi.org/10.1097/AOG.0b013e3181fdef6e.

75. Glantz, "Obstetric Variation"; J. Christopher Glantz, "Elective Induction v. Spontaneous Labor: Associations and Outcomes," *Journal of Reproductive Medicine* 50 (2005): 235–40.

76. E. R. Declercq et al., "Listening to Mothers III: Pregnancy and Birth" (New York: Childbirth Connection, May 2013), http://transform.childbirth connection.org/wp-content/uploads/2013/06/LTM-III_MajorSurveyFindings_PregnancyAndBirth.pdf.

77. See ACOG's various positions in "Labor Induction: Resource Overview—ACOG," www.acog.org/Womens-Health/Labor-Induction. See also Gaskin, *Ina May's Guide*, 207.

78. Sakala, Corry, and Milbank Memorial Fund, *Evidence-Based Maternity Care*, 36.

79. Glantz, "Obstetric Variation"; Barbara Bodner-Adler et al., "Influence of Labor Induction on Obstetric Outcomes in Patients with Prolonged Pregnancy," *Wiener Klinische Wochenschrift* 117, no. 7 (2005): 287–92, https://doi.org/10.1007/s00508-005-0330-2. See also James M. Alexander, Donald D. McIntire,

and Kenneth J. Leveno, "Forty Weeks and Beyond: Pregnancy Outcomes by Week of Gestation," *Obstetrics and Gynecology* 96, no. 2 (2000): 291–94; Aaron Caughey et al., "Maternal and Neonatal Outcomes of Elective Induction of Labor," *Evidence Report/Technology Assessment*, no. 176 (2009), https://ohsu.pure.elsevier.com/en/publications/maternal-and-neonatal-outcomes-of-elective-induction-of-labor-2. See also ACOG's report on the risks of elective induction at www.acog.org/Resources-And-Publications/Committee-Opinions/Committee-on-Obstetric-Practice/Definition-of-Term-Pregnancy.

80. See Peter Conrad, *The Medicalization of Society: On the Transformation of Human Conditions into Treatable Disorders* (Baltimore: Johns Hopkins University Press, 2007).

81. Rahul K. Nath et al., "Birth Weight and Incidence of Surgical Obstetric Brachial Plexus Injury," *Eplasty* 15 (2015): e14.

82. Declercq et al., "Listening to Mothers III."

83. J. W. Weeks, T. Pitman, and J. A. Spinnato, "Fetal Macrosomia: Does Antenatal Prediction Affect Delivery Route and Birth Outcome?," *American Journal of Obstetrics and Gynecology* 173, no. 4 (October 1995): 1215–19.

84. D. Sadeh-Mestechkin et al., "Suspected Macrosomia? Better Not Tell," *Archives of Gynecology and Obstetrics* 278, no. 3 (September 2008): 225–30, https://doi.org/10.1007/s00404-008-0566-y.

85. Sean C. Blackwell et al., "Overestimation of Fetal Weight by Ultrasound: Does It Influence the Likelihood of Cesarean Delivery for Labor Arrest?," *American Journal of Obstetrics and Gynecology* 200, no. 3 (March 2009): 340.e1–3, https://doi.org/10.1016/j.ajog.2008.12.043.

86. Sadeh-Mestechkin et al., "Suspected Macrosomia?"

87. As another obstetrician observed, "The same has been said for various diagnostic criteria for gestational diabetes mellitus (GDM). The ones that give more women a diagnosis of GDM are associated with higher cesarean rates but no significant improvement in outcome. In other words, the diagnosis of GDM leads to more interventions, despite no documented benefits."

88. Sadeh-Mestechkin et al., "Suspected Macrosomia?" Possible explanations for such inductions are discussed in chap. 6.

89. E. A. Friedman, "Primigravid Labor; a Graphicostatistical Analysis," *Obstetrics and Gynecology* 6, no. 6 (December 1955): 567–89.

90. Zhang et al., "Contemporary Patterns"; Jeremy L. Neal et al., "'Active Labor' Duration and Dilation Rates among Low-Risk, Nulliparous Women with Spontaneous Labor Onset: A Systematic Review," *Journal of Midwifery and Women's Health* 55, no. 4 (2010): 308–18, https://doi.org/10.1016/j.jmwh.2009.08.004.

91. Neal et al., "'Active Labor' Duration."

92. Zhang et al., "Contemporary Patterns."

93. Emma L. Barber et al., "Indications Contributing to the Increasing

Cesarean Delivery Rate," *Obstetrics and Gynecology* 118, no. 1 (July 2011): 29–38, https://doi.org/10.1097/AOG.0b013e31821e5f65.

94. Improving Birth, "'Kelly,' Who Had a Forced Episiotomy."

95. Hunter Schwarz, "Following Reports of Forced Sterilization of Female Prison Inmates, California Passes Ban," *Washington Post*, September 26, 2014, www.washingtonpost.com/blogs/govbeat/wp/2014/09/26/following-reports-of-forced-sterilization-of-female-prison-inmates-california-passes-ban/.

96. Sarah Yahr Tucker and Callie Beusman, "There Is a Hidden Epidemic of Doctors Abusing Women in Labor, Doulas Say," *Broadly*, May 8, 2018, https://broadly.vice.com/en_us/article/evqew7/obstetric-violence-doulas-abuse-giving-birth; Elizabeth Hlavinka, "When Docs Sexually Violate Patients," *MedPage Today*, January 24, 2019, www.medpagetoday.com/publichealthpolicy/ethics/77605.

97. Friesan, "Educational Pelvic Exams."

98. Esther Honig, "Teen Moms in Some States Are Denied Pain Relief during Childbirth," *Broadly*, accessed November 15, 2017, www.sideeffectspublic media.org/post/teen-moms-some-states-are-denied-pain-relief-during-childbirth.

99. Rinat Dray v. Staten Island University Hospital, no. 500510/2014.

100. A major difference between hospital birth and home birth is that the midwife is a guest in the mother's home and can be asked to leave at any time. Laboring women may be unable to leave hospitals either because they misunderstand what is required to leave against medical advice or because they are physically incapable of leaving as a result of the progress of labor itself.

101. Mary Briody Mahowald, *Women and Children in Health Care: An Unequal Majority* (New York: Oxford University Press, 1996), 52–53.

102. Wertz and Wertz, *Lying-In*; Emily Oster, *Expecting Better: Why the Conventional Wisdom Is Wrong—and What You Really Need to Know* (New York: Penguin, 2013), xvi.

103. Oster, *Expecting Better*, xvi.

104. Sarah C. M. Roberts and Amani Nuru-Jeter, "Universal Screening for Alcohol and Drug Use and Racial Disparities in Child Protective Services Reporting," *Journal of Behavioral Health Services and Research* 39, no. 1 (January 2012): 3–16, https://doi.org/10.1007/s11414-011-9247-x.

105. In one instance I was present for, a laboring mother and her doula were discussing options for a scheduled cesarean section with her physician. When the mother asked about whether there was a designated "stork nurse" on shift to allow her to have immediate skin-to-skin contact with her baby (an option that was explicitly mentioned by another member of the labor and delivery staff that day), the obstetrician said "right now I'm more concerned about saving the life of the mother and baby." There were no signs that either mother or child was in any distress, and previously that night the obstetrician had indicated that the surgery could safely take place the next day. The language of fear seemed to

play no role other than to hasten consent to the surgery, consent that was already forthcoming. Perhaps playing a role, the interaction occurred at the end of the physician's shift, and the parents suspected that the physician wanted to get the surgery done quickly.

106. While providers outside of hospitals can also engage in coercive or manipulative behavior, there are fewer incentives for midwives to intervene, and the close relationship between midwives and the pregnant women they assist lends itself to a less hierarchical and authoritarian relationship, which may also limit violations of patient autonomy.

107. Bryan Murray, "Informed Consent: What Must a Physician Disclose to a Patient?," *AMA Journal of Ethics* 14, no. 7 (July 1, 2012): 563–66, https://doi .org/10.1001/virtualmentor.2012.14.7.hlaw1-1207.

108. Cristen Pascucci, "You're Not Allowed to Not Allow Me," *Birth Monopoly* (blog), June 17, 2014, http://birthmonopoly.com/allowed/.

109. American College of Obstetricians and Gynecologists (ACOG) Committee on Ethics, "Refusal of Medically Recommended Treatment during Pregnancy," June 2016, www.acog.org/Clinical-Guidance-and-Publications /Committee-Opinions/Committee-on-Ethics/Refusal-of-Medically-Recom mended-Treatment-During-Pregnancy.

110. Wertz and Wertz, *Lying-In*; Ehrenreich and English, *For Her Own Good*.

111. Wertz and Wertz, *Lying-In*; Lindheim, "Birthing Centers and Hospices."

112. Robert A. Nye, "Medicine and Science as Masculine 'Fields of Honor,'" *Osiris* 12 (1997): 60–79.

113. Cristen Pascucci, "Physician Trauma: A Doctor Answers, Why Do We Sometimes Do Terrible Things?," *Birth Monopoly* (blog), August 31, 2018, http://birthmonopoly.com/physician-trauma/.

114. William F. Rayburn and American Congress of Obstetricians and Gynecologists, *The Obstetrician/Gynecologist Workforce in the United States: Facts, Figures, and Implications* (American Congress of Obstetricians and Gynecologists, 2011); Glantz, "Obstetric Variation."

115. Amy Michelle DeBaets, "From Birth Plan to Birth Partnership: Enhancing Communication in Childbirth," *American Journal of Obstetrics and Gynecology* 216, no. 1 (January 2017): 31.e1–31.e4, https://doi.org/10.1016/j .ajog.2016.09.087. See also discussions of physicians' comments on social media, some of which are discussed in Cristen Pascucci, "Birth Plans Are Never a Joke: Trust, Betrayal, and Misogyny in Maternity Care," *Birth Monopoly* (blog), November 20, 2017, http://birthmonopoly.com/plans/.

116. Sarah D McDonald et al., "A Qualitative Descriptive Study of the Group Prenatal Care Experience: Perceptions of Women with Low-Risk Pregnancies and Their Midwives," *BMC Pregnancy and Childbirth* 14 (September 26, 2014), https://doi.org/10.1186/1471-2393-14-334.

117. Bernie Divall et al., "Plans, Preferences or Going with the Flow: An Online Exploration of Women's Views and Experiences of Birth Plans," *Midwifery* 54 (November 2017): 29–34, https://doi.org/10.1016/j.midw.2017.07.020; Joanne V. Welsh and Andrew G. Symon, "Unique and Proforma Birth Plans: A Qualitative Exploration of Midwives' Experiences," *Midwifery* 30, no. 7 (July 2014): 885–91, https://doi.org/10.1016/j.midw.2014.03.004.

118. DeBaets, "From Birth Plan to Birth Partnership."

119. Doktor Schnabel, "Study: Length of Birth Plan Correlates to Length of C-Section Scar," *GomerBlog* (blog), May 12, 2014, http://gomerblog.com/2014/05/birth-plan/.

120. DeBaets, "From Birth Plan to Birth Partnership"; Divall et al., "Plans, Preferences."

121. DeBaets, "From Birth Plan to Birth Partnership."

122. Jennifer is a pseudonym.

123. Murray, "Informed Consent."

124. It is also telling that routine cervical checks during labor are an example of a standard protocol with dubious clinical benefit. There are few legitimate reasons to perform a cervical check against a woman's will during the course of a routine labor absent other clinical concerns.

125. J. P. Lenihan, "Relationship of Antepartum Pelvic Examinations to Premature Rupture of the Membranes," *Obstetrics and Gynecology* 63, no. 1 (January 1984): 33–37; R. S. McDuffie et al., "Effect of Routine Weekly Cervical Examinations at Term on Premature Rupture of the Membranes: A Randomized Controlled Trial," *Obstetrics and Gynecology* 79, no. 2 (February 1992): 219–22.

126. The desire for a tub might seem to be a relatively minor subjective preference, but laboring in water plays an important role in pain management and can limit other interventions. It therefore has both individual and clinical importance.

127. Mahowald, *Women and Children*, 50.

128. Ariadne Labs, *Designing Capacity*, 4.

Chapter 2. Medicalized Death and the Current of Centralized Care

1. Robert Schulte, Christian J. Weisman, in his capacity as Power of Attorney for, and on behalf of, Beatrice J. Weisman, Plaintiff, v. Maryland General Hospital, Inc., Health Care Provider/Defendant, no. 24-C-16-004199 (Circuit Court of Maryland, July 25, 2016).

2. *Schulte.*

3. Paula Span, "The Patients Were Saved. That's Why the Families Are Suing," *New York Times*, April 10, 2017, www.nytimes.com/2017/04/10/health/wrongful-life-lawsuit-dnr.html.

4. Kenneth A. Fisher, Lindsay E. Rockwell, and Missy Scott, *In Defiance of Death: Exposing the Real Costs of End-of-Life Care* (Westport, CT: Praeger, 2008), 1.

5. Institute of Medicine (US) and Committee on Approaching Death: Addressing Key End-of-Life Issues, *Dying in America: Improving Quality and Honoring Individual Preferences near the End of Life* (Washington, DC: National Academies Press, 2015); Jessica Nutik Zitter, *Extreme Measures: Finding a Better Path to the End of Life* (New York: Avery, 2017); Ira Byock, *Dying Well: Peace and Possibilities at the End of Life* (New York: Riverhead Books, 1999); Atul Gawande, *Being Mortal: Medicine and What Matters in the End* (New York: Henry Holt, 2014).

6. Liran Einav et al., "Predictive Modeling of U.S. Health Care Spending in Late Life," *Science* 360, no. 6396 (June 29, 2018): 1462–65, https://doi.org/10.1126/science.aar5045.

7. Melissa D. Aldridge and Amy S. Kelley, "The Myth Regarding the High Cost of End-of-Life Care," *American Journal of Public Health* 105, no. 12 (December 2015): 2411–15, https://doi.org/10.2105/AJPH.2015.302889.

8. Aldridge and Kelley, "Myth Regarding the High Cost"; Eric B. French et al., "End-of-Life Medical Spending in Last Twelve Months of Life Is Lower Than Previously Reported," *Health Affairs* 36, no. 7 (July 1, 2017): 1211–17, https://doi.org/10.1377/hlthaff.2017.0174.

9. Fisher, Rockwell, and Scott, *In Defiance of Death*, 6.

10. Alfred F. Connors, "A Controlled Trial to Improve Care for Seriously Ill Hospitalized Patients: The Study to Understand Prognoses and Preferences for Outcomes and Risks of Treatments (SUPPORT)," *Journal of the American Medical Association* 274, no. 20 (November 22, 1995): 1591, https://doi.org/10.1001/jama.1995.03530200027032.

11. Joan M. Teno et al., "Change in End-of-Life Care for Medicare Beneficiaries," *Journal of the American Medical Association* 309, no. 5 (February 6, 2013): 470–77, https://doi.org/10.1001/jama.2012.207624.

12. Teno et al., "Change in End-of-Life Care."

13. Fisher, Rockwell, and Scott, *In Defiance of Death*, 8.

14. Baohui Zhang et al., "Health Care Costs in the Last Week of Life: Associations with End-of-Life Conversations," *Archives of Internal Medicine* 169, no. 5 (March 9, 2009): 480–88, https://doi.org/10.1001/archinternmed.2008.587.

15. Zitter, *Extreme Measures*, 23.

16. Connors, "Controlled Trial."

17. Harold Y. Vanderpool, *Palliative Care: The 400-Year Quest for a Good Death* (Jefferson, NC: McFarland, 2015), 160, http://public.eblib.com/choice/publicfullrecord.aspx?p=2081810.

18. Vanderpool, *Palliative Care*, 172.

19. Gawande, *Being Mortal*; Byock, *Dying Well*; Zitter, *Extreme Measures*; Fisher, Rockwell, and Scott, *In Defiance of Death*.

20. Fisher, Rockwell, and Scott, *In Defiance of Death*, 1.

21. Susan L. Mitchell et al., "Clinical and Organizational Factors Associated with Feeding Tube Use among Nursing Home Residents with Advanced Cognitive Impairment," *Journal of the American Medical Association* 290, no. 1 (July 2, 2003): 73–80, https://doi.org/10.1001/jama.290.1.41; Paula Span, "More on CPR for the Elderly," *New Old Age* (blog), August 10, 2012, https://newoldage.blogs.nytimes.com/2012/08/10/more-on-cpr-for-the-elderly/; Kei Ouchi et al., "Prognosis after Emergency Department Intubation to Inform Shared Decision-Making," *Journal of the American Geriatrics Society* 66, no. 7 (July 2018): 1377–81, https://doi.org/10.1111/jgs.15361; Fisher, Rockwell, and Scott, *In Defiance of Death*, 43.

22. Vanderpool, *Palliative Care*, 93.

23. Vanderpool, *Palliative Care*, 92.

24. Vanderpool, *Palliative Care*, 94.

25. Sharon R. Kaufman, *Ordinary Medicine: Extraordinary Treatments, Longer Lives, and Where to Draw the Line* (Durham, NC: Duke University Press, 2015).

26. Sharon R. Kaufman, —*And a Time to Die: How American Hospitals Shape the End of Life* (Chicago: University of Chicago Press, 2006), 3.

27. M. Dollinger, "Guidelines for Hospitalization for Chemotherapy," *Oncologist* 1, nos. 1 and 2 (1996): 107–11.

28. Roslyn Lindheim, "Birthing Centers and Hospices: Reclaiming Birth and Death," *Annual Review of Public Health* 2 (1981): 1–29, https://doi.org/10.1146/annurev.pu.02.050181.000245.

29. Lindheim, "Birthing Centers and Hospices," 18.

30. Lindheim, "Birthing Centers and Hospices," 18.

31. Vanderpool, *Palliative Care*, 77.

32. American Hospital Association, "Fast Facts on U.S. Hospitals, 2019 | AHA," www.aha.org/statistics/fast-facts-us-hospitals.

33. Zitter, *Extreme Measures*, 26.

34. Institute of Medicine (US) and Committee on Approaching Death, *Dying in America*, 33.

35. Vanderpool, *Palliative Care*, 126.

36. Austin Frakt, "Medical Mystery: Something Happened to U.S. Health Spending after 1980," *New York Times*, June 9, 2018, www.nytimes.com/2018/05/14/upshot/medical-mystery-health-spending-1980.html.

37. Vanderpool, *Palliative Care*, 141.

38. However, Medicare's requirement that a patient have a terminal illness combined with a life expectancy of six months or less limited access to cancer

patients and those for whom diagnosis and prognosis were clear. See Vanderpool, *Palliative Care*, 145.

39. Ira Byock, *Best Care Possible: A Physician's Quest to Transform Care through the End of Life* (New York: Avery, 2013), 26.

40. Byock, *Best Care Possible*, 25.

41. Vanderpool, *Palliative Care*, 119.

42. Vanderpool, *Palliative Care*, 116.

43. Lindheim, "Birthing Centers and Hospices," 19.

44. Jane C. Weeks et al., "Patients' Expectations about Effects of Chemotherapy for Advanced Cancer," *New England Journal of Medicine* 367, no. 17 (October 25, 2012): 1616–25, https://doi.org/10.1056/NEJMoa1204410; Mieke Visser, Luc Deliens, and Dirk Houttekier, "Physician-Related Barriers to Communication and Patient- and Family-Centred Decision-Making towards the End of Life in Intensive Care: A Systematic Review," *Critical Care* 18 (November 18, 2014): 604, https://doi.org/10.1186/s13054-014-0604-z.

45. Gawande, *Being Mortal*, 8.

46. The prominent author and physician Sherwin Nuland described this shift, remarking that the "necessity of nature's final victory was expected and accepted in generations before our own. Doctors were far more willing to recognize the signs of defeat and far less arrogant about denying them." See Sherwin B. Nuland, *How We Die: Reflections on Life's Final Chapter* (New York: Vintage Books, 2010), 259.

47. Tammy C. Hoffmann and Chris Del Mar, "Clinicians' Expectations of the Benefits and Harms of Treatments, Screening, and Tests: A Systematic Review," *JAMA Internal Medicine* 177, no. 3 (March 1, 2017): 407–19, https://doi.org/10.1001/jamainternmed.2016.8254; Lindy Willmott et al., "Reasons Doctors Provide Futile Treatment at the End of Life: A Qualitative Study," *Journal of Medical Ethics* 42, no. 8 (August 1, 2016): 496–503, https://doi.org/10.1136/medethics-2016-103370.

48. Hoffmann and Del Mar, "Clinicians' Expectations."

49. Weeks et al., "Patients' Expectations," 1624.

50. L. D. Cripe, "Hope Is the Thing with Feathers," *Journal of the American Medical Association* 315, no. 3 (January 19, 2016): 265–66, https://doi.org/10.1001/jama.2015.18557; Darius N. Lakdawalla et al., "How Cancer Patients Value Hope and the Implications for Cost-Effectiveness Assessments of High-Cost Cancer Therapies," *Health Affairs* 31, no. 4 (April 1, 2012): 676–82, https://doi.org/10.1377/hlthaff.2011.1300.

51. John Ellershaw and Chris Ward, "Care of the Dying Patient: The Last Hours or Days of Life," *BMJ* 326, no. 7379 (January 4, 2003): 30–34.

52. Maureen Bisognano and Ellen Goodman, "Engaging Patients and Their Loved Ones in the Ultimate Conversation," *Health Affairs* 32, no. 2 (February 1, 2013): 203–6, https://doi.org/10.1377/hlthaff.2012.1174.

53. Tammy C. Hoffmann and Chris Del Mar, "Patients' Expectations of the Benefits and Harms of Treatments, Screening, and Tests: A Systematic Review," *JAMA Internal Medicine* 175, no. 2 (February 2015): 274–86, https://doi.org/10.1001/jamainternmed.2014.6016.

54. Kaufman, *Ordinary Medicine*, 42–43.

55. Richard A. Deyo, "Cascade Effects of Medical Technology," *Annual Review of Public Health* 23, no. 1 (2002): 30.

56. H. Gilbert Welch, Lisa Schwartz, and Steve Woloshin, *Overdiagnosed: Making People Sick in the Pursuit of Health*, 1st ed. (Boston: Beacon, 2011), 15–20; Christine M. Campanelli, "American Geriatrics Society Updated Beers Criteria for Potentially Inappropriate Medication Use in Older Adults," *Journal of the American Geriatrics Society* 60, no. 4 (April 2012): 616–31, https://doi.org/10.1111/j.1532-5415.2012.03923.x.

57. Campanelli, "American Geriatrics Society."

58. Zitter provides the account of the rise and fall of the Swan catheter as one example of how new innovations and techniques become widespread well before their actual efficacy is known. Zitter, *Extreme Measures*, 35.

59. Deyo, "Cascade Effects," 23.

60. Elliott S. Fisher, "Medical Care—Is More Always Better?," *New England Journal of Medicine* 349, no. 17 (October 23, 2003): 1665–67, https://doi.org/10.1056/NEJMe038149.

61. Vanderpool, *Palliative Care*, 80, 114.

62. Department of Health and Human Services, Centers for Medicare & Medicaid Services, "Cardiopulmonary Resuscitation (CPR) in Nursing Homes," October 18, 2013, www.cms.gov/Medicare/Provider-Enrollment-and-Certification/SurveyCertificationGenInfo/Downloads/Survey-and-Cert-Letter-14-01.pdf.

63. This policy is required in all facilities that receive Medicare funds. See Centers for Medicare and Medicaid Services, "CMS Manual System: Revisions to the State Operations Manual (SOM)—Appendix PP—Guidance to Surveyors for Long-Term Care Facilities" (Department of Health and Human Services, February 6, 2015), www.cms.gov/Regulations-and-Guidance/Guidance/Transmittals/downloads/R133SOMA.pdf.

64. Myke S. van Gijn et al., "The Chance of Survival and the Functional Outcome after In-Hospital Cardiopulmonary Resuscitation in Older People: A Systematic Review," *Age and Ageing* 43, no. 4 (July 1, 2014): 456–63, https://doi.org/10.1093/ageing/afu035.

65. Haider Warraich, *Modern Death: How Medicine Changed the End of Life* (New York: St. Martin's, 2017), 91.

66. Zitter, *Extreme Measures*, 6.

67. David Casarett et al., "Do Palliative Consultations Improve Patient Outcomes?," *Journal of the American Geriatrics Society* 56, no. 4 (April 2008): 593–99, https://doi.org/10.1111/j.1532-5415.2007.01610.x.

68. Lindheim, "Birthing Centers and Hospices," 18.

69. Joan M. Teno et al., "Family Perspectives on End-of-Life Care at the Last Place of Care," *Journal of the American Medical Association* 291, no. 1 (January 7, 2004): 88–93, https://doi.org/10.1001/jama.291.1.88.

70. Kaufman, —*And a Time to Die*, 96.

71. Kaufman, —*And a Time to Die*, 96.

72. Jennifer S. Temel et al., "Early Palliative Care for Patients with Metastatic Non-small-cell Lung Cancer," *New England Journal of Medicine* 363, no. 8 (August 19, 2010): 733–42, http://dx.doi.org.ezproxy.rit.edu/10.1056/NEJMoa1000678.

73. Gawande, *Being Mortal*, 9.

74. S. A. Norton et al., "Proactive Palliative Care in the Medical Intensive Care Unit: Effects on Length of Stay for Selected High-Risk Patients," *Critical Care Medicine* 35, no. 6 (2007): 1530–35.

75. Norton et al., "Proactive Palliative Care."

76. Zitter, *Extreme Measures*, 31.

77. Jonathan B. Bartels, "The Pause," *Critical Care Nurse* 34, no. 1 (February 1, 2014): 74–75, https://doi.org/10.4037/ccn2014962; Rachelle E. Bernacki and Susan D. Block, "Communication about Serious Illness Care Goals: A Review and Synthesis of Best Practices," *JAMA Internal Medicine* 174, no. 12 (December 1, 2014): 1994, https://doi.org/10.1001/jamainternmed.2014.5271.

78. Zitter, *Extreme Measures*, 242.

79. Lois Snyder and Timothy E. Quill, eds., *Physician's Guide to End-of-Life Care*, 1st ed. (Philadelphia: American College of Physicians, 2001), 146–48.

80. Snyder and Quill, *Physician's Guide*, 147.

81. Snyder and Quill, *Physician's Guide*, 147.

82. Melissa M. Garrido et al., "Chemotherapy Use in the Months before Death and Estimated Costs of Care in the Last Week of Life," *Journal of Pain and Symptom Management* 51, no. 5 (May 2016): 875–81.e2, https://doi.org/10.1016/j.jpainsymman.2015.12.323.

83. Kaufman, —*And a Time to Die*, 238–39.

84. Kaufman, —*And a Time to Die*, 238–39.

85. Alexandria J. Bear, Elizabeth A. Bukowy, and Jayshil J. Patel, "Artificial Hydration at the End of Life," *Nutrition in Clinical Practice: Official Publication of the American Society for Parenteral and Enteral Nutrition* 32, no. 5 (October 2017): 628–32, https://doi.org/10.1177/0884533617724741; Eduardo Bruera et al., "Parenteral Hydration in Patients with Advanced Cancer: A Multicenter, Double-Blind, Placebo-Controlled Randomized Trial," *Journal of Clinical Oncology* 31, no. 1 (January 1, 2013): 111–18, https://doi.org/10.1200/JCO.2012.44.6518.

86. Kaufman, —*And a Time to Die*, 238–39.

87. Temel et al., "Early Palliative Care."

88. C. Campos-Calderón et al., "Interventions and Decision-Making at the End of Life: The Effect of Establishing the Terminal Illness Situation," *BMC Palliative Care* 15 (November 7, 2016): 91, https://doi.org/10.1186/s12904-016-0162-z.

89. Hoffmann and Del Mar, "Patients' Expectations"; Campos-Calderón et al., "Interventions and Decision-Making."

90. Cripe, "Hope Is the Thing."

91. Zitter, *Extreme Measures*, 30–32.

92. Lakdawalla et al., "How Cancer Patients Value Hope."

93. Willmott et al., "Reasons Doctors Provide Futile Treatment."

94. Kathleen Ouimet Perrin and Mary Kazanowski, "Overcoming Barriers to Palliative Care Consultation," *Critical Care Nurse* 35, no. 5 (October 1, 2015): 44–52, https://doi.org/10.4037/ccn2015357.

95. Zitter, *Extreme Measures*, 73.

96. Zitter, *Extreme Measures*, 19.

97. Zitter, *Extreme Measures*, 82–84.

98. Zitter, *Extreme Measures*, 84.

99. Zitter, *Extreme Measures*, 82.

100. Courtenay R. Bruce, John E. Fetter, and J. S. Blumenthal-Barby, "Cascade Effects in Critical Care Medicine: A Call for Practice Changes," *American Journal of Respiratory and Critical Care Medicine* 188, no. 12 (December 15, 2013): 1384–85, https://doi.org/10.1164/rccm.201309-1606ED.

101. Zitter, *Extreme Measures*, 47.

102. Vanderpool, *Palliative Care*, 108.

103. Edward S. Dove et al., "Beyond Individualism: Is There a Place for Relational Autonomy in Clinical Practice and Research?," *Clinical Ethics* 12, no. 3 (September 2017): 150–65, https://doi.org/10.1177/1477750917704156; Peter I. Osuji, "Relational Autonomy in Informed Consent (RAIC) as an Ethics of Care Approach to the Concept of Informed Consent," *Medicine, Health Care, and Philosophy* 21, no. 1 (March 2018): 101–11, https://doi.org/10.1007/s11019-017-9789-7; Jennifer K. Walter and Lainie Friedman Ross, "Relational Autonomy: Moving beyond the Limits of Isolated Individualism," *Pediatrics* 133, no. S1 (February 2014): S16–23, https://doi.org/10.1542/peds.2013-3608D.

104. Zitter, *Extreme Measures*, 79–81.

105. Span, "Patients Were Saved."

Chapter 3. Safe Harbors for Demedicalized Birth and Death

1. Jane Sandall, "Place of Birth in Europe," *Entre Nous* 81 (2015), www.euro.who.int/__data/assets/pdf_file/0010/277741/Place-of-birth-in-Europe.pdf?ua=1; A. Elash, "Freestanding Hospices Ease Pressure on Physicians, Hospitals, MD Says," *Canadian Medical Association Journal* 158, no. 13 (June 30, 1998): 1757–58; Justin E. Bekelman et al., "Comparison of Site of Death,

Health Care Utilization, and Hospital Expenditures for Patients Dying with Cancer in 7 Developed Countries," *Journal of the American Medical Association* 315, no. 3 (January 19, 2016): 272, https://doi.org/10.1001/jama.2015.18603.

2. Ina May Gaskin, *Ina May's Guide to Childbirth* (New York: Bantam Books, 2003), 186; Richard W. Wertz and Dorothy C. Wertz, *Lying-in: A History of Childbirth in America* (New York: Free Press, 1977), 169.

3. Gaskin, *Ina May's Guide*, 186.

4. Elisabeth Kübler-Ross, *On Death and Dying: What the Dying Have to Teach Doctors, Nurses, Clergy and Their Own Families* (New York: Scribner, 2014), 8.

5. Kübler-Ross, *On Death and Dying*, 7. She continues, "Dying becomes lonely and impersonal because the patient is often taken out of his familiar environment and rushed to an emergency room."

6. Roslyn Lindheim, "Birthing Centers and Hospices: Reclaiming Birth and Death," *Annual Review of Public Health* 2 (1981): 25, https://doi.org/10.1146/annurev.pu.02.050181.000245.

7. Gaskin, *Ina May's Guide*, 184; Kübler-Ross, *On Death and Dying*, 6.

8. John S. Fairbairn, "Physiological Principles in Midwifery Practice," *BMJ* 1, no. 3142 (March 19, 1921): 413–15.

9. Gaskin, *Ina May's Guide*, 141, 184.

10. Cicely Saunders, "The Evolution of Palliative Care," *Journal of the Royal Society of Medicine* 94, no. 9 (September 2001): 430–32.

11. Richard A. Kalish, "The Onset of the Dying Process," *OMEGA—Journal of Death and Dying* 1, no. 1 (April 1, 1970): 57–69, https://doi.org/10.2190/HAF7-J66R-FD9V-0C76; Kübler-Ross, *On Death and Dying*.

12. Grantly Dick-Read, *Childbirth without Fear: The Principles and Practice of Natural Childbirth* (London: Pinter & Martin, 2013).

13. Fairbairn, "Physiological Principles in Midwifery Practice," 414.

14. Alexandria J. Bear, Elizabeth A. Bukowy, and Jayshil J. Patel, "Artificial Hydration at the End of Life," *Nutrition in Clinical Practice: Official Publication of the American Society for Parenteral and Enteral Nutrition* 32, no. 5 (October 2017): 628–32, https://doi.org/10.1177/0884533617724741.

15. Lois Snyder and Timothy E. Quill, eds., *Physician's Guide to End-of-Life Care*, 1st ed. (Philadelphia: American College of Physicians, 2001), 26–30.

16. Gaskin, *Ina May's Guide*.

17. Saunders, "Evolution of Palliative Care."

18. These concerns have been expanded in recent years, as research suggests that the hospital environment may impede not only the physiological processes of birth and death but also healing itself. See Harlan M. Krumholz, Kumar Dharmarajan, and Harlan M. Krumholz, "Is Posthospital Syndrome a Result of Hospitalization-Induced Allostatic Overload?," *Journal of Hospital Medicine*, May 25, 2018, https://doi.org/10.12788/jhm.2986.

19. M. C. Bushnell et al., "Effect of Environment on the Long-Term Consequences of Chronic Pain," *Pain* 156, no. S1 (April 2015): S42–49, https://doi.org/10.1097/01.j.pain.0000460347.77341.bd.

20. S. C. Segerstrom and G. E. Miller, "Psychological Stress and the Human Immune System: A Meta-analytic Study of 30 Years of Inquiry," *Psychological Bulletin* 130, no. 4 (2004): 601–30.

21. Richard A. Deyo, "Cascade Effects of Medical Technology," *Annual Review of Public Health* 23, no. 1 (2002): 23–44.

22. Jennifer S. Temel et al., "Early Palliative Care for Patients with Metastatic Non-small-cell Lung Cancer," *New England Journal of Medicine* 363, no. 8 (August 19, 2010): 733–42, http://dx.doi.org.ezproxy.rit.edu/10.1056/NEJMoa1000678.

23. Harold Y. Vanderpool, *Palliative Care: The 400-Year Quest for a Good Death* (Jefferson, NC: McFarland, 2015), 127–31; Jan Howard and Anselm Strauss, *Humanizing Health Care* (New York: John Wiley, 1975), 191–93.

24. T. Halper, "On Death, Dying, and Terminality: Today, Yesterday, and Tomorrow," *Journal of Health Politics, Policy and Law* 4, no. 1 (1979): 11–29. Quoted in Lindheim, "Birthing Centers and Hospices," 19.

25. Fairbairn, "Physiological Principles in Midwifery Practice"; Gaskin, *Ina May's Guide*; Cassandra Y. W. Wong et al., "An Integrative Literature Review on Midwives' Perceptions on the Facilitators and Barriers of Physiological Birth," *International Journal of Nursing Practice* 23, no. 6 (December 2017), https://doi.org/10.1111/ijn.12602; Jenny M. Luke, *Delivered by Midwives: African American Midwifery in the Twentieth-Century South* (Jackson: University Press of Mississippi, 2018).

26. Lindheim, "Birthing Centers and Hospices"; Howard and Strauss, *Humanizing Health Care*, 25–27.

27. Lindheim, "Birthing Centers and Hospices"; Gaskin, *Ina May's Guide*.

28. Vanderpool, *Palliative Care*; Gaskin, *Ina May's Guide*; Adrienne Rich, "The Theft of Childbirth," *New York Review of Books*, October 2, 1975, www.nybooks.com/articles/1975/10/02/the-theft-of-childbirth/.

29. Kübler-Ross, *On Death and Dying*, xii.

30. Gaskin, *Ina May's Guide*, 226–27.

31. Gaskin, *Ina May's Guide*, 99. The maneuver has subsequently been taught in obstetrics programs as a highly effective way of alleviating shoulder dystocia. See also J. P. Bruner et al., "All-Fours Maneuver for Reducing Shoulder Dystocia during Labor," *Journal of Reproductive Medicine* 43, no. 5 (May 1998): 439–43.

32. Onnie Lee Logan and Katherine Clark, *Motherwit: An Alabama Midwife's Story* (San Francisco: Untreed Reads, 2013), 91.

33. Gaskin, *Ina May's Guide*, 184.

34. Vanderpool, *Palliative Care*, 127.

35. Vanderpool, *Palliative Care*, 128.

36. However, none but Roslyn Lindheim drew clear parallels between the calls to demedicalize birth and death. See Lindheim, "Birthing Centers and Hospices."

37. Saunders, "Evolution of Palliative Care," 12.

38. Frédérick Leboyer, *Birth without Violence* (London: Pinter & Martin, 2011); Saunders, "Evolution of Palliative Care."

39. Howard and Strauss, *Humanizing Health Care*.

40. Pamela Sutherland and Laura Kaplan Shanley, "Unassisted Childbirth," *Social Science and Medicine* 42, no. 3 (1996): 477.

41. Vanderpool, *Palliative Care*; Kathleen Doherty Turkel, *Women, Power, and Childbirth: A Case Study of a Free-Standing Birth Center* (Westport, CT: Bergin & Garvey, 1996).

42. Gaskin, *Ina May's Guide*, 150–53; Kübler-Ross, *On Death and Dying*, 1–9.

43. Vanderpool, *Palliative Care*, 142–47; Sharon R. Kaufman, —*And a Time to Die: How American Hospitals Shape the End of Life* (Chicago: University of Chicago Press, 2006).

44. Theresa Morris, *Cut It Out: The C-Section Epidemic in America* (New York: New York University Press, 2013), 59.

45. Morris, *Cut It Out*, 59; Haider Warraich, *Modern Death: How Medicine Changed the End of Life* (New York: St. Martin's, 2017).

46. Ira Byock, *Best Care Possible: A Physician's Quest to Transform Care through the End of Life* (New York: Avery, 2013), 266–67.

47. US Department of Health and Human Services and Centers for Disease Control and Prevention, "Birth: Final Data for 2016," *National Vital Statistics Reports* 67, no. 1 (January 31, 2018), www.cdc.gov/nchs/data/nvsr/nvsr67 /nvsr67_01_tables.pdf.

48. Marian MacDorman, T. J. Mathews, and Eugene Declercq, "Trends in Out-of-Hospital Births in the United States, 1990–2012," Centers for Disease Control and Prevention, March 2014, www.cdc.gov/nchs/products/databriefs /db144.htm.

49. National Hospice and Palliative Care Organization, *Hospice Care in America*, April 2017, www.nhpco.org/sites/default/files/public/Statistics _Research/2017_Facts_Figures.pdf.

50. Donald H. Taylor et al., "What Length of Hospice Use Maximizes Reduction in Medical Expenditures near Death in the US Medicare Program?," *Social Science and Medicine* 65, no. 7 (October 2007): 1466–78, https://doi .org/10.1016/j.socscimed.2007.05.028.

51. National Hospice and Palliative Care Organization, *Hospice Care in America*.

52. Gaskin, *Ina May's Guide*, 226–33.

53. "About Midwives: State by State," Midwives Alliance of North America, http://mana.org/about-midwives/state-by-state.

54. Gaskin, *Ina May's Guide*, 183–85.

55. Kenneth A. Fisher, Lindsay E. Rockwell, and Missy Scott, *In Defiance of Death: Exposing the Real Costs of End-of-Life Care* (Westport, CT: Praeger, 2008), 80.

56. Sriram Yennurajalingam and Eduardo Bruera, eds., *Oxford American Handbook of Hospice and Palliative Medicine and Supportive Care*, 2nd ed. (Oxford: Oxford University Press, 2016).

57. See the International End of Life Doula Association's website, www .inelda.org/.

58. John Leland and Devin Yalkin, "The Positive Death Movement Comes to Life," *New York Times*, June 22, 2018, www.nytimes.com/2018/06/22/ny region/the-positive-death-movement-comes-to-life.html.

59. Yennurajalingam and Bruera, *Oxford American Handbook*; Vanderpool, *Palliative Care*.

60. Vanderpool, *Palliative Care*, 194.

61. Catherine Elton, "American Women: Birthing Babies at Home," *Time*, September 4, 2010, http://content.time.com/time/magazine/article/0,9171,2011 940-2,00.html.

62. Kübler-Ross, *On Death and Dying*.

63. Vera P. Sarmento et al., "Home Palliative Care Works: But How? A Meta-ethnography of the Experiences of Patients and Family Caregivers," *BMJ Supportive and Palliative Care*, February 23, 2017, https://doi.org/10.1136 /bmjspcare-2016-001141.

64. Melissa Cheyney et al., "Outcomes of Care for 16,924 Planned Home Births in the United States: The Midwives Alliance of North America Statistics Project, 2004 to 2009," *Journal of Midwifery and Women's Health* 59, no. 1 (January 1, 2014): 17–27, https://doi.org/10.1111/jmwh.12172.

65. Medicare Payment Advisory Commission, "Report to the Congress; Medicare Beneficiaries' Access to Hospice," May 2002, www.medpac.gov/docs /default-source/contractor-reports/report-to-the-congress-medicare-beneficiaries -access-to-hospice-may-2002-.pdf?sfvrsn=0.

66. "Home Health Services," Medicare.gov, www.medicare.gov/coverage /home-health-services.html.

67. Warraich, *Modern Death*, 177–78.

68. Logan and Clark, *Motherwit*, 61.

69. Ellen McCarthy, "Dying Is Hard. Death Doulas Want to Help Make It Easier," *Washington Post*, July 22, 2016, www.washingtonpost.com/lifestyle /style/dying-is-hard-death-doulas-want-to-help-make-it-easier/2016/07/22

/53d8of5c-24f7-11e6-8690-f14ca9de2972_story.html?noredirect=on&utm
_term=.b22ce4b7d8e6.

70. "Death Doulas: What We Do," Death Doulas, https://deathdoulas.com
/whatwedo/; "What Is a Doula," DONA International, www.dona.org/what-is
-a-doula/.

71. Renee Mehra et al., "Recommendations for the Pilot Expansion of
Medicaid Coverage for Doulas in New York State," *American Journal of Public
Health* 109, no. 2 (February 2019): 217–19, https://doi.org/10.2105/AJPH
.2018.304797; Deb Rawlings et al., "What Role Do Death Doulas Play in
End-of-Life Care? A Systematic Review," *Health and Social Care in the Com-
munity*, September 26, 2018, https://doi.org/10.1111/hsc.12660.

72. Mehra et al., "Recommendations for the Pilot Expansion"; Rawlings et
al., "What Role Do Death Doulas Play?"

73. These issues are addressed at length in chaps. 4, 5, and 6.

74. Susan Rutledge Stapleton, Cara Osborne, and Jessica Illuzzi, "Outcomes
of Care in Birth Centers: Demonstration of a Durable Model," *Journal of
Midwifery and Women's Health* 58, no. 1 (January 2013): 3–14, https://doi
.org/10.1111/jmwh.12003.

75. Stapleton, Osborne, and Illuzzi, "Outcomes of Care in Birth Centers."

76. Sarah de Leeuw, "A Family Way of Dying," *Canadian Family Physician*
62, no. 8 (August 2016): 660–63.

77. Alexander K. Smith et al., "The Diverse Landscape of Palliative Care
Clinics," *Journal of Palliative Medicine* 16, no. 6 (June 2013): 661–68, https://
doi.org/10.1089/jpm.2012.0469.

78. See later chapters for more in-depth discussion of homes for the dying.

79. When asked about differences between palliative care in hospitals and
in home hospice, one nurse interviewed for this book said, "There are fewer
protocols in home hospice. Nurses have a little more latitude or autonomy. And
ultimately it's the patient's wishes that generate the course of action in hospice.
In an inpatient environment they are often told what will happen."

80. Jill Alliman and Julia C. Phillippi, "Maternal Outcomes in Birth
Centers: An Integrative Review of the Literature," *Journal of Midwifery and
Women's Health* 61, no. 1 (January 2016): 21–51, https://doi.org/10.1111
/jmwh.12356.

81. Cheyney et al., "Outcomes of Care"; K. C. Johnson, "Outcomes of
Planned Home Births with Certified Professional Midwives: Large Prospective
Study in North America," *BMJ* 330, no. 7505 (June 18, 2005): 1416, https://doi
.org/10.1136/bmj.330.7505.1416.

82. Stapleton, Osborne, and Illuzzi, "Outcomes of Care in Birth Centers."

83. Mark T. Hughes and Thomas J. Smith, "The Growth of Palliative Care
in the United States," *Annual Review of Public Health* 35, no. 1 (March 18,
2014): 459–75, https://doi.org/10.1146/annurev-publhealth-032013-182406;

Edward W. Campion, Amy S. Kelley, and R. Sean Morrison, "Palliative Care for the Seriously Ill," *New England Journal of Medicine* 373, no. 8 (August 20, 2015): 747–55, https://doi.org/10.1056/NEJMra1404684.

84. Temel et al., "Early Palliative Care."

85. S. A. Norton et al., "Proactive Palliative Care in the Medical Intensive Care Unit: Effects on Length of Stay for Selected High-Risk Patients," *Critical Care Medicine* 35, no. 6 (2007): 1530–35.

86. Peter Whoriskey and Dan Keating, "Dying and Profits: The Evolution of Hospice," *Washington Post*, December 26, 2014, www.washingtonpost.com /business/economy/2014/12/26/a7d90438-692f-11e4-b053-65cea7903f2e_story .html.

87. Gayle Shier et al., "Hospice Enrollment Saves Money for Medicare and Improves Care Quality across a Number of Different Lengths-of-Stay," *Health Affairs* 32, no. 3 (March 2013): 552–61; Katherine A. Ornstein et al., "Association between Hospice Use and Depressive Symptoms in Surviving Spouses," *JAMA Internal Medicine* 175, no. 7 (July 1, 2015): 1138, https://doi.org/10 .1001/jamainternmed.2015.1722.

88. Gaskin, *Ina May's Guide*, 270; Ira Byock, *Dying Well: Peace and Possibilities at the End of Life* (New York: Riverhead Books, 1999), 36.

89. Gaskin, *Ina May's Guide*, 134–42; Kübler-Ross, *On Death and Dying*, 14–16.

90. Lauren Jansen et al., "First Do No Harm: Interventions during Childbirth," *Journal of Perinatal Education* 22, no. 2 (2013): 83–92, https://doi.org /10.1891/1058-1243.22.2.83; American College of Obstetricians and Gynecologists, "Approaches to Limit Intervention during Labor and Birth," Committee Opinion (Washington, DC, February 2017). See chap. 4 for a discussion of the growth of regulatory control over home birth and birth centers.

91. Morris, *Cut It Out*, 55–63.

92. Lindheim, "Birthing Centers and Hospices," 7–9.

93. Aleksandra S. Dain et al., "Massage, Music and Art Therapy in Hospice: Results of a National Survey," *Journal of Pain and Symptom Management* 49, no. 6 (June 2015): 1035–41, https://doi.org/10.1016/j.jpainsymman.2014.11.295.

94. Byock, *Best Care Possible*, 262–63.

95. Terri Nuss et al., "The Impact of Opening Visitation Access on Patient and Family Experience," *Journal of Nursing Administration* 44, no. 7/8 (August 2014): 403–10, https://doi.org/10.1097/NNA.0000000000000090.

96. Angelo E. Volandes, *The Conversation: A Revolutionary Plan for End-of-Life Care* (New York: Bloomsbury, 2016), 160–63.

97. Joanne Motino Bailey, Patricia Crane, and Clark E. Nugent, "Childbirth Education and Birth Plans," *Obstetrics and Gynecology Clinics of North America* 35, no. 3 (September 2008): 497–509, ix, https://doi.org/10.1016/j .ogc.2008.04.005; Byock, *Best Care Possible*, 238.

98. Some doulas provide free care or income based sliding scale fees. For more information, see www.inelda.org/; "Doula Training and Doula Certification," DONA International, www.dona.org/.

99. Byock, *Best Care Possible*, 257–58.

100. Bert N. Uchino, *Social Support and Physical Health: Understanding the Health Consequences of Relationships* (New Haven, CT: Yale University Press, 2004); Kenneth J. Gruber, Susan H. Cupito, and Christina F. Dobson, "Impact of Doulas on Healthy Birth Outcomes," *Journal of Perinatal Education* 22, no. 1 (2013): 49–58, https://doi.org/10.1891/1058-1243.22.1.49; Byock, *Best Care Possible*, 259.

101. Bailey, Crane, and Nugent, "Childbirth Education and Birth Plans."

102. Vanderpool, *Palliative Care*, 126–29; Katie Cook and Colleen Loomis, "The Impact of Choice and Control on Women's Childbirth Experiences," *Journal of Perinatal Education* 21, no. 3 (2012): 158–68, https://doi.org/10.1891/1058-1243.21.3.158.

Chapter 4. Navigating the Regulation Tributary

1. Lesley Rathbun, "Letter to Donald Clark, Secretary of the Federal Trade Commission," American Association of Birth Centers, April 30, 2014, https://c.ymcdn.com/sites/aabc.site-ym.com/resource/collection/dcbda72a-41ea-4afe-a8d1-112542f4a0bc/FTC_Letter_-_4.30.14_with_appendices.pdf?hhSearchTerms=%22burdensome%22.

2. Rathbun, "Letter to Donald Clark."

3. Rathbun, "Letter to Donald Clark," 8.

4. "CON—Certificate of Need State Laws," National Conference of State Legislatures, www.ncsl.org/research/health/con-certificate-of-need-state-laws.aspx.

5. "CON—Certificate of Need State Laws."

6. Thomas Stratmann and Steven Monaghan, "The Effect of Interest Group Pressure on Favorable Regulatory Decisions" (working paper, Mercatus Center, George Mason University, August 29, 2017), www.mercatus.org/publications/interest-group-pressure-favorable-regulatory-decisions-certificate-of-need.

7. Derek Delia et al., "Effects of Regulation and Competition on Health Care Disparities: The Case of Cardiac Angiography in New Jersey," *Journal of Health Politics, Policy and Law* 34, no. 1 (February 2009): 63–91, https://doi.org/10.1215/03616878-2008-992.

8. Thomas Stratmann and David Wille, "Certificate-of-Need Laws and Hospital Quality" (working paper, Mercatus Center, George Mason University, September 26, 2016), www.mercatus.org/publications/certificate-need-laws-and-hospital-quality.

9. "Federal Trade Commission, Department of Justice Issue Joint Statement on Certificate-of-Need Laws in Illinois," Federal Trade Commission, www.ftc

.gov/news-events/press-releases/2008/09/federal-trade-commission-department
-justice-issue-joint-statement.

10. "CON—Certificate of Need State Laws."

11. California Research Bureau, California State Library, "The Corporate Practice of Medicine in a Changing Healthcare Environment," April 2016, https://sbp.senate.ca.gov/sites/sbp.senate.ca.gov/files/CRB%202016%20CPM %20Report.pdf; Darcy Bryan, Jared Rhoads, and Robert Graboyes, "Corporate Medicine," Mercatus Center, November 30, 2016, www.mercatus.org/hoap /corporate-medicine.

12. Bryan, Rhoads, and Graboyes, "Corporate Medicine."

13. Department of Health and Human Services, Centers for Medicare and Medicaid Services, "Advanced Practice Registered Nurses, Anesthesiologist Assistants, and Physician Assistants," Medicare Learning Network, October 2016, www.cms.gov/Outreach-and-Education/Medicare-Learning-Network -MLN/MLNProducts/Downloads/Medicare-Information-for-APRNs-AAs-PAs -Booklet-ICN-901623.pdf.

14. Pauline Chen, "The Gulf between Doctors and Nurse Practitioners," *Well* (blog), June 27, 2013, https://well.blogs.nytimes.com/2013/06/27/the-gulf -between-doctors-and-nurse-practitioners/.

15. Sara Markowitz et al., "Competitive Effects of Scope of Practice Restrictions: Public Health or Public Harm?," *Journal of Health Economics* 55 (September 1, 2017): 201–18, https://doi.org/10.1016/j.jhealeco.2017.07.004.

16. Markowitz et al., "Competitive Effects."

17. Hospice Association of America, *Hospice Regulatory Blueprint for Action* (Hospice Association of America, 2018), www.nahc.org/wp-content /uploads/2018/06/2018-Hospice-Regulatory-Blueprint.pdf.

18. Department of Health and Human Services, "Advanced Practice Registered Nurses."

19. California Research Bureau, California State Library, "The Corporate Practice of Medicine in a Changing Healthcare Environment."

20. Jenny M. Luke, *Delivered by Midwives: African American Midwifery in the Twentieth-Century South* (Jackson: University Press of Mississippi, 2018), 67.

21. Confusingly, some direct-entry midwives refer to themselves as traditional midwives, though for the purposes of this discussion I will preserve the distinction above and refer to direct-entry midwives as those with some form of external certification. I follow the Midwife Alliance of North America's usage in what follows. See https://mana.org/resources/become-a-midwife for more information.

22. Referred to hereafter as "nurse midwives."

23. Quoted in Roslyn Lindheim, "Birthing Centers and Hospices: Reclaiming Birth and Death," *Annual Review of Public Health* 2 (1981): 5, https://doi .org/10.1146/annurev.pu.02.050181.000245.

24. Barbara Ehrenreich and Deirdre English, *For Her Own Good: Two Centuries of the Experts' Advice to Women* (New York: Anchor Books, 2005), 108.

25. Eugene R. Declercq, "The Trials of Hanna Porn: The Campaign to Abolish Midwifery in Massachusetts," *American Journal of Public Health* 84, no. 6 (1994): 1023.

26. "The Big Push for Midwives," http://pushformidwives.nationbuilder.com/.

27. See the Senate bill that ultimately changed that legislation (however, the health department has been slow in implementing the change). Kemp Hannon, "NY State Senate Bill S4325," Pub. L. No. S4325 (2015), www.nysenate.gov /legislation/bills/2015/s4325/amendment/original.

28. American College of Nurse-Midwives and American College of Obstetricians and Gynecologists, "Joint Statement of Practice Relations between Obstetrician-Gynecologists and Certified Nurse-Midwives / Certified Midwives," April 2018, www.acog.org/-/media/Statements-of-Policy/Public/87ACNM-College Policy-Statement—-June-2018.pdf?dmc=1&ts=20190126T1701076020.

29. Michelle Andrews, "States Vary on What They Allow Midwives to Do," NPR, February 14, 2012, www.npr.org/sections/health-shots/2012/02/14 /146859861/states-vary-on-what-they-allow-midwives-to-do.

30. Leia Dingott, "Pushing for Change: The State of Arizona Should Allow Women Greater Access to Midwifery Care," *Arizona State Law Journal* 49, no. 2 (July 29, 2017): 433–64.

31. Lazarus Wendy, Ellen S. Levine, and Lawrence S. Lewin, *Competition among Health Practitioners: The Influence of the Medical Profession on the Health Manpower Market: A Report* (US Federal Trade Commission, 1981), 2:19–20.

32. Rathbun, "Letter to Donald Clark."

33. Rathbun, "Letter to Donald Clark."

34. "Legal Status of U.S. Midwives," Midwives Alliance of North America, http://mana.org/about-midwives/legal-status-of-us-midwives.

35. "Legal Status of U.S. Midwives."

36. North American Registry of Midwives, "Direct Entry Midwifery State-by-State Legal Status," http://narm.org/pdffiles/Statechart.pdf.

37. Mary Sell and Jennifer Edwards, "Vote Is Today on Midwife Regulation Bill," *TimesDaily*, March 8, 2017, www.timesdaily.com/news/local/vote-is-today -on-midwife-regulation-bill/article_c15f3d83-b390-5247-81f2-27476d6932f7 .html; Anna Vollers, "Midwifery Is Now Legal in Alabama. When Can Midwives Start Delivering Babies?," *Advance Local*, May 25, 2017, www.al.com /news/index.ssf/2017/05/midwifery_is_now_legal_in_alab.html.

38. Rebecca Grant, "The Secret Baby Catchers of Alabama," *Huffington Post*, December 19, 2018, https://highline.huffingtonpost.com/articles/en /alabama-midwives/.

39. Karen Grigsby Bates, "In Rural Alabama, Limited Access to Obstetrics

Care," NPR, May 31, 2015, www.npr.org/2015/05/31/411044409/in-rural-alabama-limited-access-to-obstetrics-care.

40. Stefan Grzybowski, Kathrin Stoll, and Jude Kornelsen, "Distance Matters: A Population Based Study Examining Access to Maternity Services for Rural Women," *BMC Health Services Research* 11 (June 10, 2011): 147, https://doi.org/10.1186/1472-6963-11-147.

41. Andy Davis, "State Protocol on Births at Home Raises Ire; Exam Rule Snarls Midwives, Clients," *Arkansas Online*, May 9, 2018, www.arkansasonline.com/news/2018/may/09/protocol-on-births-at-home-raises-ire-2/; Andy Davis, "Little Rock Midwife's Appeal to Panel Rejected; Client Didn't Get Two Prebirth Exams," *Arkansas Online*, May 11, 2018, www.arkansasonline.com/news/2018/may/11/midwife-s-appeal-to-panel-rejected-2018-1/.

42. Chelsea Cameron, "GoFundMe Campaign: Arkansas Moms Sue Health Department," www.gofundme.com/arkansas-moms-sue-health-department.

43. Associated Press, "Arkansas Midwife Appeals At-Home Birth Violation," *AP News*, May 9, 2018, https://apnews.com/7d90b8f13a37453382fc27802540946f.

44. Joseph R. Wax et al., "Maternal and Newborn Outcomes in Planned Home Birth vs Planned Hospital Births: A Metaanalysis," *American Journal of Obstetrics and Gynecology* 203, no. 3 (September 2010): 243.e1–243.e8, https://doi.org/10.1016/j.ajog.2010.05.028. K. C. Johnson, "Outcomes of Planned Home Births with Certified Professional Midwives: Large Prospective Study in North America," *BMJ* 330, no. 7505 (June 18, 2005): 1–7, https://doi.org/10.1136/bmj.330.7505.1416.

45. The rate of neonatal death in the home birth meta-analysis commissioned by ACOG is 2 or 3 deaths per 1,000 births, while the rate for hospitals is 1 death per 1,000 births. In both cases, such deaths are quite rare, though the higher-risk population in hospitals probably does indicate an even more elevated risk for home birth than the data themselves capture.

46. American College of Obstetricians and Gynecologists, "Refusal of Medically Recommended Treatment during Pregnancy—ACOG," www.acog.org/Clinical-Guidance-and-Publications/Committee-Opinions/Committee-on-Ethics/Refusal-of-Medically-Recommended-Treatment-During-Pregnancy.

47. Nigel Bunyan, "Morecambe Bay Report Exposes 'Lethal Mix' of Failures That Led to Baby Deaths," *Guardian*, March 3, 2015, www.theguardian.com/society/2015/mar/03/morecambe-bay-report-lethal-mix-problems-baby-deaths-cumbria; Teddy Kulmala, "Jury: Death of Baby at Fort Mill Birthing Center Was Homicide," *Charlotte Observer*, June 4, 2015, www.charlotteobserver.com/news/local/crime/article23132913.html.

48. Grant, "Secret Baby Catchers of Alabama."

49. Saraswathi Vedam et al., "Mapping Integration of Midwives across the United States: Impact on Access, Equity, and Outcomes," *PLOS ONE* 13, no. 2 (February 21, 2018): e0192523, https://doi.org/10.1371/journal.pone.0192523.

50. Christopher Koopman and Anne Philpot, "The State of Certificate of-Need Laws in 2016," Mercatus Center, September 26, 2016, www.mercatus.org/publications/state-certificate-need-laws-2016; "Ambulatory Surgery Centers | Related Links | Department of Health & Senior Services," Missouri Department of Health & Senior Services, http://health.mo.gov/safety/asc/. Many thanks to Anne Philpott from the Mercatus Center for clarifying by email how states classify birth centers.

51. Rathbun, "Letter to Donald Clark."

52. Mary Akers, "Comments for Kentucky 'Modernization of the Certificate of Need Process'" (2015).

53. Akers, "Comments for Kentucky 'Modernization.'"

54. Moreover, the appeals judge ruled that the original administrative law judge, who rejected the CON application for a birth center, allowed improper evidence relating to the safety and financial stability of birth centers generally, an issue that is irrelevant to the question whether an alternative birth center is needed. Such issues, he ruled, relate to licensing, not to CONs. See J. Phillip Shepherd, The Visitation Birth and Family Wellness Center, Inc., v. Commonwealth of Kentucky, Cabinet for Health and Family Services, et al., No. 13-CI-01013 (Franklin Circuit Court, February 23, 2015).

55. *Shepherd.*

56. Onnie Lee Logan and Katherine Clark, *Motherwit: An Alabama Midwife's Story* (San Francisco: Untreed Reads, 2013), 188.

57. Logan and Clark, *Motherwit*; Bates, "In Rural Alabama."

58. Rachel Rabkin Peachman, "What You Don't Know about Your Doctor Could Hurt You," *Consumer Reports*, April 20, 2016, www.consumerreports.org/cro/health/doctors-and-hospitals/what-you-dont-know-about-your-doctor-could-hurt-you/index.htm.

59. Ehrenreich and English, *For Her Own Good.*

60. See chap. 7 for more details on health disparities. See also Vedam et al., "Mapping Integration of Midwives."

61. Hospice Association of America, *Hospice Regulatory Blueprint for Action* (2018), www.nahc.org/wp-content/uploads/2018/06/2018-Hospice-Regulatory-Blueprint.pdf.

62. It should be noted, of course, that hospitals also struggle with regulations, and many feel that an excessively burdensome regulatory environment drives defensive protocols and limits quality of care. Criticisms of regulations of community-based options should not be read as a defense of the regulations facing hospitals and other medical providers.

63. "Becoming a Hospice: The Certificate of Need Process," *Florida Trend*, August 1, 2011, www.floridatrend.com/article/1614/becoming-a-hospice-the-certificate-of-need-process.

64. Jennifer W. Thompson, Melissa D. A. Carlson, and Elizabeth H. Bradley,

"US Hospice Industry Experienced Considerable Turbulence from Changes in Ownership, Growth, and Shift to For-Profit Status," *Health Affairs* 31, no. 6 (June 1, 2012): 1286–93, https://doi.org/10.1377/hlthaff.2011.1247; Andrea Chung and Alan Sorensen, "For-Profit Entry and Market Expansion in the Hospice Industry" (working paper, 2015), www.ssc.wisc.edu/~sorensen/papers /hospice.pdf.

65. Chung and Sorensen, "For-Profit Entry."

66. Harold Y. Vanderpool, *Palliative Care: The 400-Year Quest for a Good Death* (Jefferson, NC: McFarland, 2015), 145.

67. Vanderpool, *Palliative Care*, 145.

68. Heather Wilson, "Hospice Prognosis vs Diagnosis—Can We Slow Down for a Minute Please?," *Hospice Compliance Network* (blog), accessed January 26, 2019, www.hospicecompliance.com/compliance/201542prognosis.

69. Department of Health and Human Services, Office of Inspector General, *Hospices Inappropriately Billed Medicare over $250 Million for General Inpatient Care* (Washington, DC: Department of Health and Human Services, 2016), https://oig.hhs.gov/oei/reports/oei-02-10-00491.pdf.

70. Chung and Sorensen, "For-Profit Entry."

71. Emily Rappleye, "Top 20 Healthcare Lobbyists by Spending," *Beckers Hospital Review*, August 21, 2015, www.beckershospitalreview.com/finance /top-20-healthcare-lobbyists-by-spending.html.

72. Frank A. Sloan and Chee-Ruey Hsieh, *Health Economics* (Cambridge, MA: MIT Press, 2017), 101.

73. While maternity care itself is not particularly profitable for hospitals, it is used as a marketing tool to attract patients on the assumption that women in particular are loyal to the hospitals they give birth in. See, e.g., S. Hoholik, "Hospitals Lose Now, Gain Later on Maternity," *Columbus Dispatch*, August 29, 2010, www.dispatch.com/content/stories/local/2010/08/29/hospitals-lose -now-gain-later-on-maternity.html; Gale Scott, "Birthing Biz Booms for Hospitals," *Crain's New York Business*, March 8, 2014, www.crainsnewyork.com /article/20140309/HEALTH_CARE/140309897/birthing-biz-booms-for -hospitals.

74. "Stats of the State of Alabama," Centers for Disease Control and Prevention, www.cdc.gov/nchs/pressroom/states/alabama/alabama.htm; Bates, "In Rural Alabama."

75. See a copy of the handout, archived by a birth advocate, at http:// birthmonopoly.com/bmp/wp-content/uploads/2017/05/Lay-Midwife-Statement -re-HB315-050317.pdf.

76. Vollers, "Midwifery Is Now Legal in Alabama."

77. Beth Greenfield, "Mom Who Sued Hospital for Traumatic Birth Wins $16 Million," *Yahoo News*, August 8, 2016, www.yahoo.com/beauty/mom-who -sued-hospital-for-traumatic-birth-wins-16-million-173203800.html.

78. Brandon Moseley, "Medical Association Strongly Opposes Decriminalizing Midwives," *Alabama Political Reporter* (blog), March 13, 2017, www.alreporter.com/2017/03/13/medical-association-strongly-opposes-decriminalizing-midwives/.

79. Michael Dresser, "Women Who Want to Give Birth at Home Seek to Change Restrictive Md. Law," *Baltimore Sun*, February 11, 2015, www.baltimoresun.com/news/maryland/politics/bs-md-midwines-hearings-2015 0209-story.html.

80. Elizabeth Kukura, "Choice in Birth: Preserving Access to VBAC," *Penn State Law Review* 114, no. 3 (July 25, 2010): 955–1001.

81. Dan Frosch, "Refusals Cut Options after C-Sections," *New York Times*, April 14, 2014, www.nytimes.com/2014/04/15/health/refusals-cut-options-after-c-sections.html.

82. Despite 56% of hospitals allowing a trial of labor after cesarean, the VBAC rate was only 10.8% in those hospitals, while VBAC success rates with supportive providers are generally estimated at around 70%. Mary K. Barger et al., "A Survey of Access to Trial of Labor in California Hospitals in 2012," *BMC Pregnancy and Childbirth* 13 (April 3, 2013): 83, https://doi.org/10.1186/1471-2393-13-83.

83. Ashley Hill, "Issues and Procedures in Women's Health—Vaginal Birth after Cesarean (VBAC)" (International Cesearean Awareness Network, January 2014), www.ican-online.org/wp-content/uploads/2014/06/Issues-Surrounding-VBAC.pdf.

84. Theresa Morris, *Cut It Out: The C-Section Epidemic in America* (New York: New York University Press, 2013), 128–29.

85. Marsden Wagner, *Born in the USA: How a Broken Maternity System Must Be Fixed to Put Mothers and Infants First* (Berkeley: University of California Press, 2008), 130.

86. J. Christopher Glantz, "Obstetric Variation, Intervention, and Outcomes: Doing More but Accomplishing Less," *Birth* 39, no. 4 (December 1, 2012): 286–90, https://doi.org/10.1111/birt.12002.

87. Renee Sullender and Sarah Selenich, *Financial Considerations of Hospital-Based Palliative Care* (Research Triangle Park, NC: RTI Press, 2016), https://doi.org/10.3768/rtipress.2016.rr.0027.1603.

88. One hospice director expressed concern about the growth of hospital-based palliative care, noting, "Hospitals are trying to expand their palliative care programs and own the outpatient setting and with the new Medicaid redesign there's a potential for them to redesign what the community already has." But overall she spoke positively about working with palliative care physicians in the community, and the palliative care specialists interviewed also supported community-based care over hospital-based programs for reasons laid out in chap. 2.

89. "Nursing Homes, Hospice Dropped from 'CON' Repeal," *WUSF News*, April 7, 2017, http://wusfnews.wusf.usf.edu/post/nursing-homes-hospice-dropped-con-repeal.

90. Jim Ash, "Hospice Providers Fight the Demise of 'CON,'" *WUSF News*, March 2, 2017, http://wusfnews.wusf.usf.edu/post/hospice-providers-fight-demise-con.

91. Thompson, Carlson, and Bradley, "US Hospice Industry."

92. Chadd K. Kraus and Thomas A. Suarez, "Is There a Doctor in the House? . . . Or the Senate? Physicians in US Congress, 1960–2004," *Journal of the American Medical Association* 292, no. 17 (November 3, 2004): 2125–29, https://doi.org/10.1001/jama.292.17.2125.

93. Robert Garrett, "While Texas Legislature Seats the Most Doctors, Health Care Still on Back-Burner," *Dallas News*, September 2015, www.dallasnews.com/news/politics/2015/09/04/while-texas-legislature-seats-the-most-doctors-health-care-still-on-back-burner.

94. April Weaver, "HB 344—Alabama 2017 Regular Session," Pub. L. No. HB 344 (2017), /al/bills/2017rs/HB344/.

95. Joey Holleman, "SC Birthing Center Regulations Spark Debate about Competition, Safety," *State*, April 16, 2015, www.thestate.com/news/local/article18692004.html.

96. Angie Welling, "Midwives Lobby against Restrictive Legislation," *Deseret News*, February 6, 2007, www.deseretnews.com/article/660193073/Midwives-lobby-against-restrictive-legislation.html?pg=all.

97. Alia Beard Rau, "Senate Bill Pursues Midwife Restrictions," *Republic*, February 12, 2014, http://archive.azcentral.com/news/politics/articles/20140212senate-bill-pursues-midwife-restrictions.html.

98. Wendy, Levine, and Lewin, *Competition among Health Practitioners*, 2:26.

99. Wendy, Levine, and Lewin, *Competition among Health Practitioners*, 2:27.

100. Advisory board approval was also necessary because physician opposition to demedicalized alternatives was sufficient to prevent the success of such alternatives in practice. According to the report, "if providers aren't going to cooperate in real life, it won't fly."

101. Federal Trade Commission and Department of Justice, "Improving Health Care: A Dose of Competition," July 2004, 22, www.justice.gov/sites/default/files/atr/legacy/2006/04/27/204694.pdf.

102. Rathbun was also the president of the AABC for two terms until 2017. AABC has historical connections to and still works collaboratively with the major birth center accrediting body, the CABC.

103. See, e.g., Baby+Co., www.babyandcompany.com/.

104. Chung and Sorensen, "For-Profit Entry."

Chapter 5. Swept Away on the Reimbursement Headwater

1. Barbara Ehrenreich and Deirdre English, *For Her Own Good: Two Centuries of the Experts' Advice to Women* (New York: Anchor Books, 2005).

2. Agency for Healthcare Research & Quality, "The Science of Making Better Decisions about Health: Cost-Effectiveness and Cost-Benefit Analysis," September 9, 2015, www.ahrq.gov/professionals/education/curriculum-tools /population-health/russell.html.

3. Centers for Medicare & Medicaid Services, "NHE-Fact-Sheet," April 17, 2018, www.cms.gov/research-statistics-data-and-systems/statistics-trends-and -reports/nationalhealthexpenddata/nhe-fact-sheet.html.

4. Sharon R. Kaufman, *Ordinary Medicine: Extraordinary Treatments, Longer Lives, and Where to Draw the Line* (Durham, NC: Duke University Press, 2015), 40–50.

5. Agency for Healthcare Research & Quality, "Science of Making Better Decisions."

6. Elisabeth Rosenthal, "Those Indecipherable Medical Bills? They're One Reason Health Care Costs So Much," *New York Times*, March 29, 2017, www .nytimes.com/2017/03/29/magazine/those-indecipherable-medical-bills-theyre -one-reason-health-care-costs-so-much.html.

7. Amy S. Oxentenko et al., "Time Spent on Clinical Documentation: A Survey of Internal Medicine Residents and Program Directors," *Archives of Internal Medicine* 170, no. 4 (February 22, 2010): 377–80, https://doi.org/10 .1001/archinternmed.2009.534.

8. Tait D. Shanafelt et al., "Burnout and Satisfaction with Work-Life Balance among US Physicians Relative to the General US Population," *Archives of Internal Medicine* 172, no. 18 (October 8, 2012): 1377–85, https://doi.org/10 .1001/archinternmed.2012.3199.

9. Truven Health Analytics, *The Cost of Having a Baby in the United States* (January 2013), www.chqpr.org/downloads/CostofHavingaBaby.pdf.

10. Institute of Medicine (US) and Committee on Approaching Death: Addressing Key End-of-Life Issues, *Dying in America: Improving Quality and Honoring Individual Preferences near the End of Life* (Washington, DC: National Academies Press, 2015).

11. William McGowan, quoted in Uwe E. Reinhardt, "The Pricing of U.S. Hospital Services: Chaos behind a Veil of Secrecy," *Health Affairs* 25, no. 1 (January 1, 2006): 57–69, https://doi.org/10.1377/hlthaff.25.1.57.

12. "You Can Get Your Hospital's Price List. Good Luck Making Sense of It," *NBC News*, www.nbcnews.com/news/us-news/hospital-price-list-charge master-rules-trump-mandate-2019-n959006.

13. Carol Sakala, Maureen P. Corry, and Milbank Memorial Fund, *Evidence-Based Maternity Care: What It Is and What It Can Achieve* (New York: Milbank Memorial Fund, 2008).

14. Melissa D. Aldridge and Amy S. Kelley, "The Myth regarding the High Cost of End-of-Life Care," *American Journal of Public Health* 105, no. 12 (December 2015): 2411–15, https://doi.org/10.2105/AJPH.2015.302889.

15. Centers for Medicare and Medicaid Services, "National Health Expenditures 2015 Highlights," www.cms.gov/research-statistics-data-and-systems /statistics-trends-and-reports/nationalhealthexpenddata/downloads/highlights.pdf.

16. Sakala, Corry, and Milbank Memorial Fund, *Evidence-Based Maternity Care.*

17. Sakala, Corry, and Milbank Memorial Fund, *Evidence-Based Maternity Care*; Institute of Medicine (US) and Committee on Approaching Death, *Dying in America.*

18. Derek C. Angus and Robert D. Truog, "Toward Better ICU Use at the End of Life," *Journal of the American Medical Association* 315, no. 3 (January 19, 2016): 255, https://doi.org/10.1001/jama.2015.18681; Sakala, Corry, and Milbank Memorial Fund, *Evidence-Based Maternity Care.*

19. Institute of Medicine (US) and Committee on Approaching Death, *Dying in America.*

20. Centers for Disease Control and Prevention, "Trends in Inpatient Hospital Deaths: National Hospital Discharge Survey, 2000–2010," March 2013, www.cdc.gov/nchs/products/databriefs/db118.htm.

21. Sakala, Corry, and Milbank Memorial Fund, *Evidence-Based Maternity Care.*

22. Aaron L. Schwartz et al., "Measuring Low-Value Care in Medicare," *JAMA Internal Medicine* 174, no. 7 (July 1, 2014): 1067–76, https://doi.org/10 .1001/jamainternmed.2014.1541.

23. James S. Goodwin et al., "Overuse of Screening Colonoscopy in the Medicare Population," *Archives of Internal Medicine* 171, no. 15 (August 8, 2011): 1335–43, https://doi.org/10.1001/archinternmed.2011.212; Frank van Hees et al., "The Appropriateness of More Intensive Colonoscopy Screening Than Recommended in Medicare Beneficiaries: A Modeling Study," *JAMA Internal Medicine* 174, no. 10 (October 1, 2014): 1568–76, https://doi.org/10 .1001/jamainternmed.2014.3889.

24. Truven Health Analytics, *Cost of Having a Baby*, 30–31.

25. Truven Health Analytics, *Cost of Having a Baby.*

26. Institute of Medicine (US) and Committee on Approaching Death, *Dying in America.*

27. Institute of Medicine (US) and Committee on Approaching Death, *Dying in America*; Sakala, Corry, and Milbank Memorial Fund, *Evidence-Based Maternity Care.*

28. Elisabeth Rosenthal, "Getting Insurance to Pay for Midwives," *Well* (blog), July 3, 2013, http://well.blogs.nytimes.com/2013/07/03/getting-insurance -to-pay-for-midwives/.

29. Truven Health Analytics, *Cost of Having a Baby*, 7.

30. These costs do not include costs for infant-related care, which can dramatically increase the total in the case of prematurity or other complications. Truven Health Analytics, *Cost of Having a Baby*.

31. Elisabeth Rosenthal, "American Way of Birth, Costliest in the World," *New York Times*, June 30, 2013, www.nytimes.com/2013/07/01/health/american-way-of-birth-costliest-in-the-world.html.

32. Thomas P. Sartwelle, James C. Johnston, and Berna Arda, "A Half Century of Electronic Fetal Monitoring and Bioethics: Silence Speaks Louder Than Words," *Maternal Health, Neonatology and Perinatology* 3 (November 21, 2017): 21, https://doi.org/10.1186/s40748-017-0060-2.

33. Theresa Morris, *Cut It Out: The C-Section Epidemic in America* (New York: New York University Press, 2013), 50–51.

34. Nicholas J. Kassebaum et al., "Global, Regional, and National Levels and Causes of Maternal Mortality during 1990–2013: A Systematic Analysis for the Global Burden of Disease Study 2013," *Lancet (London, England)* 384, no. 9947 (September 13, 2014): 980–1004, https://doi.org/10.1016/S0140-6736(14)60696-6.

35. Truven Health Analytics, *Cost of Having a Baby*.

36. Rosenthal, "American Way of Birth."

37. Sakala, Corry, and Milbank Memorial Fund, *Evidence-Based Maternity Care*, 60.

38. While there may be incentives for birth centers to transfer care to hospitals for prolonged labors, most birth centers have policies on the timing of such transfers precisely because long, difficult labors can put mothers and infants at risk. Thus, the incentive generally points in the same direction as evidence-based care.

39. Sakala, Corry, and Milbank Memorial Fund, *Evidence-Based Maternity Care*, 60.

40. "Essential Facts about Midwives," American College of Nurse-Midwives, www.midwife.org/Essential-Facts-about-Midwives.

41. Deborah Walker, Barbara Lannen, and Debra Rossie, "Midwifery Practice and Education: Current Challenges and Opportunities," *Online Journal of Issues in Nursing* 19, no. 2 (May 31, 2014), http://ojin.nursingworld.org/Main MenuCategories/ANAMarketplace/ANAPeriodicals/OJIN/TableofContents /Vol-19-2014/No2-May-2014/Midwifery-Practice-and-Education.html.

42. North American Registry of Midwives, "Direct Entry Midwifery State-by-State Legal Status," narm.org/pdffiles/statechart.pdf.

43. Susan Rutledge Stapleton, Cara Osborne, and Jessica Illuzzi, "Outcomes of Care in Birth Centers: Demonstration of a Durable Model," *Journal of Midwifery and Women's Health* 58, no. 1 (January 2013): 3–14, https://doi.org/10.1111/jmwh.12003.

44. See a map detailing these payment schedules by state at www.midwife
.org/acnm/files/ccLibraryFiles/Filename/000000005129/MedicaidPayment-CPT
59400.pdf.

45. State of New Jersey, "New Jersey Administrative Code, Title 10, Chapter
58," N.J.A.C 10:58, www.state.nj.us/humanservices/providers/rulefees/regs
/NJAC%2010_58%20Nurse%20Midwifery%20Services.pdf.

46. Henry J. Kaiser Family Foundation, "Medicaid Benefits: Freestanding
Birth Center Services," http://kff.org/other/state-indicator/medicaid-benefits
-freestanding-birth-center-services/.

47. Marian MacDorman, T. J. Mathews, and Eugene Declercq, "Trends in
Out-of-Hospital Births in the United States, 1990–2012," Centers for Disease
Control and Prevention, March 2014, www.cdc.gov/nchs/products/databriefs
/db144.htm. See also American Association of Birth Centers, "AABC Press
Kit—American Association of Birth Centers," www.birthcenters.org/?page
=press_kit&terms=%22aabc+and+press+and+kit%22.

48. Centers for Disease Control and Prevention, "FastStats: Birth and
Natality," www.cdc.gov/nchs/fastats/births.htm.

49. Commission for the Accreditation of Birth Centers, "Accredited Birth
Centers," www.birthcenteraccreditation.org/find-accredited-birth-centers
/#mapkeycabc.

50. On home birth and VBAC, see, e.g., Kim J. Cox et al., "Planned Home
VBAC in the United States, 2004–2009: Outcomes, Maternity Care Practices,
and Implications for Shared Decision Making," *Birth* 42, no. 4 (December 1,
2015): 299–308, https://doi.org/10.1111/birt.12188.

51. Henry Chong Lee, Yasser Y. El-Sayed, and Jeffrey B. Gould, "Population
Trends in Cesarean Delivery for Breech Presentation in the United States 1997–
2003," *American Journal of Obstetrics and Gynecology* 199, no. 1 (July 2008):
59.e1–59.e8, https://doi.org/10.1016/j.ajog.2007.11.059; Morris, *Cut It Out*.

52. Sakala, Corry, and Milbank Memorial Fund, *Evidence-Based Maternity
Care*.

53. American College of Obstetricians and Gynecologists, "ACOG Refines
Fetal Heart Rate Monitoring Guidelines," June 22, 2009, www.mnhospitals.org
/Portals/0/Documents/patientsafety/Perinatal/3a_ACOG%20Bulletin%20106.pdf.

54. Sakala, Corry, and Milbank Memorial Fund, *Evidence-Based Maternity
Care*, 35–40.

55. American College of Obstetricians and Gynecologists, "Committee
Opinion: Approaches to Limit Intervention during Labor and Birth," 2017.

56. Kenneth J. Gruber, Susan H. Cupito, and Christina F. Dobson, "Impact
of Doulas on Healthy Birth Outcomes," *Journal of Perinatal Education* 22, no. 1
(2013): 49–58, https://doi.org/10.1891/1058-1243.22.1.49; K. B. Kozhimannil
et al., "Doula Care, Birth Outcomes, and Costs among Medicaid Beneficiaries,"
American Journal of Public Health 103, no. 4 (2013): 113–21.

57. Gruber, Cupito, and Dobson, "Impact of Doulas"; Katy B. Kozhimannil and Rachel Hardeman, "How Medicaid Coverage for Doula Care Could Improve Birth Outcomes, Reduce Costs, and Improve Equity," *Health Affairs* (blog), July 1, 2015, http://healthaffairs.org/blog/2015/07/01/how-medicaid-coverage-for-doula-care-could-improve-birth-outcomes-reduce-costs-and-improve-equity/.

58. Kozhimannil and Hardeman, "How Medicaid Coverage."

59. Kozhimannil and Hardeman, "How Medicaid Coverage."

60. Kozhimannil and Hardeman, "How Medicaid Coverage."

61. "Medicaid: A Primer—Key Information on the Nation's Health Coverage Program for Low-Income People," *Henry J. Kaiser Family Foundation* (blog), March 1, 2013, www.kff.org/medicaid/issue-brief/medicaid-a-primer/.

62. "The Kaiser Family Foundation," *Dual Eligible Resources* (blog), March 13, 2013, http://kff.org/tag/dual-eligible/.

63. Though it is not clear how many Americans spend down to qualify, Medicaid is the primary payer for 60% of long-term nursing home care in the United States. Donald Redfoot and Wendy Fox-Grage, *Medicaid: A Program of Last Resort for People Who Need Long-Term Services and Supports* (Washington, DC: AARP Public Policy Institute, May 2013), www.aarp.org/content/dam/aarp/research/public_policy_institute/health/2013/medicaid-last-resort-insight-AARP-ppi-health.pdf.

64. Institute of Medicine (US) and Committee on Approaching Death, *Dying in America*, 458.

65. Institute of Medicine (US) and Committee on Approaching Death, *Dying in America*, 458.

66. Christine A. Sinsky and David C. Dugdale, "Medicare Payment for Cognitive vs Procedural Care: Minding the Gap," *JAMA Internal Medicine* 173, no. 18 (October 14, 2013): 1733–37, https://doi.org/10.1001/jamainternmed.2013.9257.

67. Sharon R. Kaufman, —And a Time to Die: How American Hospitals Shape the End of Life (Chicago: University of Chicago Press, 2006); Vincent Mor et al., "The Revolving Door of Rehospitalization from Skilled Nursing Facilities," *Health Affairs (Project Hope)* 29, no. 1 (2010): 57–64, https://doi.org/10.1377/hlthaff.2009.0629.

68. Institute of Medicine (US) and Committee on Approaching Death, *Dying in America*, 263.

69. Mor et al., "Revolving Door of Rehospitalization."

70. Institute of Medicine (US) and Committee on Approaching Death, *Dying in America*, 263.

71. Helena Temkin-Greener et al., "Rehabilitation Therapy for Nursing Home Residents at the End-of-Life," *Journal of the American Medical Directors Association* 20, no. 4 (April 2019): 476–80, https://doi.org/10.1016/j.jamda.2018.07.024.

72. Institute of Medicine (US) and Committee on Approaching Death, *Dying in America*, 265.

73. Institute of Medicine (US) and Committee on Approaching Death, *Dying in America*, 265; Mor et al., "Revolving Door of Rehospitalization."

74. Mor et al., "Revolving Door of Rehospitalization."

75. Mor et al., "Revolving Door of Rehospitalization."

76. Terence Ng, Charlene Harrington, and Martin Kitchener, "Medicare and Medicaid in Long-Term Care," *Health Affairs* 29, no. 1 (January 1, 2010): 22–28, https://doi.org/10.1377/hlthaff.2009.0494; Institute of Medicine (US) and Committee on Approaching Death, *Dying in America*, 296.

77. "Medicaid Benefits: Home Health Services, Includes Nursing Services, Home Health Aides, and Medical Supplies/Equipment," *Henry J. Kaiser Family Foundation* (blog), March 27, 2013, www.kff.org/medicaid/state-indicator /home-health-services-includes-nursing-services-home-health-aides-and -medical-suppliesequipment/.

78. "Medicaid: A Primer."

79. Katherine Aragon et al., "Use of the Medicare Posthospitalization Skilled Nursing Benefit in the Last 6 Months of Life," *Archives of Internal Medicine* 172, no. 20 (November 12, 2012): 1573, https://doi.org/10.1001/archintern med.2012.4451; Institute of Medicine (US) and Committee on Approaching Death, *Dying in America*.

80. H. Stephen Kaye, Charlene Harrington, and Mitchell P. LaPlante, "Long-Term Care: Who Gets It, Who Provides It, Who Pays, and How Much?," *Health Affairs* 29, no. 1 (January 1, 2010): 11–21, https://doi.org/10.1377/hlthaff.2009 .0535.

81. Jennifer W. Thompson, Melissa D. A. Carlson, and Elizabeth H. Bradley, "US Hospice Industry Experienced Considerable Turbulence from Changes in Ownership, Growth, and Shift to For-Profit Status," *Health Affairs* 31, no. 6 (June 1, 2012): 1286–93, https://doi.org/10.1377/hlthaff.2011.1247.

82. David Stevenson and Haiden Huskamp, "Hospice Payment Reforms Are a Modest Step Forward, but More Changes Are Needed," *Health Affairs* (blog), January 4, 2016, http://healthaffairs.org/blog/2016/01/04/hospice-payment -reforms-are-a-modest-step-forward-but-more-changes-are-needed/.

83. David J. Casarett, "Rethinking Hospice Eligibility Criteria," *Journal of the American Medical Association* 305, no. 10 (March 9, 2011): 1031–32, https://doi.org/10.1001/jama.2011.271; Institute of Medicine (US) and Committee on Approaching Death, *Dying in America*, 277.

84. Melissa Aldridge and Jean Kutner, "Improving Access to High Quality Hospice Care: What Is the Optimal Path?," *Health Affairs Blog* (blog), September 9, 2014, http://healthaffairs.org/blog/2014/09/09/improving-access-to-high -quality-hospice-care-what-is-the-optimal-path/.

85. "Medicare Begins Paying Doctors to Coordinate Chronic Care for

Seniors," *PBS NewsHour*, January 11, 2015, www.pbs.org/newshour/rundown /medicare-begins-paying-doctors-coordinate-chronic-care-seniors/.

86. Ira Byock, *Dying Well: Peace and Possibilities at the End of Life* (New York: Riverhead Books, 1999), 230–31.

87. Melinda A. Chen et al., "Patient Care Outside of Office Visits: A Primary Care Physician Time Study," *Journal of General Internal Medicine* 26, no. 1 (January 2011): 58–63, https://doi.org/10.1007/s11606-010-1494-7.

88. Nathan A. Berger et al., "Cancer in the Elderly," *Transactions of the American Clinical and Climatological Association* 117 (2006): 147.

89. "Cancer Statistics," National Cancer Institute, www.cancer.gov/about -cancer/understanding/statistics.

90. The estimate is for the total of Medicare Fee-for-Service dollars in 2013, and costs have risen since. Sean Maroongroge et al., "The Cost of Cancer-Related Physician Services to Medicare," *Yale Journal of Biology and Medicine* 88, no. 2 (June 1, 2015): 107–14.

91. Kim L. Farina, "The Economics of Cancer Care in the United States," *American Journal of Managed Care*, March 16, 2012, www.ajmc.com/journals /evidence-based-oncology/2012/2012-2-vol18-n1/the-economics-of-cancer-care -in-the-united-states-how-much-do-we-spend-and-how-can-we-spend-it-better.

92. "A Very Open Letter from an Oncologist," *Health Beat by Maggie Mahar* (blog), January 10, 2009, www.healthbeatblog.com/2009/01/a-very -open-letter-from-an-oncologist/.

93. "Very Open Letter."

94. Christine B. Weldon et al., "Barriers to the Use of Personalized Medicine in Breast Cancer," *Journal of Oncology Practice* 8, no. 4 (July 2012): e24–31, https://doi.org/10.1200/JOP.2011.000448.

95. Brock O'Neil et al., "Doing More for More: Unintended Consequences of Financial Incentives for Oncology Specialty Care," *Journal of the National Cancer Institute* 108, no. 2 (February 1, 2016), https://doi.org/10.1093/jnci/djv331.

96. Farina, "Economics of Cancer Care"; Trevor J. Royce et al., "Cancer Screening Rates in Individuals with Different Life Expectancies," *JAMA Internal Medicine* 174, no. 10 (October 1, 2014): 1558–65, https://doi.org/10.1001 /jamainternmed.2014.3895.

97. Holly G. Prigerson et al., "Chemotherapy Use, Performance Status, and Quality of Life at the End of Life," *JAMA Oncology* 1, no. 6 (September 2015): 778–84, https://doi.org/10.1001/jamaoncol.2015.2378; Melissa M. Garrido et al., "Chemotherapy Use in the Months before Death and Estimated Costs of Care in the Last Week of Life," *Journal of Pain and Symptom Management* 51, no. 5 (May 2016): 875–881.e2, https://doi.org/10.1016/j.jpainsymman.2015 .12.323.

98. Institute of Medicine (US) and Committee on Approaching Death, *Dying in America*, 61.

99. One palliative care physician pointed out in an interview that "most of the treatment people are giving up to enter hospice in the first place is not curative. When people give up dialysis it's not curative; it's not going to cure their kidney failure. Most treatments in medicine at the end of life are not curative, they're there to help you maintain something. It makes for a false dichotomy—they're giving up chemo, but that chemo was never curative." See also Institute of Medicine (US) and Committee on Approaching Death, *Dying in America.*

100. Pediatric patients, whose parents are typically loath to give up hope of a cure, are frequently allowed "concurrent care" by private insurers and most recently by Medicaid under the ACA, meaning that they are allowed access to both curative treatments and palliative care at the same time.

101. S. A. Norton et al., "Proactive Palliative Care in the Medical Intensive Care Unit: Effects on Length of Stay for Selected High-Risk Patients," *Critical Care Medicine* 35, no. 6 (2007): 1530–35.

102. J. Brian Cassel et al., "Effect of a Home-Based Palliative Care Program on Healthcare Use and Costs," *Journal of the American Geriatrics Society* 64, no. 11 (November 2016): 2288–95, https://doi.org/10.1111/jgs.14354.

103. Cassel et al., "Effect of a Home-Based Palliative Care Program"; Norton et al., "Proactive Palliative Care."

104. Institute of Medicine (US) and Committee on Approaching Death, *Dying in America*, 281; "Ambulance Services Coverage," Medicare.gov, www.medicare.gov/coverage/ambulance-services.

105. Timothy F. Platts-Mills et al., "Emergency Medical Services Use by the Elderly: Analysis of a Statewide Database," *Prehospital Emergency Care: Official Journal of the National Association of EMS Physicians and the National Association of State EMS Directors* 14, no. 3 (September 2010): 329–33, https://doi.org/10.3109/10903127.2010.481759; G. Agarwal et al., "Effectiveness of a Community Paramedic-Led Health Assessment and Education Initiative in a Seniors' Residence Building: The Community Health Assessment Program through Emergency Medical Services (CHAP-EMS)," *BMC Emergency Medicine* 17, no. 1 (09 2017): 8, https://doi.org/10.1186/s12873-017-0119-4.

106. Mark T. Hughes and Thomas J. Smith, "The Growth of Palliative Care in the United States," *Annual Review of Public Health* 35, no. 1 (March 18, 2014): 459–75, https://doi.org/10.1146/annurev-publhealth-032013-182406.

107. Richard Pérez-Peña, "Use of Midwives, a Childbirth Phenomenon, Fades in City," *New York Times*, March 15, 2004, www.nytimes.com/2004/03/15/nyregion/use-of-midwives-a-childbirth-phenomenon-fades-in-city.html.

108. Phuong Ly, "A Labor without End," *Washington Post*, May 27, 2007, www.washingtonpost.com/wp-dyn/content/article/2007/05/23/AR2007052301294.html.

109. Malpractice insurance will be discussed in more detail in chap. 6.

110. This depends, however, on the financing structure and ownership of the

hospital. Incentives are different for hospitals run by insurance companies, for example. Peter May et al., "Economics of Palliative Care for Hospitalized Adults with Serious Illness: A Meta-analysis," *JAMA Internal Medicine* 178, no. 6 (June 1, 2018): 820–29, https://doi.org/10.1001/jamainternmed.2018.0750; Kathleen Bickel and Elissa Ozanne, "Importance of Costs and Cost Effectiveness of Palliative Care," *Journal of Oncology Practice* 13, no. 5 (April 24, 2017): 287–89, https://doi.org/10.1200/JOP.2016.019943.

111. Limited weekend enrollment is one of the major barriers to prompt access to hospice care, since not all Medicare data systems are available on weekends. See Hospice Association of America, *Hospice Regulatory Blueprint for Action* (Hospice Association of America, 2018), 17, www.nahc.org/wp -content/uploads/2018/06/2018-Hospice-Regulatory-Blueprint.pdf.

112. Federal Trade Commission and Department of Justice, "Improving Health Care: A Dose of Competition," July 2004, 5, www.justice.gov/sites /default/files/atr/legacy/2006/04/27/204694.pdf.

113. Some of these reforms, including capitation, managed care, and other options, will be discussed in the conclusion.

Chapter 6. Caught in the Riptide of Risk

1. "State Medical Liability Reform," American Medical Association, www .ama-assn.org/practice-management/state-medical-liability-reform.

2. Michael B. Rothberg et al., "The Cost of Defensive Medicine on Three Hospital Medicine Services," *JAMA Internal Medicine* 174, no. 11 (November 1, 2014): 1867–68, https://doi.org/10.1001/jamainternmed.2014.4649; J. William Thomas, Erika C. Ziller, and Deborah A. Thayer, "Low Costs of Defensive Medicine, Small Savings from Tort Reform," *Health Affairs* 29, no. 9 (September 1, 2010): 1578–84, https://doi.org/10.1377/hlthaff.2010.0146.

3. Rothberg et al., "Cost of Defensive Medicine"; Thomas, Ziller, and Thayer, "Low Costs of Defensive Medicine."

4. William F. McCool et al., "Closed Claims Analysis of Medical Malpractice Lawsuits Involving Midwives: Lessons Learned regarding Safe Practices and the Avoidance of Litigation," *Journal of Midwifery and Women's Health* 60, no. 4 (August 2015): 437–44, https://doi.org/10.1111/jmwh.12310.

5. Anupam B. Jena et al., "Malpractice Risk according to Physician Specialty," *New England Journal of Medicine* 365, no. 7 (August 18, 2011): 629–36, https://doi.org/10.1056/NEJMsa1012370.

6. Stuart Selkin, "End-of-Life Liability Issues," *Ethics, Law, and Aging Review* 10 (2004): 93–107.

7. Selkin, "End-of-Life Liability Issues."

8. Rachel Rabkin Peachman, "What You Don't Know about Your Doctor Could Hurt You," *Consumer Reports*, April 20, 2016, www.consumerreports

.org/cro/health/doctors-and-hospitals/what-you-dont-know-about-your-doctor
-could-hurt-you/index.htm.

9. Selkin, "End-of-Life Liability Issues."

10. M. Sonal Sekhar and N. Vyas, "Defensive Medicine: A Bane to Health-care," *Annals of Medical and Health Sciences Research* 3, no. 2 (2013): 295–96, www.ncbi.nlm.nih.gov/pmc/articles/PMC3728884/.

11. Sekhar and Vyas, "Defensive Medicine."

12. D. M. Studdert et al., "Defensive Medicine among High-Risk Specialist Physicians in a Volatile Malpractice Environment," *Journal of the American Medical Association* 293, no. 21 (2005): 2609–17; Emily R. Carrier et al., "High Physician Concern about Malpractice Risk Predicts More Aggressive Diagnostic Testing in Office-Based Practice," *Health Affairs* 32, no. 8 (August 1, 2013): 1383–91, https://doi.org/10.1377/hlthaff.2013.0233.

13. Studdert et al., "Defensive Medicine."

14. Sidney Shapiro et al., "The Truth about Torts: Defensive Medicine and the Unsupported Case for Medical Malpractice 'Reform,' " (white paper, Center for Progressive Reform, February 2012), 2.

15. D. M. Studdert et al., "Claims, Errors, and Compensation Payments in Medical Malpractice Litigation," *New England Journal of Medicine* 354, no. 19 (2006): 2024–33.

16. Claims not involving an error are more likely to reach trial owing to the fact that the trial itself is a process of discovery that uncovers facts about fault that no one could know when the litigation begins. Those cases that were settled out of court resulted in lower overall compensation, however. See Carol Sakala, Y. Tony Yang, and Maureen P. Corry, *Maternity Care and Liability: Pressing Problems, Substantive Solutions* (New York: Childbirth Connection, January 2013), http://transform.childbirthconnection.org/wp-content/uploads/2013/01/Maternity-Care-and-Liability.pdf.

17. Don McCanne, "How Much Is Wasted on Defensive Medicine?," *Physicians for a National Health Program* (blog), September 23, 2014, http://pnhp.org/blog/2014/09/23/how-much-is-wasted-on-defensive-medicine/.

18. Martin A. Makary and Michael Daniel, "Medical Error—the Third Leading Cause of Death in the US," *BMJ* 353 (May 3, 2016): i2139, https://doi.org/10.1136/bmj.i2139.

19. Shapiro et al., "Truth about Torts," 12.

20. David Cutler et al., "Physician Beliefs and Patient Preferences: A New Look at Regional Variation in Health Care Spending" (working paper, National Bureau of Economic Research, August 2013), https://doi.org/10.3386/w19320.

21. Katherine Tormey, "Policymakers Look to Tort Reform as One Way to Lower Health Care Costs," Council of State Governments, March 1, 2010,

http://knowledgecenter.csg.org/kc/content/policymakers-look-tort-reform-one way lower health care costs.

22. Alan Levine, Robert Oshel, and Sidney Wolfe, *State Medical Boards Fail to Discipline Doctors with Hospital Actions against Them* (Public Citizen, March 2011), www.citizen.org/sites/default/files/1937.pdf; Peter Eisler and Barbara Hansen, "Thousands of Doctors Practicing despite Errors, Misconduct," *USA Today*, August 20, 2013, www.usatoday.com/story/news/nation/2013/08 /20/doctors-licenses-medical-boards/2655513/.

23. Lisa Aliferis, "A Few Doctors Account for Outsize Share of Malpractice Claims," NPR, January 28, 2016, www.npr.org/sections/health-shots/2016/01 /28/464691741/a-few-doctors-account-for-outsize-share-of-malpractice-claims.

24. Levine, Oshel, and Wolfe, *State Medical Boards*.

25. Theresa Morris, *Cut It Out: The C-Section Epidemic in America* (New York: New York University Press, 2013), 33, 38.

26. Morris, *Cut It Out*, 40.

27. Morris, *Cut It Out*, 10.

28. Sakala, Yang, and Corry, *Maternity Care and Liability*, e10.

29. Michael Frakes, "Defensive Medicine and Obstetric Practices," *Journal of Empirical Legal Studies* 9, no. 3 (September 1, 2012): 457–81, https://doi.org /10.1111/j.1740-1461.2012.01259.x.

30. Britta L. Anderson, Albert L. Strunk, and Jay Schulkin, "Study on Defensive Medicine Practices among Obstetricians and Gynecologists Who Provide Breast Care," *Journal for Healthcare Quality* 33, no. 3 (May 1, 2011): 37–43, https://doi.org/10.1111/j.1945-1474.2010.00120.x.

31. Kristen Shrader-Frechette, "Perceived Risks versus Actual Risks: Managing Hazards through Negotiation," *RISK: Health, Safety and Environment* 1, no. 4 (September 1990): 342–44.

32. Morris, *Cut It Out*.

33. Sakala, Yang, and Corry, *Maternity Care and Liability*, e9.

34. Sakala, Yang, and Corry, *Maternity Care and Liability*, e9.

35. Sakala, Yang, and Corry, *Maternity Care and Liability*, e8.

36. Sakala, Yang, and Corry, *Maternity Care and Liability*, e10.

37. Sakala, Yang, and Corry, *Maternity Care and Liability*, e10.

38. Morris, *Cut It Out*, 37–38.

39. Morris, *Cut It Out*.

40. Aaron B. Caughey, "Vaginal Birth after Cesarean Delivery: Overview, Preparation, Technique," May 11, 2018, https://emedicine.medscape.com /article/272187-overview?pa=MFwhr2mPt9pmuv4dMmJUIycNVMdTBnh5 TKdgRVrX%2Fr4y2utX6lLXlbkj7qeofltV43mU9jD%2B1DtnxY47OmyybA %3D%3D.

41. Morris, *Cut It Out*, 127–28.

42. Morris, *Cut It Out*, 114.

43. Morris, *Cut It Out*, 120.

44. Both are abnormal placements of the placenta as a result of scar tissue in the uterus.

45. Emily Oster, *Expecting Better: Why the Conventional Wisdom Is Wrong—and What You Really Need to Know* (New York: Penguin, 2013), 140–41.

46. G. Siegal, M. M. Mello, and D. M. Studdert, "Adjudicating Severe Birth Injury Claims in Florida and Virginia: The Experience of a Landmark Experiment in Personal Injury Compensation," *American Journal of Law and Medicine* 34, no. 4 (2008): 493–537.

47. Morris, *Cut It Out*, 122–23.

48. "Hospital VBAC Policy Database," International Cesarean Awareness Network, www.ican-online.org/hospital-vbac-policy-database/.

49. Chad D. Kollas, Beth Boyer-Kollas, and James W. Kollas, "Criminal Prosecutions of Physicians Providing Palliative or End-of-Life Care," *Journal of Palliative Medicine* 11, no. 2 (March 2008): 238, https://doi.org/10.1089/jpm.2007.0187.

50. Selkin, "End-of-Life Liability Issues."

51. Selkin, "End-of-Life Liability Issues."

52. June L. Dahl, "Working with Regulators to Improve the Standard of Care in Pain Management: The U.S. Experience," *Journal of Pain and Symptom Management* 24, no. 2 (2002): 137.

53. Kelly K. Dineen and James M. DuBois, "Between a Rock and a Hard Place: Can Physicians Prescribe Opioids to Treat Pain Adequately while Avoiding Legal Sanction?," *American Journal of Law and Medicine* 42, no. 1 (2016): 7–52.

54. A. Alpers, "Criminal Act or Palliative Care? Prosecutions Involving the Care of the Dying," *Journal of Law, Medicine and Ethics* 26, no. 4 (1998): 308–31, 262.

55. Kollas, Boyer-Kollas, and Kollas, "Criminal Prosecutions of Physicians," 236.

56. Selkin, "End-of-Life Liability Issues," 6–7.

57. Selkin, "End-of-Life Liability Issues," 6.

58. Timothy E. Quill, Rebecca Dresser, and Dan W. Brock, "The Rule of Double Effect—a Critique of Its Role in End-of-Life Decision Making," *New England Journal of Medicine* 337, no. 24 (December 11, 1997): 1768–71, https://doi.org/10.1056/NEJM199712113372413.

59. Quill, Dresser, and Brock, "Rule of Double Effect."

60. Quill, Dresser, and Brock, "Rule of Double Effect."

61. Kollas, Boyer-Kollas, and Kollas, "Criminal Prosecutions of Physicians."

62. D. T. Lau et al., "Perceived Barriers That Impede Provider Relations and Medication Delivery: Hospice Providers' Experiences in Nursing Homes and Private Homes," *Journal of Palliative Medicine* 13, no. 3 (2010): 305–10.

63. Lau et al., "Perceived Barriers," 308.

64. Such concerns are not entirely gone, as legislators as recently as 2017 continued to introduce legislation that would limit physicians' ability to be reimbursed by Medicare for discussions about end-of-life care. See, e.g., JoNel Aleccia, "Docs Bill Medicare for End-of-Life Advice as 'Death Panel' Fears Reemerge," *USA Today*, February 9, 2017, www.usatoday.com/story/news/2017/02/09/kaiser-docs-bill-medicare-end—life-advice-death-panel-fears-reemerge/97715784/.

65. Lindy Willmott et al., "Reasons Doctors Provide Futile Treatment at the End of Life: A Qualitative Study," *Journal of Medical Ethics* 42, no. 8 (August 1, 2016): 496–503, https://doi.org/10.1136/medethics-2016-103370.

66. Cruzan v. Director, Missouri Department of Health, 497 U.S. 261 (1990).

67. See, e.g., Paula Span, "The Trouble with Advance Directives," *New York Times*, March 13, 2015, www.nytimes.com/2015/03/17/health/the-trouble-with-advance-directives.html; Paula Span, "The Patients Were Saved. That's Why the Families Are Suing," *New York Times*, April 10, 2017, www.nytimes.com/2017/04/10/health/wrongful-life-lawsuit-dnr.html.

68. Haider Warraich, *Modern Death: How Medicine Changed the End of Life* (New York: St. Martin's, 2017), 212–14. See also Cutler et al., "Physician Beliefs and Patient Preferences."

69. Warraich, *Modern Death*, 222.

70. N. E. Goldstein et al., "Prevalence of Formal Accusations of Murder and Euthanasia against Physicians," *Journal of Palliative Medicine* 15, no. 3 (2012): 335.

71. Kollas, Boyer-Kollas, and Kollas, "Criminal Prosecutions of Physicians."

72. State of Kansas v. Naramore, 25 Kan. App. 2d 302 (1998), www.aapsonline.org/judicial/statevnaramore.pdf.

73. Sheri Fink, "Strained by Katrina, a Hospital Faced Deadly Choices," *New York Times*, August 25, 2009, www.nytimes.com/2009/08/30/magazine/30doctors.html?pagewanted=all.

74. Selkin, "End-of-Life Liability Issues."

75. Lau et al., "Perceived Barriers."

76. See Marshall Kapp, "Is There a Doctor in the House? Physician Liability Fears and Quality of Care in Nursing Homes" (California HealthCare Foundation, September 2008), www.chcf.org/publication/is-there-a-doctor-in-the-house-physician-liability-fears-and-the-quality-of-care-in-nursing-homes/; and Marshall B. Kapp, "Legal Anxieties and End-of-Life Care in Nursing Homes," *Issues in Law and Medicine* 19, no. 2 (2003): 111–34.

77. Harlan M. Krumholz, Kumar Dharmarajan, and Harlan M. Krumholz, "Is Posthospital Syndrome a Result of Hospitalization-Induced Allostatic

Overload?," *Journal of Hospital Medicine*, May 25, 2018, https://doi.org/10
.12788/jhm.2986.

78. Kapp, "Is There a Doctor in the House?," 7.

79. Kathi Levine, "Old and Overmedicated: The Real Drug Problem in Nursing Homes," NPR, December 8, 2014, www.npr.org/sections/health-shots /2014/12/08/368524824/old-and-overmedicated-the-real-drug-problem-in -nursing-homes.

80. Kapp, "Is There a Doctor in the House?," 9.

81. Sharon R. Kaufman, *Ordinary Medicine: Extraordinary Treatments, Longer Lives, and Where to Draw the Line* (Durham, NC: Duke University Press, 2015), 131.

82. Kaufman, *Ordinary Medicine*, 131.

83. Rocco J. Perla, Samuel F. Hohmann, and Karen Annis, "Whole-Patient Measure of Safety: Using Administrative Data to Assess the Probability of Highly Undesirable Events during Hospitalization," *Journal for Healthcare Quality* 35, no. 5 (September 1, 2013): 20–31, https://doi.org/10.1111/jhq .12027; Paula Span, "The Illness Is Bad Enough. The Hospital May Be Even Worse," *New York Times*, August 7, 2018, sec. Health, https://www.nytimes .com/2018/08/03/health/post-hospital-syndrome-elderly.html.

84. Willmott et al., "Reasons Doctors Provide Futile Treatment."

85. Morris, *Cut It Out*, 76.

86. Julie Haizlip et al., "Perspective: The Negativity Bias, Medical Education, and the Culture of Academic Medicine: Why Culture Change Is Hard," *Academic Medicine: Journal of the Association of American Medical Colleges* 87, no. 9 (September 2012): 1205–9, https://doi.org/10.1097/ACM.0b013e3182628f03.

87. Morris, *Cut It Out*, 127.

88. Morris, *Cut It Out*, 55.

89. Aaron E. Carroll, "To Be Sued Less, Doctors Should Consider Talking to Patients More," *New York Times*, June 1, 2015, www.nytimes.com/2015/06/02 /upshot/to-be-sued-less-doctors-should-talk-to-patients-more.html.

90. Thomas H. Gallagher et al., "Can Communication-and-Resolution Programs Achieve Their Potential? Five Key Questions," *Health Affairs (Project Hope)* 37, no. 11 (November 2018): 1845–52, https://doi.org/10.1377/hlthaff .2018.0727.

91. Richard Pérez-Peña, "Use of Midwives, a Childbirth Phenomenon, Fades in City," *New York Times*, March 15, 2004, www.nytimes.com/2004/03/15 /nyregion/use-of-midwives-a-childbirth-phenomenon-fades-in-city.html.

92. Sakala, Yang, and Corry, *Maternity Care and Liability*, e8.

93. Sakala, Yang, and Corry, *Maternity Care and Liability*, e8.

94. Kapp, "Is There a Doctor in the House?"

95. Peter Whoriskey and Dan Keating, "Terminal Neglect? How Some

Hospices Treat the Dying," *Washington Post*, May 3, 2014, www.washington
post.com/business/economy/terminal-neglect-how-some-hospices fail the dying
/2014/05/03/7d3ac8ce-b8ef-11e3-96ae-f2c36d2b1245_story.html.

Chapter 7. Black Birth and Death in the Medicalized Rapids

1. Tom L. Beauchamp and James F. Childress, *Principles of Biomedical Ethics* (New York: Oxford University Press, 2016).

2. National Center for Health Statistics, *Health, United States, 2015: With Special Feature on Racial and Ethnic Health Disparities* (Hyattsville, MD: National Center for Health Statistics, 2016).

3. David R. Williams et al., "Racial Differences in Physical and Mental Health: Socio-economic Status, Stress and Discrimination," *Journal of Health Psychology* 2, no. 3 (July 1997): 335–51, https://doi.org/10.1177/135910 539700200305; Arline T. Geronimus et al., "'Weathering' and Age Patterns of Allostatic Load Scores among Blacks and Whites in the United States," *American Journal of Public Health* 96, no. 5 (May 2006): 826–33, https://doi.org/10 .2105/AJPH.2004.060749.

4. Norman B. Anderson et al., *Significance of Perceived Racism: Toward Understanding Ethnic Group Disparities in Health, the Later Years* (Washington, DC: National Academies Press, 2004), www.ncbi.nlm.nih.gov/books/NBK 25531/.

5. National Center for Health Statistics, *Health, United States, 2015*.

6. See, e.g., the records available at "Eugenics Record Office," Archives at Cold Spring Harbor Laboratory, http://library.cshl.edu/special-collections /eugenics.

7. Institute of Medicine, *Unequal Treatment: Confronting Racial and Ethnic Disparities in Health Care*, ed. Brian Smedley, Adrienne Stith, and Alan Nelson (Washington, DC: National Academies Press, 2003), www.nap.edu/read/10260 /chapter/1; Jennifer W. Mack et al., "Black-White Disparities in the Effects of Communication on Medical Care Received Near Death," *Archives of Internal Medicine* 170, no. 17 (September 27, 2010): 1533–40, https://doi.org/10.1001 /archinternmed.2010.322.

8. Institute of Medicine, *Unequal Treatment*, 125.

9. Institute of Medicine, *Unequal Treatment*, 144–45.

10. Institute of Medicine, *Unequal Treatment*, 144–45.

11. LeRoi S. Hicks et al., "Is Hospital Service Associated with Racial and Ethnic Disparities in Experiences with Hospital Care?," *American Journal of Medicine* 118, no. 5 (May 1, 2005): 529–35, https://doi.org/10.1016/j.amjmed .2005.02.012.

12. Chet D. Schrader and Lawrence M. Lewis, "Racial Disparity in Emergency Department Triage," *Journal of Emergency Medicine* 44, no. 2 (February 2013): 511–18, https://doi.org/10.1016/j.jemermed.2012.05.010.

13. Sudeep J. Karve et al., "Racial/Ethnic Disparities in Emergency Department Waiting Time for Stroke Patients in the United States," *Journal of Stroke and Cerebrovascular Diseases: The Official Journal of National Stroke Association* 20, no. 1 (February 2011): 30–40, https://doi.org/10.1016/j.jstrokecerebro vasdis.2009.10.006.

14. Laura D. Wandner et al., "The Perception of Pain in Others: How Gender, Race, and Age Influence Pain Expectations," *Journal of Pain* 13, no. 3 (March 2012): 220–27, https://doi.org/10.1016/j.jpain.2011.10.014.

15. Institute of Medicine, *Unequal Treatment: Confronting Racial and Ethnic Disparities in Health Care*, ed. Brian Smedley, Adrienne Stith, and Alan Nelson (Washington, DC: National Academies Press, 2003), https://www.nap.edu/read/10260/chapter/1.

16. Alexis Gadson, Eloho Akpovi, and Pooja K. Mehta, "Exploring the Social Determinants of Racial/Ethnic Disparities in Prenatal Care Utilization and Maternal Outcome," *Seminars in Perinatology* 41, no. 5 (August 2017): 308–17, https://doi.org/10.1053/j.semperi.2017.04.008; Elizabeth A. Howell et al., "Black-White Differences in Severe Maternal Morbidity and Site of Care," *American Journal of Obstetrics and Gynecology* 214, no. 1 (January 2016): 122.e1–122.e7, https://doi.org/10.1016/j.ajog.2015.08.019.

17. National Center for Health Statistics, *Health, United States, 2015*.

18. Myra J. Tucker et al., "The Black–White Disparity in Pregnancy-Related Mortality from Five Conditions: Differences in Prevalence and Case-Fatality Rates," *American Journal of Public Health* 97, no. 2 (February 2007): 247–51, https://doi.org/10.2105/AJPH.2005.072975.

19. Tucker et al., "Black–White Disparity."

20. Theresa M. Beckie, "Ethnic and Racial Disparities in Hypertension Management among Women," *Seminars in Perinatology* 41, no. 5 (August 2017): 278–86, https://doi.org/10.1053/j.semperi.2017.04.004.

21. F. M. Jackson et al., "Examining the Burdens of Gendered Racism: Implications for Pregnancy Outcomes among College-Educated African American Women," *Maternal and Child Health Journal* 5, no. 2 (June 2001): 95–107.

22. E. Brondolo et al., "Racism and Hypertension: A Review of the Empirical Evidence and Implications for Clinical Practice," *American Journal of Hypertension* 24, no. 5 (May 1, 2011): 518–29, https://doi.org/10.1038/ajh.2011.9.

23. Tyan Parker Dominguez et al., "Racial Differences in Birth Outcomes: The Role of General, Pregnancy, and Racism Stress," *Health Psychology* 27, no. 2 (2008): 194–203, https://doi.org/10.1037/0278-6133.27.2.194.

24. Manuck, "Racial and Ethnic Differences."

25. Heather H. Burris and Michele R. Hacker, "Birth Outcome Racial Disparities: A Result of Intersecting Social and Environmental Factors," *Seminars in Perinatology* 41, no. 6 (October 2017): 360–66, https://doi.org/10.1053/j.semperi.2017.07.002.

26. Manuck, "Racial and Ethnic Differences."

27. Louise Marie Roth and Megan M. Henley, "Unequal Motherhood: Racial-Ethnic and Socioeconomic Disparities in Cesarean Sections in the United States," *Social Problems* 59, no. 2 (May 2012): 207–27, https://doi.org/10.1525/sp.2012.59.2.207.

28. Gadson, Akpovi, and Mehta, "Exploring the Social Determinants."

29. The proportion of nonelderly black women using Medicaid for health coverage was estimated at 34% in 2017 compared to 16% for nonelderly white women. The fraction for maternity care may be higher than 30%, since the income requirements for Medicaid coverage for pregnancy and birth are higher than for other medical needs. Kaiser Family Foundation, "Medicaid Coverage Rates for the Non-elderly by Race and Ethnicity" (2017), www.kff.org/medicaid/state-indicator/rate-by-raceethnicity-3/?currentTimeframe=0&selectedRows=%7B%22wrapups%22:%7B%22united-states%22:%7B%7D%7D%7D. See also Gadson, Akpovi, and Mehta, "Exploring the Social Determinants."

30. V. E. Kolder, J. Gallagher, and M. T. Parsons, "Court-Ordered Obstetrical Interventions," *New England Journal of Medicine* 316, no. 19 (May 7, 1987): 1192–96, https://doi.org/10.1056/NEJM198705073161905.

31. Ira J. Chasnoff, Harvey J. Landress, and Mark E. Barrett, "The Prevalence of Illicit-Drug or Alcohol Use during Pregnancy and Discrepancies in Mandatory Reporting in Pinellas County, Florida," *New England Journal of Medicine* 322, no. 17 (April 26, 1990): 1202–6, https://doi.org/10.1056/NEJM199004263221706; Sarah C. M. Roberts and Amani Nuru-Jeter, "Universal Screening for Alcohol and Drug Use and Racial Disparities in Child Protective Services Reporting," *Journal of Behavioral Health Services and Research* 39, no. 1 (January 2012): 3–16, https://doi.org/10.1007/s11414-011-9247-x.

32. Monica R. McLemore et al., "Health Care Experiences of Pregnant, Birthing and Postnatal Women of Color at Risk for Preterm Birth," *Social Science and Medicine (1982)* 201 (2018): 127–35, https://doi.org/10.1016/j.socscimed.2018.02.013.

33. Hannah Yoder and Lynda R. Hardy, "Midwifery and Antenatal Care for Black Women: A Narrative Review," *SAGE Open* 8, no. 1 (January 1, 2018): 2158244017752220, https://doi.org/10.1177/2158244017752220.

34. Gadson, Akpovi, and Mehta, "Exploring the Social Determinants."

35. Howell et al., "Black-White Differences."

36. Susan Mann et al., "What We Can Do about Maternal Mortality—and How to Do It Quickly," *New England Journal of Medicine* 379, no. 18 (November 1, 2018): 1689–91, https://doi.org/10.1056/NEJMp1810649.

37. Cynthia Prather et al., "The Impact of Racism on the Sexual and Reproductive Health of African American Women," *Journal of Women's Health* 25, no. 7 (July 2016): 664–71, https://doi.org/10.1089/jwh.2015.5637.

38. Gertrude Jacinta Fraser, *African American Midwifery in the South: Dialogues of Birth, Race, and Memory* (Cambridge, MA: Harvard University Press, 2009).

39. Fraser, *African American Midwifery*, 32–35.

40. Jenny M. Luke, *Delivered by Midwives: African American Midwifery in the Twentieth-Century South* (Jackson: University Press of Mississippi, 2018), 46–47.

41. Alicia D. Bonaparte, "'The Satisfactory Midwife Bag': Midwifery Regulation in South Carolina, Past and Present Considerations," *Social Science History* 38, no. 1–2 (2014): 155–82, https://doi.org/10.1017/ssh.2015.14.

42. Luke, *Delivered by Midwives*.

43. Rochaun Meadows-Fernandez, "Just So We're Clear: Black Mothers Aren't to Blame for High Infant Mortality," *YES! Magazine*, May 4, 2017, www.yesmagazine.org/peace-justice/black-mothers-arent-to-blame-for-high -infant-mortality-20170504.

44. Yoder and Hardy, "Midwifery and Antenatal Care."

45. Jodi DeLibertis, "Shifting the Frame: A Report on Diversity and Inclusion in the American College of Nurse-Midwives" (Silver Spring, MD: American College of Nurse-Midwives, June 2015), www.midwife.org/acnm/files/cc LibraryFiles/Filename/000000005329/Shifting-the-Frame-June-2015.pdf.

46. Luke, *Delivered by Midwives*, 112.

47. Fraser, *African American Midwifery*; Onnie Lee Logan and Katherine Clark, *Motherwit: An Alabama Midwife's Story* (San Francisco: Untreed Reads, 2013).

48. Fraser, *African American Midwifery*.

49. Logan and Clark, *Motherwit*, 61.

50. Luke, *Delivered by Midwives*, 51.

51. Logan and Clark, *Motherwit*, 59.

52. Luke, *Delivered by Midwives*, 47.

53. Fraser, *African American Midwifery*.

54. Luke, *Delivered by Midwives*, 51.

55. Luke, *Delivered by Midwives*, 113.

56. Luke, *Delivered by Midwives*, 113.

57. Luke, *Delivered by Midwives*, 115.

58. Luke, *Delivered by Midwives*, 48, 115.

59. Rob Haskell, "Serena Williams on Motherhood, Marriage, and Making Her Comeback," *Vogue*, January 10, 2018, www.vogue.com/article/serena -williams-vogue-cover-interview-february-2018.

60. Tressie McMillan Cottom, "I Was Pregnant and in Crisis. All the Nurses and Doctors Saw Was an Incompetent Black Woman," *Time*, January 8, 2019, http://time.com/5494404/tressie-mcmillan-cottom-thick-pregnancy-competent/.

61. Liana Aghajanian, "Los Angeles Midwives Aim to End Racial Disparities at Birth," *Aljazeera America*, September 5, 2015, http://america.aljazeera.com /articles/2015/9/5/to-los-angeles-midwives-racial-disparities-birth.html.

62. See, e.g., http://blackmamasmatter.org/, www.blackwomenbirthing justice.org/birth-justice-allies, http://sistersong.net/, and https://blackdoulas .org/.

63. Lucia Guerra-Reyes and Lydia J. Hamilton, "Racial Disparities in Birth Care: Exploring the Perceived Role of African-American Women Providing Mid-wifery Care and Birth Support in the United States," *Women and Birth* 30, no. 1 (February 2017): e9–16, https://doi.org/10.1016/j.wombi.2016.06.004.

64. Guerra-Reyes and Hamilton, "Racial Disparities in Birth Care."

65. Sarah Benatar et al., "Midwifery Care at a Freestanding Birth Center: A Safe and Effective Alternative to Conventional Maternity Care," *Health Services Research*, April 2013, https://doi.org/10.1111/1475-6773.12061.

66. Benatar et al., "Midwifery Care."

67. Brownsyne Tucker Edmonds, Marjie Mogul, and Judy A. Shea, "Under-standing Low-Income African American Women's Expectations, Preferences, and Priorities in Prenatal Care," *Family and Community Health* 38, no. 2 (2015): 149–57, https://doi.org/10.1097/FCH.0000000000000066.

68. Aghajanian, "Los Angeles Midwives."

69. See www.birthingbeautiful.org/.

70. Heide Aungst, "Fighting Infant Mortality Requires a Neighborhood Approach," *Cleveland Magazine*, May 10, 2017, https://clevelandmagazine .com/in-the-cle/commentary/articles/fighting-infant-mortality-requires-a -neighborhood-approach.

71. Shayna D. Cunningham et al., "*Expect with Me*: Development and Evaluation Design for an Innovative Model of Group Prenatal Care to Improve Perinatal Outcomes," *BMC Pregnancy and Childbirth* 17, no. 1 (May 18, 2017): 147, https://doi.org/10.1186/s12884-017-1327-3.

72. See, e.g., a variety of initiatives run by midwives of color at http://nacpm .org/for-cpms/social-justice/initiatives/, as well as the National Association of Birth Centers of Color at www.facebook.com/NABCCC/.

73. Benatar et al., "Midwifery Care."

74. Benatar et al., "Midwifery Care," 1763.

75. Benatar et al., "Midwifery Care."

76. Phuong Ly, "A Labor without End," *Washington Post*, May 27, 2007, www.washingtonpost.com/wp-dyn/content/article/2007/05/23/AR200705230 1294.html.

77. Kimberly S. Johnson, "Racial and Ethnic Disparities in Palliative Care," *Journal of Palliative Medicine* 16, no. 11 (November 2013): 1329–34, https:// doi.org/10.1089/jpm.2013.9468.

78. Sarah Muni et al., "The Influence of Race/Ethnicity and Socioeconomic

Status on End-of-Life Care in the ICU," *Chest* 139, no. 5 (May 2011): 1025–33, https://doi.org/10.1378/chest.10-3011.

79. Amresh Hanchate et al., "Racial and Ethnic Differences in End-of-Life Costs: Why Do Minorities Cost More Than Whites?," *Archives of Internal Medicine* 169, no. 5 (March 9, 2009): 493–501, https://doi.org/10.1001/arch internmed.2008.616.

80. Charles S. Cleeland, "Pain and Treatment of Pain in Minority Patients with Cancer: The Eastern Cooperative Oncology Group Minority Outpatient Pain Study," *Annals of Internal Medicine* 127, no. 9 (November 1, 1997): 813, https://doi.org/10.7326/0003-4819-127-9-199711010-00006; Kelly M. Hoffman et al., "Racial Bias in Pain Assessment and Treatment Recommendations, and False Beliefs about Biological Differences between Blacks and Whites," *Proceedings of the National Academy of Sciences* 113, no. 16 (April 19, 2016): 4296–301, https://doi.org/10.1073/pnas.1516047113.

81. Marcella Alsan and Marianne Wanamaker, "Tuskegee and the Health of Black Men" (NBER Working Paper Series, Cambridge, MA: National Bureau of Economic Research, June 2016), https://doi.org/10.3386/w22323.

82. Muni et al., "Influence of Race/Ethnicity."

83. Jane C. Weeks et al., "Patients' Expectations about Effects of Chemotherapy for Advanced Cancer," *New England Journal of Medicine* 367, no. 17 (October 25, 2012): 1616–25, https://doi.org/10.1056/NEJMoa1204410.

84. Hoffman et al., "Racial Bias in Pain Assessment."

85. Wandner et al., "Perception of Pain in Others."

86. Andrea M. Elliott et al., "Differences in Physicians' Verbal and Nonverbal Communication with Black and White Patients at the End of Life," *Journal of Pain and Symptom Management* 51, no. 1 (January 1, 2016): 1–8, https://doi.org/10.1016/j.jpainsymman.2015.07.008.

87. Lois Snyder and Timothy E. Quill, eds., *Physician's Guide to End-of-Life Care*, 1st ed. (Philadelphia: American College of Physicians, 2001), 35–53.

88. José F. Figueroa et al., "Across US Hospitals, Black Patients Report Comparable or Better Experiences Than White Patients," *Health Affairs (Project Hope)* 35, no. 8 (August 1, 2016): 1391–98, https://doi.org/10.1377/hlthaff.2015.1426.

89. Vincent Mor, George Papandonatos, and Susan C. Miller, "End-of-Life Hospitalization for African American and Non-Latino White Nursing Home Residents: Variation by Race and a Facility's Racial Composition," *Journal of Palliative Medicine* 8, no. 1 (February 2005): 58–68, https://doi.org/10.1089/jpm.2005.8.58.

90. Nan Tracy Zheng et al., "Racial Disparities in In-Hospital Death and Hospice Use among Nursing Home Residents at the End of Life," *Medical Care* 49, no. 11 (November 2011): 992–98, https://doi.org/10.1097/MLR.0b013e318236384e.

91. Jung Kwak, William E. Haley, and David A. Chiriboga, "Racial Differences in Hospice Use and In-Hospital Death among Medicare and Medicaid Dual-Eligible Nursing Home Residents," *Gerontologist* 48, no. 1 (February 1, 2008): 32–41, https://doi.org/10.1093/geront/48.1.32.

92. Institute of Medicine, *Unequal Treatment*, 104.

93. Institute of Medicine, *Unequal Treatment*, 104.

94. Institute of Medicine and National Research Council, *Improving Palliative Care for Cancer* (Washington, DC: National Academies Press, 2001), 104.

95. Institute of Medicine, *Unequal Treatment*, 106.

96. Institute of Medicine, *Unequal Treatment*, 107.

97. Institute of Medicine, *Unequal Treatment*, 108.

98. Institute of Medicine, *Unequal Treatment*, 105.

99. Institute of Medicine, *Unequal Treatment*, 109.

100. Ashish K. Jha et al., "Concentration and Quality of Hospitals That Care for Elderly Black Patients," *Archives of Internal Medicine* 167, no. 11 (June 11, 2007): 1177, https://doi.org/10.1001/archinte.167.11.1177.

101. Philip N. Okafor et al., "African Americans Have Better Outcomes for Five Common Gastrointestinal Diagnoses in Hospitals with More Racially Diverse Patients," *American Journal of Gastroenterology* 111, no. 5 (May 2016): 649–57, https://doi.org/10.1038/ajg.2016.64.

102. Johnson, "Racial and Ethnic Disparities."

103. Mack et al., "Black-White Disparities."

104. Patrick Dillon, "African Americans and Hospice: A Culture-Centered Exploration of Disparities in End-of-Life Care" (PhD diss., University of South Florida, 2013), 14, http://scholarcommons.usf.edu/cgi/viewcontent.cgi?article=5859&context=etd; Jane L. Givens, "Racial and Ethnic Differences in Hospice Use among Patients with Heart Failure," *Archives of Internal Medicine* 170, no. 5 (March 8, 2010): 427, https://doi.org/10.1001/archinternmed.2009.547.

105. Sarah Varney, "A Racial Gap in Attitudes toward Hospice Care," *New York Times*, August 21, 2015, www.nytimes.com/2015/08/25/health/a-racial-gap-in-attitudes-toward-hospice-care.html.

106. Dillon, "African Americans and Hospice," 62.

107. Dillon, "African Americans and Hospice."

108. Dillon, "African Americans and Hospice," 63.

109. Malcolm A. Cort, "Cultural Mistrust and Use of Hospice Care: Challenges and Remedies," *Journal of Palliative Medicine* 7, no. 1 (February 2004): 63–71, https://doi.org/10.1089/109662104322737269.

110. Dillon, "African Americans and Hospice," 63.

111. Varney, "Racial Gap in Attitudes."

112. Susan Enguidanos et al., "Use of Role Model Stories to Overcome Barriers to Hospice among African Americans," *Journal of Palliative Medicine* 14, no. 2 (February 2011): 161–68, https://doi.org/10.1089/jpm.2010.0380.

113. Enguidanos et al., "Use of Role Model Stories."

114. Sheronda Drisdom, "Barriers to Using Palliative Care: Insight into African American Culture," *Clinical Journal of Oncology Nursing* 17, no. 4 (August 1, 2013): 376–80, https://doi.org/10.1188/13.CJON.376-380.

115. Abigail P. H. Holley et al., "Palliative Access through Care at Home: Experiences with an Urban, Geriatric Home Palliative Care Program: Geriatrics Home Palliative Care," *Journal of the American Geriatrics Society* 57, no. 10 (October 2009): 1925–31, https://doi.org/10.1111/j.1532-5415.2009.02452.x.

116. Elizabeth L. Ciemins et al., "An Evaluation of the Advanced Illness Management (AIM) Program: Increasing Hospice Utilization in the San Francisco Bay Area," *Journal of Palliative Medicine* 9, no. 6 (December 2006): 1401–11, https://doi.org/10.1089/jpm.2006.9.1401.

117. Glenn B. Zaide et al., "Ethnicity, Race, and Advance Directives in an Inpatient Palliative Care Consultation Service," *Palliative and Supportive Care* 11, no. 1 (February 2013): 5–11, https://doi.org/10.1017/S1478951511200041 7.

118. Varney, "Racial Gap in Attitudes."

119. Varney, "Racial Gap in Attitudes."

120. Benatar et al., "Midwifery Care."

121. Benatar et al., "Midwifery Care."

122. Ly, "Labor without End."

123. Julie Fairman, "'Go to Ruth's House': The Social Activism of Ruth Lubic and the Family Health and Birth Center," *Nursing History Review: Official Journal of the American Association for the History of Nursing* 18 (2010): 118–29.

124. Fairman, "Go to Ruth's House."

125. Miriam Zoila Pérez, "How This DC Birth Center Is Building the 'Answer for Black Women,'" *Rewire.News*, July 31, 2018, www.community ofhopedc.org/news-events/how-dc-birth-center-building-answer-black-women; see also Ly, "Labor without End."

126. Fairman, "Go to Ruth's House."

127. Karen A. Scott et al., "An Inconvenient Truth: You Have No Answer That Black Women Don't Already Possess," *ourbwbj*, October 31, 2018, www .blackwomenbirthingjustice.org/single-post/2018/10/31/An-inconvenient-truth -You-have-no-answer-that-Black-women-don%E2%80%99t-already-possess.

128. Scott et al., "Inconvenient Truth."

129. Jenny Hall et al., "Dignity and Respect during Pregnancy and Child-birth: A Survey of the Experience of Disabled Women," *BMC Pregnancy and Childbirth* 18 (August 13, 2018): 328, https://doi.org/10.1186/s12884-018 -1950-7; Reem Malouf, Jane Henderson, and Maggie Redshaw, "Access and Quality of Maternity Care for Disabled Women during Pregnancy, Birth and the Postnatal Period in England: Data from a National Survey," *BMJ Open* 7, no. 7 (20 2017): e016757, https://doi.org/10.1136/bmjopen-2017-016757.

130. Juno Obedin-Maliver and Harvey J. Makadon, "Transgender Men and Pregnancy," *Obstetric Medicine* 9, no. 1 (March 2016): 4–8, https://doi.org/10 .1177/1753495X15612658; Tomas L. Griebling, "Sexuality and Aging: A Focus on Lesbian, Gay, Bisexual, and Transgender (LGBT) Needs in Palliative and End of Life Care," *Current Opinion in Supportive and Palliative Care* 10, no. 1 (March 2016): 95–101, https://doi.org/10.1097/SPC.0000000000000196.

131. Snyder and Quill, *Physician's Guide*, 41.

132. Snyder and Quill, *Physician's Guide*, 52.

133. Snyder and Quill, *Physician's Guide*, 43.

Conclusion. Reshaping the Watershed

1. Ira Byock, *Best Care Possible: A Physician's Quest to Transform Care through the End of Life* (New York: Avery, 2013).

2. Hamilton Moses et al., "The Anatomy of Health Care in the United States," *Journal of the American Medical Association* 310, no. 18 (November 13, 2013): 1947, https://doi.org/10.1001/jama.2013.281425.

3. Moses et al., "Anatomy of Health Care," 1955.

4. Moses et al., "Anatomy of Health Care," 1950.

5. Moses et al., "Anatomy of Health Care," 1952.

6. Peiyin Hung et al., "Access to Obstetric Services in Rural Counties Still Declining, with 9 Percent Losing Services, 2004–14," *Health Affairs* 36, no. 9 (September 1, 2017): 1663–71, https://doi.org/10.1377/hlthaff.2017.0338; Sara Markowitz et al., "Competitive Effects of Scope of Practice Restrictions: Public Health or Public Harm?," *Journal of Health Economics* 55 (September 1, 2017): 201–18, https://doi.org/10.1016/j.jhealeco.2017.07.004.

7. "State Practice Environment," American Association of Nurse Practitioners, www.aanp.org/legislation-regulation/state-legislation/state-practice -environment.

8. Elizabeth Kukura, "Obstetric Violence," *Georgetown Law Journal* 106 (May 2018): 721–801.

9. Markowitz et al., "Competitive Effects."

10. Kyoungrae Jung and Daniel Polsky, "Competition and Quality in Home Health Care Markets," *Health Economics* 23, no. 3 (March 2014): 298–313, https://doi.org/10.1002/hec.2938.

11. Moses et al., "Anatomy of Health Care," 1957.

12. M. D. Brent, C. James, and Gregory P. Poulsen, "The Case for Capitation," *Harvard Business Review*, July–August 2016, https://hbr.org/2016/07 /the-case-for-capitation.

13. Michael E. Porter, "What Is Value in Health Care?," *New England Journal of Medicine* 363, no. 26 (December 23, 2010): 2477–81, http://dx.doi .org.ezproxy.rit.edu/10.1056/NEJMp1011024.

14. Institute of Medicine (US) and Committee on Approaching Death:

Addressing Key End-of-Life Issues, *Dying in America: Improving Quality and Honoring Individual Preferences near the End of Life* (Washington, DC: National Academies Press, 2015), 47–48.

15. Diane E. Meier, "Measuring Care Quality for the Sickest Patients," *NEJM Catalyst*, February 9, 2016, https://catalyst.nejm.org/measuring-quality -of-care-for-the-sickest-patients/.

16. Moses et al., "Anatomy of Health Care," 1961.

17. Paul Starr, *The Social Transformation of American Medicine: The Rise of a Sovereign Profession and the Making of a Vast Industry*, rev. ed. (New York: Basic Books, 1984), 491.

18. Porter, "What Is Value in Health Care?"

19. "The Value Modifier (VM) Program," Centers for Medicare & Medicaid Services, www.cms.gov/Medicare/Quality-Initiatives-Patient-Assessment-Instru ments/Value-Based-Programs/VMP/Value-Modifier-VM-or-PVBM.html.

20. Michael E. Porter and Thomas H. Lee, "The Strategy That Will Fix Health Care," *Harvard Business Review*, October 2013, https://hbr.org/2013 /10/the-strategy-that-will-fix-health-care.

21. Thomas H. Lee, "Putting the Value Framework to Work," *New England Journal of Medicine* 363, no. 26 (December 23, 2010): 2481–83, http://dx.doi .org.ezproxy.rit.edu/10.1056/NEJMp1013111.

22. See, e.g., the documentation supporting the BirthBundle at https://aspe .hhs.gov/system/files/pdf/255731/BundledPaymentMNBirthingCenter.pdf.

23. Joshua M. Wiener and Jane Tilly, "End-of-Life Care in the United States: Policy Issues and Model Programs of Integrated Care," *International Journal of Integrated Care* 3 (2003): e24.

24. Shayna D. Cunningham et al., "*Expect with Me*: Development and Evaluation Design for an Innovative Model of Group Prenatal Care to Improve Perinatal Outcomes," *BMC Pregnancy and Childbirth* 17, no. 1 (May 18, 2017): 147, https://doi.org/10.1186/s12884-017-1327-3.

25. Institute of Medicine (US) and Committee on Approaching Death, *Dying in America*, 45–55.

26. Constance Gustke, "Concierge Medicine: Not Just for the Rich, Any-more," CNBC, December 14, 2012, www.cnbc.com/id/100314847; Starr, *Social Transformation of American Medicine*, 490.

27. Starr, *Social Transformation of American Medicine*, 490.

28. See, e.g., "Concierge Medical Clinic," Geriatric Concierge Center, http:// geriatricsconcierge.com/concierge-clinic.html.

29. Bruce Leff, "Why I Believe in Hospital at Home," *NEJM Catalyst*, February 5, 2017, https://catalyst.nejm.org/why-i-believe-in-hospital-at-home/; Gideon A. Caplan et al., "A Meta-analysis of 'Hospital in the Home,'" *Medical Journal of Australia* 197, no. 9 (November 5, 2012): 512–19.

30. Nina Bernstein, "Fighting to Honor a Father's Last Wish: To Die at

Home," *New York Times*, September 25, 2014, www.nytimes.com/2014/09/26
/nyregion/family-fights-health-care-system-for-simple-request-to-die-at-home.
html.

31. Steven H. Landers and Ashwini R. Sehgal, "Health Care Lobbying in
the United States," *American Journal of Medicine* 116, no. 7 (April 1, 2004):
474–77, https://doi.org/10.1016/j.amjmed.2003.10.037; "Physician Payment
and Delivery Models," AMA, www.ama-assn.org/about/scope-practice.

32. Jonathan Oberlander and Joseph White, "Public Attitudes toward Health
Care Spending Aren't the Problem; Prices Are," *Health Affairs* 28, no. 5 (September 1, 2009): 1285–93, https://doi.org/10.1377/hlthaff.28.5.1285; Uwe E.
Reinhardt, "The Pricing of U.S. Hospital Services: Chaos behind a Veil of
Secrecy," *Health Affairs* 25, no. 1 (January 1, 2006): 57–69, https://doi.org/10
.1377/hlthaff.25.1.57.

33. "The Home Health Value-Based Purchasing (HHVBP) Model," Centers
for Medicare & Medicaid Services, www.cms.gov/Medicare/Quality-Initiatives
-Patient-Assessment-Instruments/Value-Based-Programs/Other-VBPs/HHVBP
.html.

34. "Medicare and Medicaid Programs; CY 2016 Home Health Prospective
Payment System Rate Update; Home Health Value-Based Purchasing Model;
and Home Health Quality Reporting Requirements," *Federal Register*, November 5, 2015, www.federalregister.gov/documents/2015/11/05/2015-27931
/medicare-and-medicaid-programs-cy-2016-home-health-prospective-payment
-system-rate-update-home.

35. See, e.g., "Early Elective Deliveries," California Maternal Quality Care
Collaborative, www.cmqcc.org/qi-initiatives/early-elective-deliveries.

36. For one discussion see Barbara S. Levy and Debjani Mukherjee, "Changes
in Obstetrics and Gynecologic Care Healthcare Triple Aims: Moving Women's
Healthcare from Volume to Value," *Clinical Obstetrics and Gynecology* 58,
no. 2 (June 2015): 355–61, https://doi.org/10.1097/GRF.0000000000000099.

37. See, e.g., the most recent opinion: American College of Obstetricians
and Gynecologists, "Approaches to Limit Intervention during Labor and Birth,"
Committee Opinion (Washington, DC, February 2017).

38. American Medical Association, "Medical Liability Reform NOW!"
(2019), 29, www.ama-assn.org/system/files/2019-03/mlr-now.pdf.

39. Allen Kachalia, "Liability Claims and Costs before and after Implementation of a Medical Error Disclosure Program," *Annals of Internal Medicine*
153, no. 4 (August 17, 2010): 213, https://doi.org/10.7326/0003-4819-153-4
-201008170-00002.

40. One study found that 20% of the patients who filed suits did so simply
to get access to information about their case. Mark A. Rothstein, "Health Care
Reform and Medical Malpractice Claims," *Journal of Law, Medicine and Ethics*
38, no. 4 (2010): 871–74, https://doi.org/10.1111/j.1748-720X.2010.00540.x.

41. Avital Nathman, "Another Nurse Held My Baby's Head into My Vagina to Prevent Him from Being Delivered," *Cosmopolitan*, August 10, 2016, www .cosmopolitan.com/lifestyle/news/a62592/caroline-malatesta-brookwood -childbirth-lawsuit/.

42. Vikki Entwistle, Michelle Mello, and Troyen A. Brennan, "Advising Patients about Patient Safety: Current Initiatives Risk Shifting Responsibility," *Joint Commission Journal on Quality and Patient Safety* 31, no. 9 (September 2005).

43. Joseph S. Kass and Rachel V. Rose, "Medical Malpractice Reform— Historical Approaches, Alternative Models, and Communication and Resolution Programs," *AMA Journal of Ethics* 18, no. 3 (March 1, 2016): 299, https://doi .org/10.1001/journalofethics.2016.18.3.pfor6-1603.

44. Emme Deland, "Let's Talk about Improving Communication in Health-care," *Columbia Medical Review* 1, no. 1 (June 22, 2015): 23–27, https://doi .org/10.7916/D8RF5T5D; Thomas H. Gallagher et al., "Can Communication-and-Resolution Programs Achieve Their Potential? Five Key Questions," *Health Affairs (Project Hope)* 37, no. 11 (November 2018): 1845–52, https://doi.org /10.1377/hlthaff.2018.0727.

45. Amy S. Oxentenko et al., "Time Spent on Clinical Documentation: A Survey of Internal Medicine Residents and Program Directors," *Archives of Internal Medicine* 170, no. 4 (February 22, 2010): 377–80, https://doi.org/10 .1001/archinternmed.2009.534; James E. Siegler, Neha N. Patel, and C. Jessica Dine, "Prioritizing Paperwork over Patient Care: Why Can't We Do Both?," *Journal of Graduate Medical Education* 7, no. 1 (March 2015): 16–18, https:// doi.org/10.4300/JGME-D-14-00494.1.

46. PricewaterhouseCoopers, *Patients or Paperwork? The Regulatory Burden Facing America's Hospitals* (Chicago: American Hospital Association, 2001).

47. Christine Sinsky et al., "Allocation of Physician Time in Ambulatory Practice: A Time and Motion Study in 4 Specialties," *Annals of Internal Medicine* 165, no. 11 (December 6, 2016): 753, https://doi.org/10.7326/M16-0961.

48. M. Leonard, S. Graham, and D. Bonacum, "The Human Factor: The Critical Importance of Effective Teamwork and Communication in Providing Safe Care," *Quality and Safety in Health Care* 13, no. S1 (October 2004): i85–90, https://doi.org/10.1136/qhc.13.suppl_1.i85; Deland, "Let's Talk about Improving Communication."

49. A. Alpers, "Criminal Act or Palliative Care? Prosecutions Involving the Care of the Dying," *Journal of Law, Medicine and Ethics* 26, no. 4 (1998): 308–31.

50. Ellen McCarthy, "Dying Is Hard. Death Doulas Want to Help Make It Easier," *Washington Post*, July 22, 2016, www.washingtonpost.com/lifestyle /style/dying-is-hard-death-doulas-want-to-help-make-it-easier/2016/07/22

/53d80f5c-24f7-11e6-8690-f14ca9de2972_story.html?noredirect=on&utm _term=.b22ce4b7d8e6.

51. Kenneth J. Gruber, Susan H. Cupito, and Christina F. Dobson, "Impact of Doulas on Healthy Birth Outcomes," *Journal of Perinatal Education* 22, no. 1 (2013): 49–58, https://doi.org/10.1891/1058-1243.22.1.49.

California, 110, 111, 128, 144, 147, 231
California Maternal Quality Care
  Collaborative program, 240
Canada, 97
cancer, 54, 55, 62, 72, 75, 86, 156–57,
  182, 211, 212, 216. *See also*
  oncologists
Carder, Angela, 202
cardiopulmonary resuscitation (CPR),
  10, 55, 56, 64, 65, 68, 70, 143
care, high-intensity, 7, 8, 23, 31, 75–76,
  152, 195, 212, 226, 233, 235; and
  consolidation of care, 229; and
  end-of-life care, 52, 55, 94, 98;
  and hospitals, 23, 32, 36, 70, 144;
  and malpractice risks, 170, 175; and
  quality care, 24, 55; and reimbursement, 139, 143, 144, 232; and risks,
  176, 188. *See also* intensive care units
  (ICUs)
care, individualized, 53, 70, 85, 123,
  136–37, 221, 226, 233, 245, 246;
  and African Americans, 197, 203,
  208, 209, 219, 222, 223–24, 225; and
  birth centers, 97, 99, 102; and decentralization, 238; and demedicalization,
  83, 86, 89, 90, 91; for dying patients,
  58, 59–60, 68, 72, 77, 78, 79, 101;
  and Family Health and Birth Center,
  220; and home birth, 93, 97, 99; and
  hospice, 88, 93, 126; in hospitals, 69,
  77, 78, 86, 102, 146, 193; and midwifery, 87, 88, 209; and reforms, 227,
  228, 229; and reimbursement, 139,
  140, 141, 146, 164; and risk, 167,
  191, 193; and standardization, 87,
  234, 247
care plans, 32, 69, 235, 244–45
CenteringPregnancy, 100, 210
centralization, 90–91, 108, 126, 136,
  169, 214, 215, 222, 229; and end-of-
  life care, 56–57; and Hill-Burton Act,
  107; and maternity care, 26–32; and
  Medicare, 12–13, 152; and reforms,
  230–31, 238. *See also under* hospitals
certificate-of-need (CON) laws, 6, 105,
  106–8, 109, 118–20, 123–24, 126,
  130, 136, 154, 228, 230, 231–32

cesarean sections, 2, 3, 21, 22, 34–35,
  41, 49, 105, 149, 150, 172, 228, 246;
  and African Americans, 200, 202; and
  birth centers, 210; and breech delivery,
  191; cost of, 23, 144; and defensive
  medicine, 174, 188; financial incentives in, 145; forced, 25, 42; and
  macrosomia, 15, 40, 177; and midwives, 132, 231; rates of, 9, 10, 24,
  36, 110, 160, 178, 220, 231, 234;
  reduction of incidence of, 240; risk of,
  24, 191; trial of labor after, 128–29;
  and uterine rupture, 24. *See also* labor
  and delivery
comfort care, 13, 69, 111, 157
comfort care homes, 121, 122–23, 154,
  227
Commission for the Accreditation of
  Birth Centers (CABC), 134, 148
communication, 1, 2, 9, 22, 44–45,
  48–49, 64, 74, 76–77, 89, 152, 224;
  about goals of care, 100, 101, 102–3,
  140, 153; and African Americans,
  196, 198, 199, 204, 212–13, 215, 216,
  218; and community-based providers,
  242–43; and hospice, 94, 243; and
  hospitals, 192, 241–43; and liability,
  167, 192, 241–43, 245; and Medicare
  and Medicaid, 219; and palliative
  care, 65, 66, 67; pause points for, 7,
  19, 71, 77, 245; reimbursement for,
  155–56, 219, 242, 308n64; training
  in, 7, 244, 247. *See also* end-of-life
  care; informed consent
communication-and-resolution programs (CRPs), 241–42
community-based care, 50, 106, 195,
  221, 239; and African Americans,
  207, 208, 210, 222–23; and CON
  laws, 107, 108; and end-of-life, 98;
  hospitals vs., 99, 105, 129, 159; and
  maternity care, 22, 28, 98, 129, 208,
  210; and Medicare, 152, 159; and
  regulations, 105–11, 149; and risk,
  187, 191–94
community-based providers, 81–82,
  104, 193, 229, 242–43; and CPM
  laws, 108; and liability, 191–94, 243;

and low-risk populations, 191–93;
and Medicaid, 140; and palliative
care, 157–58; and reforms, 230; and
reimbursement, 138, 195; start-up
costs of, 109; underestimation of risk
by, 189
corporate practice of medicine (CPM)
laws, 6, 105, 106, 108–9, 123, 124,
126, 230
costs, 6–7, 18, 80, 81, 140, 226; and
advanced practice nurses, 110; and
African Americans, 211; and birth
centers, 131, 135, 144, 162, 210; and
cancer treatment, 156; of cesarean
sections, 23, 144; and comfort care
homes, 122–23; and community-
based care, 106, 239; and CON laws,
107, 108, 109, 123; and CPM laws,
109; and decentralized birth, 98; and
demedicalization, 105; of end-of-life
care, 10, 54, 142–43; and Family
Health and Birth Center, 220; of
high-intensity care, 23; and high-
touch care, 100; of home birth, 144;
and home healthcare, 153, 239; and
hospice, 121, 122, 123, 125, 130–31,
239; of hospital care, 10, 23, 98,
141–43, 144, 210; of maternity care,
3, 10, 142, 143, 144–50; and Medicaid, 122; and Medicare, 122, 125,
143, 152; out-of-pocket, 3, 53, 161,
162; and physicians' collaboration or
oversight, 114, 115; and regulations,
106, 239; and reimbursement, 139,
141–43; of unnecessary care, 143.
See also malpractice; reimbursement
Cottom, Tressie McMillan, 208
CPR. See cardiopulmonary resuscitation
Cruzan v. Director, Missouri Department of Health (1990), 183

death, physiological, 63, 78, 83, 84, 85,
89, 90, 187, 188, 246
"death panels," 155, 179, 183
decentralization, 26, 82, 96, 102, 113,
127, 228; and African Americans,
200, 204, 217–18, 219, 223; and birth
centers, 97, 98; and CON laws, 106;

and death at home, 91–92; and
demechanized care, 99–100; and
demedicalization, 86, 89–91; and
destandardization, 99; and home
birth, 89, 91, 92, 97, 98, 192; and
hospice, 130; and informed consent,
101; and Medicare, 13, 130; and
midwifery, 28; and patient autonomy,
100–101; and reforms, 238, 239; and
reimbursement, 146; and state repre-
sentatives, 132; triage approach to, 89
DeLee, Robert, 28, 32
demedicalization, 81–82, 83, 84, 92, 96,
97, 104, 121, 136, 138, 227; and
advanced practice nurses, 110; and
CPM laws, 109; and decentralization,
86, 89–91; and hospitals, 79, 102,
105, 106, 158–59, 160–61; movement
for, 89–90; and physicians, 131–32
destandardization, 86–87, 90, 99–100
disabled individuals, 151, 196
disease, 15, 27, 57, 59, 73, 87, 102
Do Not Resuscitate (DNR) orders, 65,
69–70, 77–78, 183, 211, 213. See also
end-of-life care
doulas, 153, 209–10, 220, 235, 245–47;
birth, 91, 95, 96, 100, 150, 246;
death, 91, 93, 95, 96, 100, 218–19,
246
drugs/medications, 30, 52, 55–56, 73,
114, 118, 125–26, 201, 202. See also
narcotics; opiates; pain management

elderly people, 56, 57, 61, 63, 65, 68, 81,
216, 245–46; and end-of-life care, 60,
73; and intensive rehabilitation, 152;
and intervention cascades, 5; and long-
term care, 154; and Medicaid, 153;
and Medicare, 153, 158; payment for
care for, 150–51; and standardization,
69; and tests, 64; transfers of, 10. See
also end-of-life care
end-of-life care, 183–84, 197, 211–19;
and appetite loss, 15, 85, 246; and
artificial hydration, 58, 73, 85, 87, 99,
179, 185; and artificial nutrition, 10,
52, 54, 55, 58, 64, 73, 85, 87, 99, 179,
185, 213; and communication, 10, 52,

89–90; and individualized care, 93, 99; and insurance, 92, 161; and medications, 114; and midwives, 203; numbers of, 91, 92; out-of-pocket payment for, 146, 147, 162; and regulations, 115–18; reimbursement for, 146, 147, 160; risk of, 116–17, 189–90; and VBAC, 31, 129. *See also* maternity care

home care, 3, 4, 86, 87, 89, 143, 153, 158, 238, 239

home death, 7, 10, 83, 90, 94–95, 96. *See also* end-of-life care

home health aides, 3, 91, 153, 154, 158

homes: end-of-life care in, 53, 54, 55, 151, 183; palliative care in, 101–2

homes for the dying, 97, 122, 154

hospice, 4, 10, 54, 243; and African Americans, 197, 211, 213–14, 216–19; and bundled care, 236; competition as improving, 231–32; and concurrent care, 236–37; and CON laws, 108, 130–31, 230; and costs, 121, 122, 123, 125, 130–31, 239; and CPM laws, 108; and curative treatment, 86, 121, 159, 303n99; and families, 87, 94, 98, 99, 153, 154; for-profit, 98, 123, 126, 130–31, 136, 155, 230; history of, 87, 88; home, 81–82, 91, 93–95, 153–54, 183; and hospitals, 58, 93, 98, 121, 122, 130, 154, 158, 159; ideal length of stay in, 234; and individualized care, 87, 88, 93, 126; interdisciplinary nature of, 194; and low-risk populations, 191–92; and Medicaid, 131; and medical equipment, 96, 105, 154; and Medicare, 92, 104, 110, 121, 122, 143, 153–55, 157, 163, 213; and nursing homes, 97, 153; pain management in, 69, 93, 94, 182–83; and palliative care, 66, 67, 92, 97, 130, 158, 159; and physicians, 121–22, 124; qualification for, 121, 159; rates of use of, 92, 151; and regulations, 105, 110, 121–26, 130, 154–55; rehabilitative care vs., 157;

reimbursement for, 130, 154–55, 163, 194; residential, 81–82, 89, 91, 92, 96–97, 153, 154, 223, 239; and risk, 187, 188, 191, 192; and six-month diagnosis, 124, 157, 159; staffing requirements of, 105–6, 122, 154–55; and stress, 85–86; and terminal diagnosis, 74, 122, 125; and weekend admissions, 163, 304n111. *See also* end-of-life care; Medicare Hospice Benefit (MHB)

hospice nurses, 93, 96, 97, 132

Hospital at Home, 238

hospitalizations: as incentivized, 153; long-term, 151; and Medicare, 152, 153; and nursing homes, 153; post-acute care after, 151

hospitals: activity bias in, 63, 64, 70–73; and African Americans, 197, 199–200, 202–4, 207–8, 211, 213–15, 217, 218, 219, 222; ambulance delivery restricted to, 158, 211; artificial hydration in, 85; and birth centers, 97–98, 102, 105, 106, 119, 122, 127, 145, 148, 149; birth in, 7, 13, 22–23, 26, 28, 70, 142, 144; births outside of, 20, 91, 92; centralization in, 6, 11–13, 16, 22, 26–32, 50, 53, 80, 90, 108, 112, 141, 164, 187, 200, 225, 226, 230; cesareans in, 149, 160; and communication, 192, 241–43; community-based options vs., 99, 105, 129, 159; complex environment of, 68, 76–77, 78–79; concentration of providers in, 188; and CON laws, 107, 108, 119–20; control in, 29, 32–34, 44, 50, 70; cost of care in, 10, 141–43, 144, 162, 210; and CPM laws, 108, 109; culture of cure in, 62–63, 68, 86; death in, 7, 10, 13, 70, 142–43; as dehumanizing, 12, 31, 56, 58, 68, 82–83, 208; and demedicalization, 79, 102, 105, 106, 158–59, 160–61; design of, 36, 37; end-of-life care in, 16, 51–79, 82, 127, 142–43; and fee-for-service care, 26, 144; full code vs. comfort care in, 69;

hospitals (*cont.*)

growth of, 11–14, 57; as hierarchical, 33–34, 64, 74–75, 79, 101; high-intensity care in, 23, 32, 36, 70, 144; and Hill-Burton Act, 107; and hospices, 58, 93, 98, 121, 122, 130, 154, 158, 159; and individualized care, 69, 77, 78, 86, 102, 146, 193; infections contracted in, 27, 29, 31, 187; and insurance codes, 146; and insurance coverage, 161–62; intervention rates in, 97, 116; as isolating, 29, 56, 58, 68, 77, 79; and liability concerns, 185, 187, 188, 190, 194, 240, 241; lobbying by, 104, 126–30, 228, 238; maternity care in, 12, 16, 22, 29, 32–50, 82, 127, 145, 158, 293n73; maternity wards in, 29–30, 32, 199, 203; mechanized care in, 9, 11, 12, 30, 83, 90–91, 99–100; and Medicaid, 148, 159, 162, 194; and medicalization, 159; and Medicare, 12–13, 127, 143, 157–58, 159, 194; and midwives, 33–34, 86, 113, 117, 118, 129, 146, 189, 190; pain management in, 29, 69; palliative care in, 66–68, 101–2, 130, 157–58, 159, 294n88; and patient autonomy, 25, 77, 117; physicians in, 13, 172, 188; policy control by, 228–29; readmissions to, 10, 152, 153, 234; and regulations, 104, 105; and reimbursement, 144, 145, 160–61, 187, 233; and risk, 33–37, 68–69, 91, 166, 187–91, 194; and rural areas, 12, 178, 227; specialists in, 11, 56, 57; standardized care in, 9, 12, 32, 36–41, 60–61, 68–69, 70, 83, 86–87, 199, 242; standardized design of, 12, 29–30; and standardized protocols, 71–72, 247–48; and technology, 12, 26, 37, 86; transfers to, 10, 63, 96, 113, 114, 118, 135, 148, 185, 189–90, 236, 243, 298n38; and VBAC, 128–29, 178. *See also* intensive care units (ICUs); malpractice liability

Improving Birth #breakthesilence campaign, 26

infant mortality, 27, 117, 196, 200, 208, 233, 235; rates of, 9, 23, 29, 120, 142, 209

infants, 10, 23, 29, 90, 145, 234; birth weight of, 177, 178, 201, 210, 220; injuries to, 173, 174–75, 176; risks to, 117–18, 172; and shoulder dystocia, 39–40, 87, 173, 177–78

informed consent, 2, 8, 52, 76, 78, 89, 226, 231, 240, 247; communication about, 243; and competition, 231; and decentralized care, 101; and end-of-life care, 60, 73–78, 184; ethical commitments to, 17, 18; and hospitals, 101; lack of, 43, 49, 140; and liability, 192, 241; and maternity care, 21, 25, 26, 43, 46–47, 231. *See also* communication

insurance, 42, 138, 139, 146–47, 192; and African Americans, 211, 217; and birth centers, 114, 148, 159, 160, 193, 194, 221; and coding systems, 140; confusion over, 144, 145; and doulas, 95, 96, 150, 218; and end-of-life care, 122, 150, 151, 161, 163; and global fee policies, 162; and home birth, 92, 161; and home care, 3; and hospice, 153, 163; and hospitals, 146, 161–62; malpractice, 169, 174, 175, 176, 180, 194, 195, 221; for maternity care, 144, 161–62; and midwives, 147, 148, 160; private, 2, 141, 143, 153, 158, 162, 163. *See also* reimbursement

insurers, 2, 109, 124, 132–33, 140, 164, 227, 229; and birth centers vs. hospitals, 159; and care plan conversations, 245; and codes for care, 146; and community-based providers, 193; and hospice, 154; and incentives to physicians, 139–40; and individualized care, 164, 233; limited options from, 232; and medical procedures vs. nonmedical care, 149–50; policy control by, 228–29; private, 23, 159; treatment options covered by, 139–40. *See also* reimbursement

intensive care units (ICUs), 10, 11, 36, 76, 143, 153, 199, 211; action bias in,

75; and end-of-life care, 54, 56, 57, 64, 69–71, 72, 74, 151; hospice enrollment after, 157; as isolating, 77; and palliative care, 98; and terminal diagnosis, 75. *See also* care, high-intensity

intervention cascades, 5–6

Jim Crow, 205, 214
Journal of the American Medical Association (JAMA), 27, 112, 229; SUPPORT study, 54, 59

Kentucky, 118–19

labor, induction of, 38–40, 43, 48, 149; and African Americans, 200; financial incentives in, 145; and macrosomia, 15, 39–40, 177; rates of, 9, 22, 24, 110, 231
labor and delivery, 46–49, 226; augmentation of, 9, 24, 35, 36, 38, 145, 149; and breaking of amniotic sac, 24, 40; and breech birth, 28, 33–34, 145–46, 149, 191; and epidurals, 99; and episiotomies, 9, 22, 24, 25, 30, 41, 42, 234; financial incentives in, 145; and forceps deliveries, 9, 22, 28, 30, 41; and home birth, 94; length of, 38, 40–41, 99; movement during, 25, 29, 30, 36, 47, 190; pain at end of, 246; position for, 38, 84; and preterm births, 10, 24, 200, 201, 202, 210, 220; range of normal responses during, 37; restraint during, 25, 30, 31, 82; and vacuum extraction, 22, 30; and vaginal birth, 21, 23, 40, 97, 105, 144, 145, 172; water and food during, 25, 36, 47. *See also* cesarean sections; fetal monitoring; maternity care; vaginal birth after cesarean (VBAC)
laws, 102, 106, 111, 136, 180–83, 223. *See also* state laws and regulations
Lewin Report, 114, 132–33
LGBT (lesbian, gay, bisexual, and transgender) individuals, 15, 196, 224
licensing, 136, 146, 172, 223
living wills, 211, 245

lobbying, 26, 104, 126–31, 140, 228, 238–39
Logan, Onnie Lee, 87–88, 95, 120, 206
Louisiana, 144
low-income individuals, 120, 140, 150, 151, 153, 154, 196, 219, 237. *See also* poverty
Lubic, Ruth, 219, 220, 221

macrosomia. *See* fetal size
malpractice, 171, 305n16; award amounts in, 173, 175; and birth centers, 160, 194, 221; and California Maternal Quality Care Collaborative, 240; and cesarean sections, 188; and community-based care, 195, 221; costs from, 114, 160, 167, 171, 173–74, 175, 180; and end-of-life care, 52, 179–80, 186, 240; and fetal monitoring, 35; and hospices, 194; and hospitals, 167, 194; insurance for, 169, 174, 175, 176, 180, 194, 195, 221; and medical complexity, 168; and midwives, 160, 168, 173, 174, 192; and negligent injuries, 174–75; and nurses, 173; and obstetrics, 160, 168, 173–78, 192; and opioids, 180–81; and overtreatment, 169, 170, 177; and reform, 243; and standardization of care, 90; and undertreatment, 177; and VBAC, 169, 174, 176–77, 178. *See also* physicians; tort system
malpractice liability, 22, 42, 50; administrative, 166, 168–69; and communication, 241–43, 245; and community-based providers, 191–94, 243; and documentation burdens, 242; and hospitals, 185, 187, 188, 190, 194, 240, 241; and likelihood of error, 190; and reform, 239–44; and standard of care, 191
Manhattan Birth Center, 114, 132–33, 160, 193
Massachusetts, 112
maternal mortality, 27, 31, 117, 177, 196, 200–201, 208, 233, 235, 240; rates of, 9–10, 23–24, 29, 120, 142

maternity care, 2–3, 21–32; and African Americans, 196, 199, 200–211, 219–21; and birth as physiological vs. pathological, 7, 28; and birth plans, 7, 44–45, 244, 245; and centralized care, 26–32; and communication, 243; and community-based care, 22, 28, 98, 129, 208, 210; complications in, 10, 172; costs of, 3, 10, 142, 143, 144–50; in hospitals, 12, 16, 22, 29–30, 32–50, 82, 127, 145, 158, 199, 203, 293n73; and informed consent, 21, 25, 26, 43, 46–47, 231; insurance coverage for, 161–62; integrated options for, 237; interventions in, 5, 32–41, 233–34; language of control in, 42, 43; and liability, 240; low-risk, 22, 24, 28, 30, 31, 32, 50, 98, 99, 119, 144, 145, 149, 172, 200, 202, 235–36; and Medicaid, 10, 22; and medicalization, 22–26; and Minnesota Birth Center BirthBundle, 235–36; and out-of-pocket costs, 3, 144; and overtreatment, 7, 22; reimbursement for, 139; and reimbursement reform, 233–36; and related costs, 144–50; and risk, 168, 172–78, 189–91; and shoulder dystocia, 39–40, 87, 173, 177–78; unrealistic expectations in, 244. *See also* birth centers; home births; labor and delivery; pregnancy; prenatal care

Medicaid, 159, 162; and ACA, 146–47; and advanced practice nurses, 111; and African Americans, 198, 200, 202, 203, 213–14, 312n29; assets spent down for, 151; and assisted living care, 151; and birth centers, 148, 149, 159, 210–11, 221, 238; birth spending under, 23; and bundled care, 236; and childbirth, 144; and communication, 219; and community-based providers, 140; coordination of with Medicare, 151, 153; and documentation burdens, 242; and doulas, 150; and dual eligibility, 151, 152; and elderly people, 153; and end-of-life care, 4, 52, 57, 150–51, 153–54, 213–14, 219, 236; and Family Health

and Birth Center, 221; and global fee, 148; and home care, 153; and home health coverage, 4; and hospices, 131; and hospitals, 148, 159, 162, 194; and individualized care, 221, 223; low payment rates of, 147–48; and maternity care, 10, 22; and midwifery, 115, 147, 148, 210, 221, 238; and Minnesota Birth Center BirthBundle, 236; and nursing homes, 151, 152, 153; and pregnancy, 23, 141; and prenatal care, 148; reimbursement policies of, 6, 152; and states, 148, 151, 153; and terminally ill patients, 121; and vaginal birth and and cesarean sections, 144; and value-based care, 233. *See also* reimbursement

Medical Association of the State of Alabama, 128

medical associations, 6, 11, 13, 26, 30, 126–30, 207, 240

medical innovations, 18, 56, 57, 58, 61, 139, 140

medicalization, 9, 14–17, 169, 226; and defensive medicine, 170; defined, 7, 14; and end-of-life care, 53–55; and ethics, 17–19; increase in, 90–91; and maternity care, 22–26

Medicare, 139, 161, 228; and advanced practice nurses, 111; and African Americans, 213–14; and ambulances, 158, 211; bias toward hospital-based care in, 157–58; and bundled care, 236; and cancer treatment, 156–57; and centralized care, 12–13, 152; and codes for care, 152; and comfort care homes, 122–23; and communication, 219; and community-based care, 152, 159; and CON laws, 123; coordination of with Medicaid, 151, 153; and costs, 122, 125, 143, 152; and costs for beneficiaries in last years of life, 143; and CPR, 65; and curative and palliative treatment, 157, 158; and death, 53–54; and decentralization, 13, 130; and documentation burdens, 242; and dual eligibility, 151, 152; and elderly people, 153, 158; and end-of-life care, 3–4, 10, 57–58, 122, 141, 150–58, 171–72, 213–14, 219, 236; and end-of-life care conversations, 155–56, 308n64; and fee-for-service, 12–13, 152, 232–33; and high-intensity care, 152; and home care, 158; Home Health Benefit, 236–37; and home healthcare, 143, 239; and Home Health Value-Based Purchasing Model, 239; and hospice, 92, 104, 110, 121, 122, 143, 153–55, 157, 163, 213; and hospitalizations, 153; and hospitals, 12–13, 127, 143, 157–58, 159, 194; and ICU, 153; and individualized care, 221, 223; and mechanized care, 152; and medical technology, 13; and nursing homes, 3–4, 152, 153; and outpatient care, 13; and physicians, 152; reform of, 230, 232–33; and regulations, 104; reimbursement policies of, 6, 122, 147, 152; and skilled nursing care, 152, 157; and terminally ill patients, 121; and unnecessary testing, 143; and value-based care, 233, 235; and weekend hospice admissions, 304n111. *See also* reimbursement

Medicare D, 126

Medicare Hospice Benefit (MHB), 4, 94–95, 121, 122, 124–26, 153, 236; and African Americans, 217; and curative treatment, 121, 157, 217, 219; and drugs, 125–26; and hospitals vs. community-based care, 159; incentives vs. care under, 126; and individualized care, 58; and palliative care, 157; as protecting hospice, 130; qualification for, 121, 124–25, 157, 219; and terminal and related diagnoses, 125

midwifery, 85–86, 144, 146, 188, 219, 243; and African Americans, 200, 204–7, 208, 209, 210, 214, 218; history of, 87–88; and hospital environment, 32; and infant and maternal mortality, 27; and Medicaid, 115, 147, 148, 210, 221, 238; and Minnesota Birth Center BirthBundle,

235; personalized care in, 209; and physiology vs. pathology, 83–84; prosecutions for, 112; and regulations, 27, 28, 97

midwives, 29, 38, 44, 91, 99, 153, 203, 220, 227; African American, 112, 204–7; in Alabama, 87, 115–16, 120, 127–28, 132; and birth centers, 96, 113; and birth plans, 45; and black birth workers, 208, 209; and cesareans, 132, 231; direct-entry, 112, 113, 114, 115, 117, 127, 134, 135, 147, 148; eradication of, 26–28; granny, 87, 95, 120, 200, 204–5, 206, 208, 209, 223; home birth, 160, 162; and hospitals, 33–34, 86, 113, 117, 118, 129, 146, 189, 190; and induction rates, 231; and infant resuscitation equipment, 92; and informed consent, 46–47; and insurance, 147, 148, 160; licensing of, 112, 113, 115, 117, 120; lobbying against, 127–28; and low-risk patients, 92; and malpractice, 160, 168, 173, 174, 192; and Medicaid, 115, 147, 148, 238; and medications, 114, 118; and Minnesota Birth Center BirthBundle, 235; and motherwit, 87–88; nonmedical, 117–18; and physicians, 109, 111–12, 113–15, 118; regulation of, 105, 109, 110, 111–20, 127–28, 208; reimbursement of, 113, 146–47, 160; and risk, 92, 117, 188, 189–90; and scope of practice, 239; in South Carolina, 129, 134; and standardization, 87; and states, 11, 113, 132, 146–47; traditional, 87–88, 90, 95, 111, 112, 113, 114, 120, 204–7; training of, 97, 111–13, 205; without medical training, 117, 120

midwives, nurse, 97, 113, 115, 134, 205, 231; and birth centers, 113, 147; and CPM laws, 108; estimation of risk by, 189; and folk healers, 111; in hospitals, 146; and Medicaid, 148; as medical directors, 110; and medical training, 111; and physicians, 112, 117–18, 134; and reimbursements, 146;

midwives, nurse (*cont.*)
  and scope of practice regulations, 109,
  110. *See also* nurses
Minnesota, 150
Minnesota Birth Center, 235–36
minorities, 120, 140, 150, 211
MOLST (medical order for life-
  sustaining treatment) form, 51

Naramore, Lloyd Stanley, 184–85
narcotics, 180–83, 185. *See also* drugs/
  medications; opiates; opioids; pain
  management; palliative care
National Institutes of Health (NIH), 10,
  11, 55
natural birth movement, 84
natural childbirth, 31–32, 83
Nebraska, 148
New Jersey, 147
New York, 113, 121, 122, 124
North Dakota, 151
nurse practitioners (NPs), 105, 108, 109,
  110–11, 231
nurses, 33, 123, 154, 156, 166, 173,
  182, 188; advanced practice, 106,
  109–11, 135, 231; hospice, 93, 96,
  97, 132; and integrated practice units,
  235; and palliative care, 66–67; physician oversight of, 11, 56; physicians
  vs., 109–11; and scope of practice, 11,
  106, 239. *See also* midwives, nurse;
  skilled nursing care
nursing homes, 69, 77, 97, 130, 185–86,
  187; and CPR, 65; end-of-life care in,
  52, 57–58, 182–83, 213; and hospice,
  97, 153; and Medicaid, 151, 152, 153;
  and Medicare, 3–4, 152, 153; and
  opioids, 182–83; and transfers to
  hospitals, 10, 185

obstetricians, 2, 3, 21, 22, 112, 235; and
  birth centers, 96; and birth plans, 45;
  and defensive medicine, 175; and
  demedicalized providers, 193–94;
  female, 44; and liability costs, 175;
  scarcity of, 176; training of, 191; and
  VBAC, 178. *See also* physicians
obstetrics: and gender, 44; and malprac-

tice, 160, 168, 173–78, 181, 192;
  midwifery vs., 209; progress in, 34;
  trust in, 209; undertreatment in, 181,
  211; violence in, 25, 26, 231
oncologists, 60, 62, 74, 156, 180. *See
  also* cancer
opiates, 69, 179
opioids, 179, 180–81, 182, 183, 185,
  243. *See also* drugs/medications;
  narcotics
Oregon, 150
overtreatment, 5, 7, 52, 53, 66, 98, 166,
  174, 195, 223, 226, 233, 243; and
  African Americans, 199, 202, 211,
  213; defined, 14; in end-of-life care,
  55, 179, 183–86; and malpractice,
  169, 170, 177; and maternity care, 7,
  22; medicalization vs., 14; and
  standardization, 86–87

pain management, 9, 24, 29, 85, 89,
  90, 96, 142, 144, 234; and African
  Americans, 197, 199, 207, 208, 211,
  212, 215; in end-of-life care, 10, 54,
  178, 180–83, 186; and hospice, 69,
  93, 94, 182; in hospitals, 29, 69; and
  opioids, 180; and palliative care, 68;
  and undertreatment, 179, 180–83. *See
  also* drugs/medications; palliative care
Palin, Sarah, 155, 183
palliative care, 54–55, 75, 93, 228, 237;
  and African Americans, 197, 211,
  216, 217, 218; and communication,
  65, 66, 67; community-based, 157–58;
  and concurrent care, 236; curative
  care vs., 157, 158; and depression, 98;
  and double effect, 182; and end-of-life
  care, 70–71, 73, 151, 158; growth in,
  90; home-based, 101–2; and hospice,
  66, 67, 92, 97, 130, 158, 159; in hospitals, 66–68, 101–2, 130, 157–58,
  159, 294n88; and ICU, 98; integration
  of, 69; interdisciplinary nature of, 66;
  and legal risk, 180; and MHB, 157;
  moral and emotional support from,
  72; and opioids, 183; as opt-in, 68;
  patient satisfaction with, 98; rates of
  use of, 151; reimbursement of, 130,